Teenage Pregnancy in a Family Context

Teenage Pregnancy

in a Family Context

Implications for policy

Edited by
Theodora Ooms

Temple University Press
Philadelphia

HQ
759.4
T44

Temple University Press, Philadelphia 19122
© 1981 by Temple University. All rights reserved
Published 1981
Printed in the United States of America

Library of Congress Cataloging in Publication Data

Main entry under title:
Teenage pregnancy in a family context.

(Family Impact Seminar series)
Bibliography: p.
Includes index.
1. Adolescent mothers—United States—Congresses. 2. Pregnant school-girls—United States—Congresses. 3. Youth—United States—Family relations—Congresses. 4. Youth—United States—Sexual behavior. 5. Birth control—United States—Congresses. 6. Abortion—United States—Congresses. I. Ooms, Theodora, 1939– . II. Series.
HQ759.4.T44   362.7'96   80-39714
ISBN 0-87722-204-5

To all the families who contributed to this book

Family Impact Seminar Series

The Family Impact Seminar Series is a series of books deriving from the research of the Family Impact Seminar, which is part of the Institute for Educational Leadership at George Washington University.

Balancing Jobs and Family Life: Do Flexible Work Schedules Help?
by Halcyone H. Bohen and Anamaria Viveros-Long

Foster Care and Families: Conflicting Values and Policies
by Ruth Hubbell

Teenage Pregnancy in a Family Context: Implications for Policy
edited by Theodora Ooms

Family Impact Seminar Members

WALTER ALLEN, Assistant Professor of Sociology, University of Michigan

NANCY AMIDEI, Director, Food Research and Action Center, Inc.

MARY JO BANE, Deputy Assistant Secretary for Program Planning and Budget Analysis, U.S. Department of Education

TERREL BELL, Commissioner, Utah System of Higher Education

URIE BRONFENBRENNER, Professor of Human Development and Family Studies, Cornell University

WILBUR COHEN, Professor of Public Affairs, University of Texas at Austin

BEVERLY CRABTREE, Dean, College of Home Economics, Oklahoma State University

WILLIAM DANIEL, JR., Professor of Pediatrics, University of Alabama Medical Center

JOHN DEMOS, Professor of History, Brandeis University

PATRICIA FLEMING, Deputy Assistant Secretary for Legislation, U.S. Department of Education

ROBERT HILL, Director, Research Division, National Urban League

NICHOLAS HOBBS, Professor of Psychology, Emeritus, Vanderbilt University

A. SIDNEY JOHNSON, III, Director, Family Impact Seminar

JEROME KAGAN, Professor of Psychology, Harvard University

SHEILA KAMERMAN, Associate Professor of Social Policy and Planning, Columbia University School of Social Work

ROSABETH MOSS KANTER, Professor of Sociology, Yale University

LUIS LAOSA, Senior Research Scientist, Educational Testing Service, Princeton

ROBERT LEIK, Director, Family Study Center, University of Minnesota

SALVADOR MINUCHIN, Professor of Child Psychiatry and Pediatrics, University of Pennsylvania

FAMILY IMPACT SEMINAR MEMBERS

ROBERT MNOOKIN, Professor of Law, University of California at Berkeley

MARTHA PHILLIPS, Assistant Minority Counsel, Ways and Means Committee, U.S. House of Representatives

CHESTER PIERCE, Professor of Psychiatry and Education, Harvard University

ISABEL SAWHILL, Program Director, Employment & Labor Policy, The Urban Institute

CAROL STACK, Director, Center for the Study of Family and the State, Duke University

Preface

The Family Impact Seminar

There is a myth in our country that government is somehow neutral to families. In fact, all levels of government have policies and programs that affect families deeply.

Any family that has paid taxes, contributed to or received benefits from Social Security, married or divorced, benefited from the G.I. bill, or been involved with public school, foster care, welfare, or the court system knows that government affects families. Family Impact Seminar studies have identified 268 federal domestic assistance programs alone—administered by seventeen different departments and agencies—that have a potential for direct impact on American families. The question is not, Does government affect families? but rather, How does government affect families and how can policies that hurt families be repealed or reformed?

The Family Impact Seminar was created in 1976 to explore these kinds of questions. The Seminar is composed of twenty-four of the country's leading scholars and public policymakers concerned with families. They convene several times a year to provide leadership and guidance to the work of the Seminar's staff.

The Seminar is founded on a respect for the integrity, diversity, and privacy of American families; a conviction that government policies should strengthen families rather than weaken them; and a commitment to the idea that families themselves should participate in the decisions that affect them.

The original interest in family impact analysis—which subsequently led to the creation of the Family Impact Seminar—came from the 1973 Senate hearings on "American Families: Trends and Pressures." Vice President Mondale, then chairman of the Senate Subcommittee on Children and Youth stated: "We must start by asking to what extent government policies are helping or hurting families." Many of those who testified at the hearings recommended that family impact statements be developed for all public policies. Although intrigued by the idea, the Subcommittee concluded that legislation would be premature before the new concept had been tested. I left my position as staff director of the Mondale Subcommittee to found the Family Impact Seminar in order to undertake this testing in an independent, nongovernmental setting.

Family impact analysis, as we define it, is a process of assessing the effects of public or private policies on families. Its objective is to make policies and practices more sensitive to the needs and aspirations of families. It is designed to provide practical policy recommendations in a relatively short period of time.

The process of family impact analysis includes reviewing laws and regulations, interviewing policymakers and service providers, and learning directly from families how policies affect them. It lays considerable emphasis on assessing how programs really work. Examples of important family impact questions to ask about policies and programs are:

- Does the policy encourage or discourage marital stability?

- Do families have real opportunities to participate in the decisions that affect them?

- Does the policy encourage caring for family members by families themselves or by institutions? Does it use or ignore existing family support systems, such as extended families and kinship ties?

- Is the program sensitive to the traditions, values, and practices of families from varied racial, ethnic, and religious backgrounds?

PREFACE

This volume presents an in-depth review of teenage pregnancy policies in terms of questions like these. It is one of three family impact case studies conducted by the Seminar. The Seminar's other two case studies analyze the effect of foster care policies and work schedule policies on families.

These case studies are the first comprehensive efforts to test the value of our evolving framework for family impact analysis. They are our attempt to take some promising concepts, apply them to existing public policies, and discover if they yield useful findings and recommendations.

The results of this work have far exceeded our expectations. The talents, insights, and dedication of each study director—backed up by generous support from interested funding sources—transformed the projects from relatively short-term policy reviews to long-term, in-depth studies. Each study uses a different design and methodology: survey questionnaires and group interviews in the work schedules study; interviews at the service delivery level in the foster care study; and commissioned papers and a conference in the teenage pregnancy study. But these studies have fundamental elements in common, including: a focus on the diversity of families, an appreciation of the different levels of policy implementation, an emphasis on obtaining the views of the families being served, and a reliance on a family impact perspective and framework.

The present study was directed by Theodora Ooms, deputy director of the Family Impact Seminar, with valuable assistance from the book's thirteen contributors, Seminar members, and other experts in the field. The overall design of this book and Theodora's own chapters reflect a combination of her experiences as a social worker, family therapist, and administrator at the Philadelphia Child Guidance Clinic on the one hand, with her skills in policy analysis, which she has sharpened in Washington, on the other. In addition, as an employed mother of adolescent and pre-adolescent children, she brought a valuable, personal dimension to this study, which she identifies and discusses explicitly. The resulting book, by reflecting these different experiences and sensitivities, presents a set of thoughtful findings and suggestions that, above all, acknowledge and respect the complexities and diversity of families who experience teenage pregnancy.

Too often discussions of controversial and sensitive policy issues, such as those involved in teenage pregnancy, are unbalanced and incomplete: they either lean too heavily on the presentation of dry facts or become strident and value-laden vehicles for advocacy. By contrast, this volume presents a rich and balanced picture; a rare combination of careful scholarship and measured discussion of values and issues. Standing alone, this volume is impressive. Against the backdrop of other studies dealing with controversial issues, it is remarkable.

To my knowledge, this is the first book in the United States that has applied a family impact perspective to an examination of how teenage pregnancy policies affect families. It was designed to produce recommendations that would make teenage pregnancy policies more supportive of families, and to model and improve our approach to family impact analysis. It has fulfilled both objectives.

Our case studies provide three different promising models of family impact analysis for organizations with a national perspective and considerable resources of time, funds, and expertise. Based on the case study experiences, we have also developed a family impact approach for individuals and organizations who work with families on a daily basis, but have limited time and resources to devote to policy analysis. With the help of twelve organizations across the country—four PTAs, four anti-poverty agencies, three children's agencies, and one hospital—we have explored whether family impact analysis is also a useful tool for state and local agencies. Policymakers, service providers, and families themselves were interviewed; laws, regulations guidelines, and memoranda were dissected and analyzed. We are encouraged by the results of this field project. We gained insights into how policies are affecting families in different communities, as well as ideas about how policies may be reshaped in order to be more helpful to families.

Based on our work over the last four years in case studies and field projects, the Seminar recommends several steps to make public and private policies more responsive to the needs and aspirations of families. We propose that: (1) independent Commissions for Families be created at several levels of government to conduct family impact studies, and help ensure that public policies help rather than hurt families; (2) public and private organizations and agencies examine and improve the ways in which their own policies and practices affect families; and (3) more organizations of families themselves assess and improve the impact of policies or programs on families.

Although these suggestions alone will not solve all the problems that face families, they can be a first step toward the day when decision-makers consciously and consistently ask, "What effect will this policy have on families?"

> A. Sidney Johnson, III
> Director, Family Impact Seminar
> December 1980

Contents

	Acknowledgments	xxi
	Contributors	xxv
	Five Families	3
1	Introduction *by Theodora Ooms*	9
2	Teenage Women in the United States: Sex, Contraception, Pregnancy, Fertility, and Maternal and Infant Health *by Audrey E. Jones and Paul J. Placek*	49
3	The Family's Role in Adolescent Sexual Behavior *by Greer Litton Fox*	73
4	Implicating the Family: Teenage Parenthood and Kinship Involvement *by Frank F. Furstenberg, Jr.*	131
5	Government Policies Related to Teenage Family Formation and Functioning: An Inventory *by Kristin A. Moore*	165
6	Sex Education and the Prevention of Teenage Pregnancy: An Overview of Policies and Programs in the United States *by Peter Scales*	213
7	Adolescent Parent Programs and Family Involvement *by Janet Bell Forbush, with the assistance of Teresa Maciocha*	254
8	Ethical and Legal Issues in Teenage Pregnancies *by Margaret O'Brien Steinfels*	277
9	Adolescent Sexuality and Teenage Pregnancy from a Black Perspective *by June Dobbs Butts*	307

10	The Impact of Adolescent Pregnancy on Hispanic Adolescents and Their Families *by Angel Luis Martinez*	326
11	Bringing in the Family: Kinship Support and Contraceptive Behavior *by Frank F. Furstenberg, Jr., Roberta Herceg-Baron, and Jay Jemail*	345
12	Family Involvement, Notification, and Responsibility: A Personal Essay *by Theodora Ooms*	371
	Afterword: Family Impact Analysis	399
	Index	415

Figures and Tables

Figures

1. Central Birth Rates for Women Aged Fourteen to Nineteen, By Age, By Color: United States, 1917–1977   52
2. Number of Births Per 1,000 Females Aged Fifteen to Nineteen, Selected Countries, 1970s   54
3. Percent of Sexually Experienced Never-Married Women Aged Fifteen to Nineteen, According to Method Used at Last Intercourse, 1976 and 1971   58
4. Parents as Sources of Sex Education for Teens in Relation to Three Most Frequently Cited Sources   78
5. Features, Outcomes, and Goals of Sex Education Programs   218
6. Evolving Framework: Public Policy Dimensions   404
7. Evolving Framework: Family Impact Dimensions   406

Tables

1. Total Live Births for Women, 10–19 Years of Age, of Mother and Race, 1966–1975   50
2. Percent of Never-Married Women Aged 15–19 Who Have Ever Had Intercourse, by Age and Race, 1976 and 1971   56
3. Percent Distribution of All First Pregnancies to Women Age 15–19 at Interview, According to Pregnancy Outcome and Race, 1976 and 1971   60
4. Percent Distribution of Premaritally Pregnant Young Women, by Whether Contraception was Used at Time of Conception, According to Race   64
5. Summary of Characteristics of State Plans for Aid to Families with Dependent Children (AFDC), as of April 1978   170

Acknowledgments

My first and deepest debt is to my family. Together they have taught me most of what I know and value about families. My special thanks to them: Jessie, Norman, Derek, Joanna, and Tom Parfit in England and Van Doorn, Katrina, Alexander, and Tamara Ooms in Maryland.

Two persons have inspired and sustained me professionally in the past decade and have greatly influenced the focus and shape of this volume. Salvador Minuchin first taught me that teenage pregnancy—and other problems—must be viewed through a family lens. Sidney Johnson, my guide to the world of policy, suggested the format of commissioned papers which permitted the study to maintain a broad policy focus. To both I owe profound thanks for their steady support, encouragement and friendship.

It has been my good fortune to work with a superb team of colleagues at the Family Impact Seminar. They consistently provided a most congenial and flexible work environment, making it possible for me to balance both work and family responsibilities. Teresa Maciocha enthusiastically carried a major burden of the project in its first year, providing invaluable research assistance and coordinating the conference singlehandedly. Her persistent questioning from her youthful perspective provided a healthy counterbalance to those arising from my middle years. Elizabeth Bode exercised her many and varied editorial skills critically, deftly and patiently, helping me to think more clearly. Ruth Hubbell shared many helpful ideas as we together explored the new field of family impact analysis. Darlene Craddock provided constant sunshine and quiet efficiency even on the most stressful days. Mary Eng, Edward Metz, Amy Novick and John Sheldon attended to the tedious detailed tasks efficiently and cheerfully. I enjoyed long collegial discussions with Halcy Bohen, Susan Brown, Susan Farkas, and their friendship. Lynne Roney was the intelligent indexer. At the Institute for Educational Leadership Dietra Hallums smoothed over many a potential obstacle and Sam Halperin facilitated the Seminar's work. My many thanks to them all for the part each played in the production of this book.

The core of this volume is the work of thirteen contributors. I am very grateful for their collaboration and their patience throughout the long process of seeing the manuscript through to publication. Frank Furstenberg deserves special thanks for contributing, with Roberta Herceg-Baron and Jay Jemail, an additional chapter, and for helping me puzzle over a number of issues in my own chapters.

I have benefitted enormously in the last four years from our relationship with all of our Seminar members. In particular, this study received invaluable advice from Nancy Amidei, Beverly Crabtree, William Daniel, Luis Laosa, Salvador Minuchin, Martha Phillips, and Chester Pierce.

Several of my former colleagues at the Philadelphia Child Guidance Clinic collaboratd in the pilot project described in chapter four. My thanks to the following clinic staff for the time and skills they gave to the project: Barbara Bryant, Lynda Butler, Jay Jemail, Barbara Penn, and Iolie Wallbridge. And thanks to Harry Aponte for agreeing to it and for teaching me to understand the ecological context of families.

Many others generously contributed their expertise at different stages of the project in interviews with Teresa Maciocha and myself, participation at the invitational conference in October 1978, and/or reactions to drafts of the preliminary report and final manuscript. I wish space permitted me to recognize the specific ways in which each of them added to our knowledge, and suggested new questions, and new perspectives. The expe-

ACKNOWLEDGMENTS   xxiii

rience of Congressional staff was shared by: Tom Birch, Christine Burch, Rhonda Einhorn, George Hardy, Terence Lierman, Patricia Markey, and Maris Vinovskis. A number of persons from various units of DHEW gave advice and assistance: May Aaronson, Wendy Baldwin, Gerald Britten, Jack Dempsey, Mary Harper, Pamela Johnson, Stanley Kruger, Lynda Mellgren, Maurice Moore, Lana Muraskin, Lulu Mae Nix, William Pratt, Peter Schuck, Cecelia Sudia, Samuel Taylor, and Vivian Washington. The view from the regional and state level came from Elizabeth Bershears (OK), Dennis Coughlin (NY), Alexandra Douglas (NY), Christina Hale (AL), and Frances Hamermersh (MI). The experiences of those in service delivery were shared by Carl Coan (Los Angeles), Julie Hofheimer (Gainesville, FL), Faustina Knoll (Detroit), Tony Peterson (Washington, DC), Lana Smith (Washington, DC), Mary Tatum (Falls Church, VA), and George Thoms (Falls Church, VA).

A wealth of expertise and research about teenage pregnancy and parenthood and related laws and policy was shared by: Sharon Alexander, Judy Areen, Joan Bennesch, Callie Braxton, Catherine Chilman, Ray DeBlasio, Judith Jones, Asta Kenney, Lorraine Klerman, James Lieberman, Marjory Mecklenburg, Audrey Moore, Celia Ogden, Susan Philliber, Ray Hudson Rosen, Jeannie Rosoff, Marie Santosusso, and Basile Uddo.

I am most grateful to the Charles Stewart Mott Foundation which provided the primary financial support for the study and to Marilyn Steele, of the Foundation, for her steady encouragement, substantive advice and dedication to the needs of teenage parents. I also wish to thank the following for their contributions to the study and the Seminar: the Foundation for Child Development, Lilly Endowment, Inc., Ford Foundation, Mary Reynolds Babcock Foundation, Robert Sterling Clark Foundation, Needmor Fund, Edna McConnell Clark Foundation, General Mills Foundation, Levi Strauss Foundation, Chichester duPont Foundation, Administration for Children, Youth and Families, Community Services Administration, National Institute of Mental Health, Department of Commerce, and Carnegie Corporation of New York.

Last, but far from least, my thanks are due to Michael Ames, Doris Brandel, and Suzanna Thornton of Temple University Press for wise advice and patient assistance while guiding me through all the complexities of putting together this volume.

Contributors

JUNE DOBBS BUTTS, Ed.D., is a family life educator who currently has a joint appointment with Howard University's Department of Psychiatry and Department of Pediatrics and Child Health, where she is collaborating in a longitudinal study of the sexual learning process and development of black pre-adolescents. She is the first black person to be trained as a sex therapist by Masters and Johnson. She is also the author of several articles.

JANET BELL FORBUSH is president of JBF Associates, a national consultant service specializing in the provision of technical assistance regarding high risk adolescents, with particular emphasis on sexually active youth, pregnant teens, young parents, and their families. In the past ten years, Ms. Forbush has provided assistance to programs and agencies in over forty states, and has testified frequently before congressional committees on issues related to adolescent pregnancy.

GREER LITTON FOX, Ph.D., is associate professor of sociology at Wayne State University in Detroit, and director of their family research program. She has written extensively on many aspects of gender roles. She is just completing a research project entitled "Mother-Daughter Communication Patterns Regarding Sexuality."

FRANK F. FURSTENBERG, JR., Ph.D., is professor of sociology at the University of Pennsylvania. He is the author of the well-known book, *Unplanned Parenthood: The Social Consequences of Teenage Childbearing*, which is based on an extensive five-year longitudinal study of teenage mothers in Baltimore. He has published widely on this topic, and has testified several times at congressional hearings. Along with Richard Lincoln and Jane Menken, he is the editor of a collection of articles entitled *Teenage Sexuality, Pregnancy, and Childbearing*. In his current research, he is exploring the impact of remarriage on family life.

ROBERTA HERCEG-BARON, M.A., is a research analyst at the Family Planning Council of Southeastern Pennsylvania. Her work with the Council includes evaluational studies of family planning services and training programs in human sexuality.

JAY JEMAIL, Ph.D., is a clinical psychologist at the Philadelphia Child Guidance Clinic. She has a grant from the National Institute of Child Health and Human Development to do a longitudinal study of adolescent pregnancy and parenthood in the context of the family. She has done work in the fields of human sexuality and family therapy, and is currently involved in the clinical training of family planning counselors.

AUDREY E. JONES is a statistician at the Division of Vital Statistics, National Center for Health Statistics, HHS, in Hyattsville, Maryland. She is working on the National Natality Survey and the National Fetal Mortality Survey. Her previous work was with the Bureau of the Census.

TERESA MACIOCHA was program assistant on the Family Impact Seminar's case study of teenage pregnancy. Since leaving the Seminar, she has joined the staff of *Community Jobs*, a monthly publication geared towards people who work at community organizing.

ANGEL LUIS MARTINEZ has worked in Latin America and all over the United States, developing and implementing a variety of programs concerning adolescent sexuality and health, family planning, sex education, and health professional training. He prepares educational materials for the media, and most recently completed a film, "What Can a Guy Do?" He lives in San Francisco.

KRISTIN A. MOORE, Ph.D., is a sociological psychologist at the Program of Research on Women and Family Policy at the Urban Institute in Washington, D.C. Her most recent research has been on the social and economic consequences of teenage childbearing, and the impact of the federal welfare system on out-of-wedlock and adolescent fertility. She has written numerous articles and testified before Congress.

THEODORA OOMS, M.S.W., is deputy director of the Family Impact Seminar, Washington, D.C. As a social worker and family therapist she worked with children, teenagers and their families in many different situations primarily in New Haven, Connecticut, and Philadelphia. She directed the Seminar's family impact study on policies concerning teenage pregnancy and is now working on the Seminar's next book on families and public policy.

PAUL J. PLACEK, Ph.D., is a statistician at the Division of Vital Statistics, National Center for Health Statistics, HHS, in Hyattsville, Maryland. He is the Project Director of the 1980 National Natality and Fetal Mortality Surveys, and has published a number of articles in fertility and maternal and infant health. He is co-editor (with Gerry Hendershot) of a new book, *Predicting Fertility: Demographic Studies of Birth Expectations*.

CONTRIBUTORS

PETER SCALES, Ph.D., is a researcher, author, and lecturer in human sexuality, with a special interest in teenagers and family relationships. He is co-author with Sol Gordon and Kathleen Everly of *The Sexual Adolescent: Communicating with Teenagers about Sex*. Scales is a consultant on youth affairs for many groups, and is currently a senior research analyst at Mathtech, Inc., in Bethesda, Maryland, where he is also director of the Project on Barriers to Sex Education.

MARGARET O'BRIEN STEINFELS is an editor at Basic Books. She served as editor of *The Hastings Center Report*, published by the Hastings Center, Institute of Society, Ethics, and the Life Sciences. She is also the author of *Who's Minding the Children?: The History and Politics of Day Care in America*.

Teenage Pregnancy in a Family Context

Five Families

This volume begins with brief vignettes of five families whose school-age daughter became pregnant and in four cases had a baby. They provide vivid, real-life examples of some of the immediate ways in which teenage pregnancy has an impact on families. (Minor changes have been made to protect their identity.)

Tina's Family

The Sullivans, a white suburban family, have four children, aged ten to eighteen. Two of their three daughters became pregnant while attending high school. Tina, the second oldest, became pregnant when she was sixteen. She suspected both parents would be upset, but her father simply "hit the roof." One night he smashed their new hi-fi equipment in a rage; he then went into a depression for two months, going into his bedroom every night and not talking to anyone. The tension at home was felt by everyone. Tina told her mother that she thought she should leave home. Her mother encouraged her to have a talk with her father, which she did, and it was very emotional for them both.

After that, things changed for the better, and the whole family became involved in helping Tina with her pregnancy and caring for the new baby. The baby has changed many things for the family.

Tina's father is now a proud grandfather. So that Tina could continue in school, her mother has quit her part-time job to look after the baby. Her brother Jimmy, who had been the baby of the family until then, feels displaced; his grades have started dropping in school. However, both he and his sister Arlene take turns caring for the baby.

Tina's older sister, Annie, who had been living across town and with her girlfriends, came home one day to announce that she, too, was pregnant. Annie has now moved back home for a while but thinks that maybe one day she will marry the baby's father and move out on her own.

Angela's Family

"My God, you're pregnant!" exclaimed Mrs. Rogers.

Angela had attempted to conceal her condition but was betrayed by her "morning sickness." Upon the recommendation of her girlfriend, she had even tried home remedies—epsom salts, a mixture of Clorox and milk, quinine—in an effort to resume her menstrual period. But she had only become sicker and more afraid of a confrontation with her mother.

Following several days of disbelief and inertia, Mrs. Rogers sought counseling and medical assistance for her fifteen-year-old daughter. She discovered that such help was not covered by her health insurance and that neither she nor her daughter qualified for local human resources programs, because she earned too much money. Frustrated and anxious, she approached her family, her ex-husband and Angela's boyfriend's family for financial help. She and Angela were not prepared for the less than polite rejection they received.

Finally, Mrs. Rogers succeeded in obtaining counseling on a sliding-fee scale, through a family services agency. Following several costly and emotional sessions, Angela decided upon a therapeutic abortion. Mrs. Rogers was relieved by the decision, and grateful for the availability of a highly recommended and relatively inexpensive abortion clinic that would perform the same-day procedure. Hospitalization, which would have cost five times the amount charged by the clinic, was simply beyond her reach. And Angela could not bear the thought of a full-term pregnancy that would separate her from her friends and interrupt her schooling.

Following the abortion the household returned to an uneasy "business as usual." Angela was relieved to know that her friends did not shun her. As a matter of fact, they wanted to know all of the details of the experience! And her ten-year-old sister's scorn was short-lived. Her boyfriend resumed his visits —which had stopped when his mother reneged on her promise of assistance—much to the chagrin of Mrs. Rogers. Now all she could do was pray that Angela would follow the birth control plan suggested at the clinic.

Carmelita's Family

Carmelita Rodriguez's parents came from Puerto Rico fifteen years ago. They had eight children and several grandchildren. Carmelita, the second youngest child, became pregnant for the first time when she was sixteen. Her father was terribly upset and embarrassed: he was a deeply religious man, and the year had been hard on him. He had lost two of his sons in a car accident the previous year.

Mr. Rodriguez always made the decisions in their family. He insisted that Carmelita marry her boyfriend, Pedro. He reminded his daughter that one day he and his wife wanted to return home to Puerto Rico and said how important it was for the baby to look on Carmelita as his mother, and Pedro as his father.

Carmelita and Pedro moved into a small apartment around the corner. Each morning Carmelita brought Angelo with her to her parents' home. Mrs. Rodriguez raised Angelo. She fed him, bathed him, and played with him under her husband's constant, watchful instruction. Angelo became a member of their family, while Carmelita napped or went out. Each night Carmelita took Angelo back to her place. Carmelita became pregnant again when Angelo was a year old. Pedro left her. She moved back into her parents' home.

Gloria's Family

Mrs. Williams, a divorced black woman, suspected that her very attractive and somewhat rebellious sixteen-year-old daughter, Gloria, was having sex when she stayed out late. She told Gloria that she must not get into "trouble," and was pleased that Gloria followed her advice and went to a family planning clinic and got birth control pills. Mrs. Williams was very angry, but not surprised, when Gloria told her she thought she was pregnant. After all, Gloria could never remember to do anything every day. She thought the solution was obvious—she would help Gloria to get an abortion.

But Gloria was not so sure. The school counselor told her it was Gloria's decision, not her mother's. The doctor at the clinic said the same. Her boyfriend didn't want her to have an abortion either. She was confused, upset, and angry at her mother.

Gloria and her mother had some bad scenes. Mrs. Williams wanted to know who would take care of the baby. She couldn't help because she had a chronic illness that required frequent hospitalizations and left her tired and weak. The school counselor and the clinic social worker suggested a foster home. Mrs. Williams wouldn't hear of such a thing. She had known too many bad ones and wouldn't have a stranger taking care of her grandchild. But she added that Gloria was too young to take care of the baby and needed to finish school. Mrs. Williams pointed out that neither Gloria's boyfriend nor her boyfriend's family had offered any help beyond paying for the crib.

Finally Gloria agreed to an abortion. But by this time it was too late. The doctor confirmed it would no longer be safe.

Mrs. Williams and Gloria then went through a honeymoon period, becoming much closer during the pregnancy and early months of the baby's life as they shared in the care of Tommy. Then Gloria tired of being a mother and wanted to "party" again. She did not want to return to school. She left home from time to time, returning to shower Tommy with love, but never staying around for long. Mrs. Williams managed by first asking her eighty-year-old mother to move in with her. Then, when her mother had to return to other responsibilities, Mrs. Williams luckily found a neighbor to care for Tommy when she could not. She wonders what would happen to Tommy if her health seriously deteriorated. She now realizes that her dream of Gloria going to college will never come true.

June's Family

Mr. and Mrs. Fletcher, a white family living in a large city, were proud of June, their eldest child, who had always been competent, resourceful, and independent. Yet, there were many times when she was a complete mystery to them. When she was fourteen years old, she suddenly took off and left home. Three anxious weeks later, the Fletchers learned that she was across town, living with Mrs. Fletcher's mother. She didn't come home for several months. June was an "A" student, but left school early because of boredom. She got an excellent office job and made plans to go to night school and enroll in a community college. Her parents couldn't understand what she saw in her boyfriend, Larry. He was unemployed, several years older, and unmotivated. They spent all their time together. After a pregnancy scare, June went with her mother to the birth control clinic. Still, by the age of seventeen, she was pregnant.

June decided she wanted the baby, and her parents supported her decision. But Mrs. Fletcher insisted that June support herself financially and take care of the baby. In order to qualify for welfare and Medicaid payments for childbirth, and the like, June had to leave home and set up her own household. Larry was never officially a resident, but in fact, he turned out to be a devoted father. June went back to work when Iris was six months old; Larry took care of Iris. The Fletchers didn't really approve of June and Larry's hippie lifestyle, but had to admit that their granddaughter was healthy, beautiful, and as bright as a button. Three years later June found herself pregnant again. She didn't want the baby, as she and Larry had just started a new life out of state. She gave it up for adoption. The Fletchers were embarrassed and told all their friends that the baby was stillborn. However, June is glad she only has one child now and feels sorry for her younger friends who are tied down by three or four.

1

Introduction

Theodora Ooms

> I would there were no age between sixteen and three and twenty or that youth would sleep out the rest: for there is nothing in the between but getting wenches with child, wronging the ancientry, stealing, fighting.
>
> Shepherd, *The Winter's Tale*
> (Act III, Scene 3)

The shepherd's complaint about the between years—which we now call adolescence—has a familiar ring, though many parents would say the problems start well before sixteen. It takes only the addition of statistics about teenage auto accidents, suicides, and drug and alcohol abuse to bring Shakespeare's litany of complaints into the modern era. No wonder then that parents anxiously anticipate the adolescent years, wondering if their teenager will survive the passage to adulthood without floundering somewhere along the way.

Teenage pregnancy is not a new problem for adolescents and their families, but it has only recently become recognized as a problem for public policy. In the last few years a spate of newspaper stories, magazine and journal articles, books, and television and radio programs has made what is termed the "epidemic" of teenage pregnancy into a public issue. Although 1978 was a lean year for new social programs, the ninety-fifth Congress enacted the first federal legislation specifically designed to combat the problem.

A wide range of policies and programs that aim to affect adolescent sexual behavior, pregnancy, and parenting is discussed in this volume. Each chapter critically examines some aspect of policy from a new perspective, that of its impact on families. A family perspective maintains that adolescents are influenced by many factors in their environment: family, peers, school, media, church, and neighborhood. Yet, although its relative influence may be diminishing, the family remains the teenager's primary source of long-term caring and support, just as the family is often the primary source of most intense conflict. The family perspective holds that adolescents can best be understood, and served, within their family context.

To date policy discussions and research about teenage sex and fertility have almost totally neglected the adolescent's family. This assertion may seem surprising since, clearly, anyone interested in teenage pregnancy is primarily concerned about the well-being of the family unit of teenage mother and child. This focus is too narrow. It neglects the other family members in the teenager's life—mother, father, siblings, and others—and also ignores the role of the teenage boy and his family.[1] All these family members may contribute to the teenager's pattern of sexual behavior, and all can be profoundly affected if a birth occurs as a consequence of the behavior.

This volume is the final product of the Family Impact Seminar's study of teenage pregnancy, which consisted primarily of nine commissioned papers from experts. These papers were presented and discussed at an invitational conference held in Washington, D.C., in October 1978. The edited papers, with one additional paper, form the core of this book. Our study had a two-fold purpose. First, it sought new insights into how policy makers and professionals should approach the problems of teenage pregnancy. Second, it aimed to test a process called family impact analysis, which is designed to help make policies more sensitive to families.

The book focuses on the range of policies concerned with

teenage pregnancy, from those aimed at prevention, such as sex education and family planning programs, to those providing health care, economic support, and social services to the pregnant adolescent and young parent.

The contributors were asked, where possible, to address themselves to teenagers of school age. It is the under-eighteen-year-old for whom the consequences of pregnancy can be most devastating and long term. It is also for school-age teenagers, who, for the most part, are living with their families, that the family issues are most relevant.

The design for this study arose out of a review of the Seminar's ecological framework, from which a series of family impact questions were developed. The questions became the basis on which we commissioned the individual papers. (The framework, study design, and general methodology are briefly described and assessed in the Afterword.) These central family impact questions were: What do we know about the ways in which family members influence teenage sexual behavior? How do families respond to a teenager's pregnancy and parenthood? How do policy and programs affect and involve family members? This focus on the family context of teenage pregnancy and its implications for policy and services is this volume's unique contribution to the growing body of writing on the topic.

A related question, which arises directly from the family perspective, is whether parents should need to give their consent for (or be notified of) sex-related medical care provided to their minor children. Although rarely addressed in the professional literature in any depth, this question raises difficult and sensitive ethical and legal issues that are being actively debated in the media, and in courts and legislatures at federal and state levels.

Values and Paradoxes

As a society, we are very confused about the relationship, especially with regard to teenagers' sexual behavior, of parents to teenagers, and teenagers to parents. Attitudes expressed in policies of both the government and private sector convey contradictory messages to both generations about their roles and responsibilities in these matters.

Consider some of the paradoxes that families may encounter:

- In most states, a fifteen-year-old girl needs her parent's signed permission for an excused absence from school, to have her ears pierced, get a broken arm set, take a blood test, be interviewed for a survey, or get a job. She is not allowed to sign contracts, drink liquor, or drive a car. Yet she may walk into a clinic and be treated for venereal disease (VD), get a prescription for birth control pills, have an intrauterine device (IUD) inserted, or obtain an abortion, without her parents ever being informed.[2]
- A seventeen-year-old boy, encouraged by peers and the media to "score," is not expected to be responsible for using contraceptives. If his partner becomes pregnant but the two do not marry, he does not have a right to be involved in any decisions about the pregnancy or care of his baby. He has apparently no recourse if the teenage mother decides that she or her family does not want him to visit the baby. Yet, if she is to receive welfare assistance for her child, she has to identify him as the father; and if paternity is established, he is obliged to provide her with child support payments for years to come.
- Television, radio, and pop songs daily present themes of premarital sex, unwed pregnancy, and adultery. In Jesse Jackson's words, these media messages "encourage adolescents into premature heat." Advertisements of all kinds of feminine hygiene products abound, including pregnancy test kits. And yet the voluntary code followed by the National Association of Broadcasters does not allow advertisements of contraceptives which might encourage responsible teenage sexual behavior.[3]
- Surveys report that 80 percent of parents want schools to provide sex education to their children; and of these, 70 percent are willing for that education to include instruction about birth control. Yet it is estimated that only one-third of the schools offer

INTRODUCTION   13

any kind of sex education, even on an optional basis; and only 6 percent of school students are receiving any kind of comprehensive sex education. High school biology textbooks may carefully avoid teaching the basic facts about human reproduction;[4] and special sex education courses that teach about the perils of venereal disease often omit any reference to how to avoid catching it.

- A fifteen-year-old mother lives with her parents who took care of her during pregnancy, and now provide shelter, food, and care for her baby while she attends school. But these parents were not allowed to be with their daughter during her labor, nor visit her in the hospital. They have yet to meet any of the doctors or nurses at the well-baby clinic and parent education program their daughter attends weekly. They have no legal rights to or responsibilities for their grandchild, even though they are legally responsible for their daughter's expenses. (Their daughter may collect a welfare assistance check for her baby irrespective of her parents' income.)

The topics of teenage sex, pregnancy, and parenting involve intensely felt, but seldom articulated, feelings, attitudes, and moral values. With the exception of debates about abortion, there has been little effort in various policy discussions to make these issues explicit. Two kinds of ethical issues are involved here: those concerned with sexuality in general, especially for the young and unmarried, and those relating specifically to parental roles in teenage sexual behavior. Some, a minority, believe so strongly that teenagers should not engage in sex outside of marriage that they oppose sex education in schools—for fear that it may encourage such activity. This fear may also explain some of the opposition to abortion, since it is believed that making abortion available may encourage premarital sex. Others may be accepting of teenage sex, or at least accept its inevitability, but believe it is immoral to have an unwanted baby. Thus they advocate programs that teach "responsible" sexual behavior, usually meaning teaching teenagers to use contraceptives.

Some feel that teenagers should not be punished for engaging in sex, and that they, and especially their babies, need all the help they can get to avoid some of the risks and hardships of young parenthood. These advocates concentrate their efforts on establishing programs to provide income, health, education, and other services to the teen mother and child. Others feel that providing welfare assistance and special programs to this group somehow gives sanction to teenage pregnancy and may serve to encourage teenage parenthood as a valid way of life. As an example, a recent letter to the *Washington Post* suggesting that the material incentives should be reversed proposed a "deferred motherhood" plan whereby single girls, age fourteen to twenty-one, would receive annual cash payments irrespective of income if they did *not* get pregnant or give birth.[5]

Some feel that since the consequences of engaging in sex bear most heavily on the woman, she should be the one to take the responsibility for contraception, and it is she who needs the services. Others perceive this as a sexist attitude that may perpetuate the problem and lay the responsibility and the blame equally on the girl's partner; this group advocates more education and programs that address male teenagers.[6]

The critical ethical issue that a family perspective leads one to consider, however, is the appropriate role of the state—and its representatives—in intervening in an area of family life that has, until recently, been considered to be the family's own affair. (See Margaret O'Brien Steinfels, Chapter 8.) Courts, currently struggling with this question, are finding it very difficult to resolve, largely because of the ambiguous role of adolescents in relationship to society and to their parents. The dilemmas are particularly acute because an individual's sexual behavior is generally considered to be a private, personal area of life in which the intrusion of others, even family members, is inappropriate. Perhaps one reason that policy is confused and inconsistent in this area is that it is seldom grounded in a firm understanding of the nature of adolescents or of their families.

Adolescents and Their Families

A great deal has been written about the stage of life that is now called adolescence, but not very much has been said about the experience from the perspective of others in the family. Adolescence is the stage of transition between childhood and adulthood, or dependence to independence. Its age boundaries are not distinct: some may achieve a good measure of adulthood when they reach the age of legal majority at eighteen; others may take much longer. Early adolescence especially, from eleven to sixteen, is perhaps the period of greatest concern to parents, but ironically is least well understood by experts.[7]

Policy discussions, and this book is no exception, inevitably run the risk of overemphasizing the problem side of any stage of life. Yet it is important to remember that adolescence is not mostly a time of problems. It is a time of astonishing growth and change, of many new skills and achievements, and a time for testing one's wings. All of these developments are as much a source of pride, pleasure, and delight to teenagers themselves, their families, teachers, and others as they can be a source of worry and exasperation.

We are familiar with the years from ten to sixteen as a period of rapid growth and physical change stimulated by hormonal activity. Perhaps less well appreciated is the range of individual variation in both the onset and duration of this growth spurt. One teenage girl can have completed her physical maturation by the age of thirteen before another, the same age, has even begun hers. Variations in growth rates are comparable for boys. J. M. Tanner, who has meticulously documented these variations within normally developing adolescents, maintains that "the statement that a boy is fourteen is in most contexts hopelessly vague," and thus, it is impossible on the basis of age alone to consider how grown up he is either physically or socially, "since much behavior is conditioned by physical status."[8] This variation in both sexes poses considerable problems for programs and policies related to chronological age (such as most education programs), and for the definition of legal maturity.

Two other biological facts are pertinent here. On the average, girls start the maturation process two years earlier than boys; and both sexes now begin physical maturation much earlier than in previous generations, apparently because of improved nutrition. The onset of menstruation (menarche), for example, now occurs almost two years earlier than it did forty to fifty years ago. The average age was fifteen in the 1930s, compared to thirteen in the 1970s. This earlier biological maturation may account, in part, both for the earlier initiation of sexual activity among adolescents today and for the rise in pregnancies among eleven-to-fourteen-year-olds.

Erik Erikson characterizes adolescence as a critical stage in the development of identity and autonomy. He attributes this to complex development on several fronts at once: sexual, vocational, and peer group.[9] Sexual maturation signals that the young person is on the threshold of adulthood; indeed, a pregnant young girl is assigned some adult legal rights by virtue of her biological maturity alone. (If she marries she automatically gains full majority status.) Yet, as the average age for initiating sexual activity falls, society raises the age at which most young people assume adult economic responsibilities. Entry into the labor force today is postponed either through the requirement of education or the scarcity of jobs for youth.

Other writers have emphasized adolescence as a period in which young people become less guided by parental values and concerns and more dependent both on the views and approval of peers and on other influences, such as the media. It is a time for much experimenting and risk taking. Piagetian theory emphasizes that the period of adolescence should accomplish the last stage of cognitive development, where one becomes capable of *formal operational* thinking, meaning the ability to reason logically and abstractly. Until this stage is completed, adolescents may continue to be present-oriented, not future-oriented, believing in their own immortality and deliberately courting danger. (Some believe this explains why adolescents take risks such as having "unprotected" sex: They simply don't believe "it can happen to them," and many are not used to planning ahead but believe in living "for the moment.")[10]

While adolescent years are clearly a time of much questioning and testing of adult values and concerns, many argue that the great majority of young people make the necessary transition without overt rebellion or traumatic stress in their relationships with their parents. Discussions of the steps that adolescents take to gain independence from their parents and family are one-sided. The emphasis is usually on the teenager "getting away" from parents. There is rarely mention of the complex two-way process by which this independence is achieved or of the steps taken by parents to "let go." Very few studies examine the impact of adolescence on parents or siblings, or the effects of the adolescent youth culture invading the family home. The literature on adolescence seldom discusses how parents, facing their own physical aging, are affected by their teenagers' blossoming sexuality. For, at the same time they are having to deal with their teenagers, parents are often facing the pressures of their own mid-life crises. For example, parents may find themselves struggling to balance their economic and psychological responsibilities to their elderly and ailing parents with the demands and economic needs of their vigorous, often college-bound adolescents. Greer Litton Fox in Chapter 3 speculates on additional tasks and tensions within families at this stage of life.

The life-stages approach to understanding the development of individual adults and children has gained considerable popular attention in the last few years,[11] yet no similar recognition is given to the fact that families, too, undergo development. In 1964, Reuben Hill laid out an interesting typology of families in terms of life cycle stages.[12] But there has been little published since then about the evolution families experience as they cope with and adjust to what Jay Haley calls the "ordinary affairs" or main events of life: courtship and marriage; the birth of a child; children entering school; children leaving home; the death of a parent; retirement and old age; and the variations on this schema, such as divorce and remarriage, or remaining childless.[13]

One of the few is Haley's review of the family life cycle (in his book about the therapist Milton Erickson), in which he discusses the stage of families with adolescents in a chapter entitled "Weaning Parents from Children."[14] Haley writes that the renegotiation of family rules that is necessary at this stage—to give teenagers both more freedom and more responsibility—has been somewhat misunderstood. Adolescents do not need or want complete separation, Haley notes; they must become separated from the family and yet remain involved with them. Similarly, parents must learn to let go, but not completely; they must shift to treating their children more as peers.

Disputes and conflicts between parents and adolescents are necessary and normal. They are usually resolved by mutual negotiation which can, as John Gagnon describes in a college textbook, "be rational and thoughtful, angry and explosive, or it can entail agreements to overlook behavior or avoid confrontation."[15] The family is a complex system of relationships involving several individuals whose feelings about each other change, depending upon mood and topic. As Gagnon says, parents may be delighted with their son's progress in school or on the athletic field, arguing constantly about his use of the car, but tacitly agreeing to avoid the subject of whether he is having sex with his girlfriend. Both Fox and Frank Furstenberg in this volume describe the oblique patterns of communication and contradictory messages that most parents give their teenagers about sex (Chapters 3 and 4, respectively). And in Chapter 8, Steinfels writes of how professionals and the courts warily regard the family conflicts that may follow from a teenager's pregnancy.

This backdrop of the family context of adolescence is important to setting the stage for any discussion of policy regarding adolescent sexuality, pregnancy, and parenting. Sexual maturity immediately sets up new boundaries between parents and children. When the adolescent engages in sexual activity, more than any other activity, it perhaps symbolizes a separation from par-

INTRODUCTION   19

ents. And yet parents still have the duty, while respecting the need for privacy, to help their children understand the responsibilities and consequences of engaging in sex. Paradoxically, pregnancy dramatically signals to the family and the world outside that, in one dimension at least, adult status has been achieved; at the same time, it usually thrusts the teenager into renewed dependence on parents, sexual partner, or other adults (doctors, counselors, etc.).

The Teenage Pregnancy Problem

Many will argue that teenage pregnancy does not belong in the catalogue of such serious social problems as drug and alcohol abuse, delinquency, and auto accidents. After all, pregnancy can be the result of a positive loving relationship; giving birth is a creative act; and babies themselves, even when unplanned, are usually cherished and loved. Many people who are living successfully today were born to teenage mothers.

Each contributor to this volume would disagree with such a complacent view and insist that teenage pregnancy is often a serious problem for both the individuals and families involved and certainly for society at large. The five family vignettes, adapted from real life, that open this book provide a small sample of the most immediate ways in which the pregnancy of an adolescent affects the other family members. It is important also to grasp a sense of the overall numbers: how many adolescents and their families experience this problem nationwide. (Of course, in many situations, when she does not tell them of her abortion, parents may never know that their adolescent daughter became pregnant.)

The statistics on adolescent childbearing, a recent book states succinctly, "can provide either some degree of reassurance or considerable cause for alarm . . . depending on which indicator, which specific time period and which age segment we examine."[16] Since this study is primarily concerned with teenagers of school age, the following five facts relating to those under eighteen years of age are especially compelling (see Audrey Jones and Paul Placek, Chapter 2):[17]

- Forty percent of women age seventeen had had sexual intercourse in 1976, as compared with only 26 percent in 1971.
- Approximately one-third of sexually active girls under the age of seventeen never use contraceptives. (Only one in three sexually active teenage women, age fifteen to nineteen, always use birth control.)
- One in five of today's fourteen-year-old girls can expect to become pregnant before she reaches eighteen. Most of these pregnancies occur within the first six months of becoming sexually active.
- One-third of more than a million abortions each year are performed on teenagers, approximately one half of these on the under-eighteen-year-olds.
- In 1977 more than half a million births occurred among women under the age of twenty. Of these, 39 percent were to teenagers of school age.

Although the current rates of teenage pregnancy and births have been labeled "epidemic," the historical data presented in Chapter 2, Figure 1, indicate that the overall rate of teenage births has declined from a high in the 1950s and is now about the same level as it was in the 1930s. However, other indicators do show cause for concern: sexual activity continues to rise, putting more teenagers at risk of pregnancy; teenage pregnancy and abortion rates are rising, and childbearing rates are climbing for the youngest ages. Further, although birth control is more available and becoming more successfully used by adolescents, pregnancies and birth rates are not declining among school-age adolescents as they are for the eighteen- and nineteen-year-olds.

There is clearly no simple explanation for the present rates of teenage pregnancy. The research on this topic is, according to one authority, quite inadequate.[18] The causes cited range from basic ignorance about the facts of sex and contraception through psychological reluctance to use contraceptives; from the passivity of girls in submitting to boys urging them to have sex, and vice versa, to poor education and unemployment. When surveyed nationally most teenage pregnancies are said to be unwanted. Other evidence suggests some of them are desired, or at least passively "backed into," probably because parenthood has more attractions than a life of school failure and unemployment.[19]

Parental roles in providing information, guidance, or seeking to control children's sexual behavior have seldom been explored. In Chapter 3, Fox reviews the available evidence on the family determinants of teenage pregnancy, and suggests that the family is still the crucible of much sexual learning, however much its role is undervalued or undermined by various institutions in our society.

There is little doubt that, to a girl of school age, pregnancy is a crisis—for both her and her family. In the short run, she faces a number of difficult choices. She may choose abortion, formal or informal adoption, or keeping the baby. Choosing the latter, she has to make some major readjustments in her life, as usually does her family. In Chapter 4, Furstenberg points out that in the long run, many teenage mothers do surmount the difficulties, especially those who receive the assistance and support of their families. However, considerable evidence indicates that the teenage mother is at much greater risk than her peers of dropping out of school, being unemployed over the years, getting pregnant again quickly, and/or receiving welfare assistance.[20] There is not much evidence about how her children fare in the long run, although a recent review of ongoing research on the subject also suggests that the availability of family support seems to improve the long-term effects of early motherhood on her child's development.[21]

The various contributors to this volume confirm how little emphasis there has been on the role of the male in teenage sex or how he is affected by his partner's pregnancy, or reacts to parenthood. In addition to his being ignored by research, it is still the exceptional family planning or parenting program that reaches out to include him; and government policy—in attempting to claim financial support from him—undoubtedly contributes to his seeking to stay firmly out of the picture.

The above arguments make it clear that teenage pregnancy is a serious problem for many teenagers and families, but why is it also considered a problem for society? In particular, why does it receive increasing public attention at a time when statistics indicate the problem is, in many respects, not getting worse?

Social historian Maris Vinovskis believes that teenage pregnancy has become more visible for three demographic reasons: first, teenage births are now a considerably larger proportion of overall births because of the dramatic declining fertility in older women; second, fewer teenage mothers are getting married; third, many more are keeping their babies rather than giving them up for adoption.[22] The latter two trends have been particularly striking in the white population; for pregnant black teenagers, neither marriage nor adoption had been as common as for whites. Thus, the rates of unwed motherhood have risen substantially, especially in white, middle-class communities.

Although society no longer regards illegitimacy to be as immoral as it once did—hence the current term "out of wedlock"—we are beginning to reckon how costly it can be to public budgets. A recent estimate by Stanford Research Institute International calculates that the present rate of teenage births may cost federal, state, and local governments as much as $8.3 billion a year in welfare and medical costs alone.[23] This staggering figure, taken together with the list of forty-three federal programs described by Kristin Moore (in Chapter 5) as having potential or actual effect on adolescent family formation and parenthood, indicates that teenage pregnancy has been considered a public responsibility for at least the past decade.

What accounts for the largely unacknowledged growth of such public programs? and, why has policy been concerned

INTRODUCTION

only with the adolescent girl? While it is true that most social policy in the United States is developed in terms of specific categories of individuals (by age or need), three historical themes account for the particularly strong focus on the individual teenage girl: the traditional stigma and double standard attached to illegitimacy and extramarital sex, which affected the way services have been offered; the dominance of medical leadership in defining the nature of the problem; and the development of the women's rights and children's rights movements.

Historical Perspectives

Several decades before national attention was focused on the problems of teenage pregnancy, several community-based, private sector agencies—such as the Florence Crittenton and Salvation Army's Booth maternity homes, and the Jewish and Catholic counseling and adoption agencies—were quietly offering counseling, shelter, and other services to pregnant teenagers as part of their overall program for unmarried pregnant women. The primary concern in those years was not the age of clients but their unmarried status. Attitudes towards out-of-wedlock pregnancy have shifted dramatically in the last two decades. In the fifties, Leontine Young, a social worker, wrote vividly about how Americans responded with condemnation and punitive attitudes to public evidence of premarital, or extramarital, sex.[24] When a girl found herself pregnant, the most common recourse was a hasty marriage. If this was not possible or desired, rather than submit herself to the harsh judgment of her family and community—and subject her child to the unenvied state of bastardy—many thousands of girls, particularly white girls from lower- and middle-class homes, fled their communities and sought refuge elsewhere, particularly in large cities. If the girls were lucky, they would obtain counseling, some financial assistance, shelter, and help in giving up their babies for adoption—the outcome preferred by the agencies and chosen by most women. The girls were often regarded as "fallen women," and, according to Young, agencies tended to be excessively punitive in some of the ways they treated them.

The stigma attached to illegitimacy influenced not only the nature of some of the services, but also society's view about its cause. Young's book presents a surprisingly dogmatic and simplified explanation of unwed pregnancy. In reflecting the views of much of the clinical literature of the period, her book, in turn, clearly influenced the thinking of a generation of social workers.[25] In Young's experience, when a young, unmarried woman became pregnant, it was no accident, but a result of a pathological relationship with her parents. "In every case the girl had unhappiness and problems in her life which led directly to this action."[26] Young, unlike most recent writers, was very conscious of the powerful influence of the family, but viewed this influence in entirely negative terms. She characterized the families as: mother-dominated, with the father passive and seductive; dominated by a tyrannical, cruel, and abusive father; or as insufficiently attentive, with both parents being remote and rejecting. In her view, a girl would get pregnant, either consciously or unconsciously, to give a "gift" to her mother, to shame and hurt her father, or to have someone of her own to love and receive love from.

It is no surprise, then, that staff of these agencies rarely viewed the family of their clients as a positive resource to their pregnant clients. Nor is it surprising that their counseling efforts were largely directed to helping the pregnant women become psychologically and economically independent of their parents. Although few agency staff would currently subscribe to the theories or attitudes prevalent in the forties and fifties, Janet Forbush and Teresa Maciocha in Chapter 7 note that agencies' individual casework approach to service delivery has not substantially altered. However, the variety of services offered has changed. A recent report of the Child Welfare League describes how, as more young white women decided to keep their babies, programs reoriented their services to include more counseling and education programs but fewer maternity shelters and adoption services.[27]

Young also discusses the cultural factors that influence the ways in which teenage pregnancy is treated. She notes that in certain European countries and "in Negro cultures, . . . which have fewer taboos about sex, . . . out-of-wedlock children are born without guilt or conflict and happily accepted into the family."[28] One consequence of this racial difference in America is that traditionally out-of-wedlock pregnancy and teenage pregnancy were most visible in the black community, and regarded by whites as symptoms of immorality and broken homes.[29] Public debates centered on whether unwed mothers deserved welfare assistance; some even suggested they should be sterilized. (See June Dobbs Butts' Chapter 9.) Joyce Ladner points out that when a problem once ascribed to the black community becomes openly recognized as a problem of the white community, our terms become less pejorative: "illegitimacy" becomes "out-of-wedlock"; "broken homes" becomes "single parenting"; common law marriage, "alternative life style"; bastards, "love children"; and, most recently, venereal disease, "socially transmitted disease."[30] The increased recognition of teenage parenting as a fact of life in white and middle-class communities may help to account for the fact that, in 1978, Congress passed the teenage pregnancy legislation.

In the early sixties, another series of events and trends contributed to thrusting the needs of pregnant teenagers into public consciousness. The technological revolution in birth control methods and the emerging women's movement led to a much greater interest in questions of fertility control. It is easy to forget that, only two decades ago, there was a raging debate about public funding of family planning services. Welfare workers in many states were not allowed to even mention the subject to their public assistance clients, even when they already had six children. Several states had laws forbidding the use or sale of contraceptives. Court battles were successfully fought against these laws, leading to the establishment of family planning clinics, many of which later affiliated with the Planned Parenthood Federation of America. (Planned Parenthood—originally started in 1914 by Margaret Sanger, then known as the National Birth Control League—was renamed in 1946.)

Family planning services grew phenomenally from the mid-60s to the mid-70s. In 1964, the federal government made its first family planning grant, which served only married women. By 1970, Congress had passed the first national family planning and population legislation. Federal expenditures grew from $16 million to close to $200 million. In 1969, there were less than a quarter of a million teenagers using family planning clinics; by 1976 this had swollen to 1.2 million.[31]

Obstetricians and pediatricians drew attention to the increased health risks and complications accompanying too early pregnancy and childbearing. In 1972, the findings of the first Kantner and Zelnik national survey of adolescent girls were published; they showed that nearly three in ten unwed teens were sexually active, and more than half were not using contraception. Hospital-based demonstration and research programs that were established (sometimes with federal funds) focused on the problems of young mothers, who typically did not have access to adequate family planning, prenatal, and maternity and child health services. These programs were usually situated in large inner-city areas and served a predominantly black population.

The medical orientation of most of these programs was another factor in focusing attention solely on the adolescent girl. Although the revolutionary discovery of the "pill" helped to liberate women from unwanted childbearing, it had several unfortunate consequences, one of which is rarely mentioned: it absolved males from responsibility for contraception.[32] Thus, even the prevention of adolescent pregnancy became a female issue, to be solved through ensuring that teenage girls had access to contraceptives provided under medical auspices. Further, teenage pregnancy and childbearing were regarded as posing a challenge primarily for prenatal, obstetrical, and pediatric services.

INTRODUCTION

Typically, doctors and other health care personnel are protective of the confidentiality of their individual patients. Yet, in the case of minors, state laws required parental consent for medical treatment. Many professions became concerned that such consent acted as a barrier to teenagers seeking the sex-related treatment they needed. What was to become the most influential professional journal in the field of fertility, *Family Planning Perspectives*, was first published by the Alan Guttmacher Institute in the spring of 1969. In its first few years of publication, the journal seldom addressed the problems of teenagers as if they were distinct from women in general; however, parental consent requirements and the changing status of the law on this issue was the subject of two major and often-quoted articles by Harriet Pilpel (1969 and 1971).[33] In the second article, Pilpel notes the dramatic change that had occurred in the attitude of the professional medical associations towards parental consent since her first article. By 1971, the American Medical Association (AMA), the American College of Obstetrics and Gynecology, the American Academy of Pediatrics, and the American Association of Family Physicians had all adopted statements recommending that doctors be allowed to prescribe contraceptives for sexually active minors without parental consent (although doctors were encouraged to try to obtain the parents' consent).

Access to effective fertility control as a basic human and constitutional right was next argued by civil liberty lawyers and other women's rights advocates. Contraceptive services became more available for women, especially poor women; and this movement culminated in the Supreme Court decision of 1973, *Roe v. Wade*, legalizing abortion. At first, it was not clear that minors were to be accorded adult status in obtaining abortions. However, these decades also saw the emergence of the children's rights movement, which began with decisions in the juvenile court arena, and soon extended to other constitutional rights. Relevant here was the extension of adult rights to adolescents in the area of venereal disease and drug-related treatment, and later, in many states, to any treatment related to sexuality.

By 1979, the American Bar Association had adopted a set of standards that recommended "that minors of any age be able to consent to their own sex-related care without notification or consent of parents being necessary," unless the adolescent's life was clearly endangered. This position was justified on several grounds, including that "the overriding importance of the minor's and infant's health and society's welfare requires the subordination of parental interests despite the potentially adverse impact on the family."[34] After the *Bellotti v. Baird* Supreme Court decision in July 1979, the American Civil Liberties Union declared that it "opposed any impediment be it parental or judicial, in the path of a minor's right to obtain an abortion."[35]

In 1976, the Alan Guttmacher Institute, Planned Parenthood's research arm, published a booklet—*11 Million Teenagers*—that has been widely distributed, and is the single most influential publication on the topic of teenage pregnancy.[36] This report summarizes a great deal of information, data, and research, and takes a strong advocacy stand. It urges the public to become more aware of the large numbers of teenagers at risk of pregnancy (eleven million adolescents—including married teens, eleven through nineteen years of age—are sexually active), and refers to the rates of teenage pregnancy as "an epidemic." It portrays the economic and social consequences of teenage childbearing in dire terms; a pregnant girl has her "life's script written for her." Insofar as the booklet proposes solutions, it emphasizes the need to improve the quantity, quality, and accessibility of medical services, especially family planning and abortion. The booklet's bias towards a medical perspective on teenage pregnancy also dominates all the articles on the topic until quite recently.

The success of the movement towards reproductive freedom and improving the availability of contraceptive services was not accomplished easily. Butts, in Chapter 9, alludes to the accusations of genocide made by some members of the black community during this period. Not unexpectedly, various religious groups—in particular, Roman Catholic and certain fundamentalist groups—also strongly opposed the growth of family planning clinics. In part, this was a question of their belief in the immorality of artificial methods of contraception. In part, there was the fear that such attempts to "control" population represented efforts on the part of the dominant, upper class, Protestants to repress the growth of the Catholic and lower-class populations.[37]

Although the health care professions took the lead in being concerned about teenage pregnancy, educators during the sixties were also alerted to the fact that teenage pregnancy was the single highest known cause of school dropout among girls. In Chapter 7, Forbush and Maciocha describe the origins (from 1963 on) of school-based programs that attempt to provide alternative education and related services that enable pregnant adolescents and adolescent parents to complete high school. This process was aided by the passage of Title IX of the Education Amendments in 1972, which made it illegal to exclude pregnant students from school.

The most successful efforts at prevention of teenage pregnancy during these years were in the family planning field. By contrast, as Peter Scales describes in Chapter 6, efforts to implement sex education programs in schools have been only sporadically successful and have evoked some intensely vocal opposition. However, sex education as a field of knowledge has grown substantially and was nurtured by the establishment of two professional advocacy organizations: the Sex Information and Education Council of the United States (SIECUS), founded in 1964; and the American Association of Sex Educators, Counselors, and Therapists (AASECT), founded in 1964.

Although a few very innovative and successful models of sex education programs in schools and in private sector organizations have been established during the last decade, estimates of their number vary, with only between 10 and 30 percent of the schools offering any kind of sex education at all; moreover, the instruction may consist of only a couple of sessions on menstruation (see Chapter 6).

Federal Legislation

During the late sixties and the seventies, as Forbush and Maciocha have described, a loosely organized network of organizations and individuals began to advocate energetically—with some federal encouragement—for the recognition of the multiple needs of adolescent parents (mothers) and the provision of comprehensive services. A first attempt to legislate a federal program was made when Senator Edward Kennedy introduced the National School Age Mother and Child Act in 1975, but it did not get out of committee. Three years later these efforts bore fruit in the Carter Administration.

The Carter Administration's Teenage Pregnancy Initiative, 1978

On the last day of the Ninety-fifth Congress, October 15, 1978, Congress passed the Health Services and Centers Amendments Act. Titles VI, VII and VIII of this legislation established the first federal grants program to focus specifically on the problems of teenage pregnancy. This legislation was drafted and sponsored by the Administration, and was originally introduced as a separate bill, S.2910, in the spring. It was described by HEW* Secretary Califano on April 13, 1978, as "the centerpiece of President Carter's strategy to deal with the urgent problem of teenage pregnancy across the nation."

Julius Richmond, the Assistant Secretary for Health, outlined the other components of the policy initiative in testimony to the Senate: "In fiscal year 1979 we have requested a total of $344 mil-

*Since most of the writing of this book was undertaken in 1978 and 1979, references throughout are to the Department of Health, Education, and Welfare (HEW) prior to its reorganization: On May 6, 1980, the new Department of Education came into being, and HEW became the Department of Health and Human Services (HHS).

INTRODUCTION 31

lion for programs to address the pressing problems of teenage pregnancy. This represents an increase of $148 million over current efforts." In addition to $60 million requested to fund the grants program, the package of additional funds included a $24 million expansion in Medicaid coverage for adolescents through the proposed Child Health Assessment Program, which would enable pregnant and nonpregnant adolescents to receive family planning and other health services, and monies to support increases and specific targeting for existing family planning programs, maternal and child health services research, and health education curricula.

The new policy initiative had been developed by an HEW task force that worked for a number of months to develop a series of policy options. Some commentators have pointed out that this package was initially referred to as the "Alternatives to Abortion" initiative, signifying that both members of the Administration and Congress felt a need to do something positive in this area in reaction to the government's recent negative stand on public funding of abortion.[38]

Secretary Califano asked each major division of HEW to develop plans for increased efforts to deal with the problems of adolescent pregnancy. Through a series of public meetings the Administration sought advice from a variety of experts and organizations. In selecting the particular package, Califano strongly favored maintaining a balance between support of primary prevention, including sex education, and secondary prevention, mostly improved services for teenage parents.

Legislative History

Preparatory to the introduction of the adolescent pregnancy bill, the House Select Committee on Population, chaired by Representative James H. Scheuer, held three days of hearings on "Adolescent and Pre-adolescent Pregnancy." Maris Vinovskis, a member of the staff of the Select Committee on Population during this period, and a close observer of the legislative process of this bill, comments that many congressmen received the rather misleading impression that teenage births were on the rise, and hence misconstrued the reasons for the legislation. He notes that if demographics were the only justification for such a program, then legislation should have been passed under the Eisenhower Administration, when teenage fertility rates were at their peak.[39] He feels that the humanitarian concerns for teenage parents were in fact the dominant influence in achieving passage of the bill—not the desire to prevent teenage pregnancy.

Leadership of the Administration's original bill in the Senate was provided by Senators Kennedy and Williams. Co-sponsors were Senators Javits, Hathaway, Humphrey (Muriel), Leahy, Randolph, Riegle, and Pell. The House sponsors were Representatives Rogers and Brademas. Secretary Califano personally testified in favor of the bill, and was known to be a strong supporter, as were Sargent and Eunice Shriver of the Joseph P. Kennedy, Jr., Foundation.

A wide variety of experts, service and organizational representatives, as well as a few teenagers testified at the hearings. Significantly, parents of adolescents did not testify. Most witnesses welcomed the bill, and praised its intent. A number of witnesses criticised the scope and purposes of the bill; for example, the lack of attention to sex education and primary prevention. Other criticisms focused on the low level of funding requested to achieve such ambitious goals. In general, however, those testifying agreed that there was a substantial unmet need for services, and strongly urged passage of the bill. An ad hoc coalition of service organizations worked hard for the bill's passage and made several criticisms and suggestions, some of which were incorporated in the final version.

A major controversial issue was whether grantees should be either required or allowed to offer abortion counseling. A compromise was reached that stipulated that grantees are to be asked to provide an assurance that each pregnant adolescent will be "informed of the availability of counseling on all options regarding her pregnancy." This counseling is to be provided ei-

INTRODUCTION   33

ther by the agency itself or through referral. A second major controversy concerned whether the bill should have an equal focus on primary prevention and secondary prevention (which was the Administration's original intent), or should give priority to teenage parents—that is, secondary prevention. The Senate rewrote the bill, de-emphasizing the primary prevention aspects. A third, somewhat muted controversy was over whether the program should be administratively located in HEW in the Office of the Assistant Secretary for Health or in the Office for Human Development Services, a debate that symbolized the divergence between the medical and social models of teenage pregnancy. In the months to come, most of the other parts of the initiative package were not approved by Congress.

It is interesting to note which organizations were involved in the ad hoc coalition working for the passage of the bill, and which were not. Those in the coalition represented a broad spectrum of services and points of view: the Child Welfare League, National Conference of Catholic Charities, Alan Guttmacher Institute/Planned Parenthood, American Academy of Child Psychiatry, National Alliance Concerned with School-Age Parents, American Academy of Pediatrics, Joseph P. Kennedy, Jr., Foundation, and the National Association of State Boards of Education. Strikingly absent from this group, and from previous advocacy efforts, were any organized women's and feminist groups, or black and Hispanic organizations. As this volume emphasizes, teenage pregnancy has been largely defined to date as a woman's problem. Yet most organized women's groups have not viewed the needs or rights of adolescent women as any different from those of women in general (whose reproductive rights they have lobbied for intensively and successfully). An exception is the Project on Equal Education Rights (PEER), which has made special efforts to draw attention to the exclusion of pregnant teenagers from school in their efforts to monitor enforcement of Title IX (of the 1972 Education Amendments).

Furthermore, given the well-advertised higher rate of adolescent pregnancy in the black community, and its association with poverty and welfare dependency, it is also surprising that the major black organizations have not placed teenage pregnancy on their national agenda. Nor have the national Hispanic organizations. However, in their case, as Angel Martinez points out (Chapter 10), there are no data on the extent to which adolescent pregnancy is a problem in Hispanic communities. There are signs that leaders of both minorities are beginning to address the issue as a serious one for them. The National Urban League and the National Council on Negro Women have recently started small demonstration programs designed to help black teenage parents. The National Council of La Raza's 1980 conference on Hispanic Youth Employment identified teenage pregnancy as a leading cause of the high Hispanic school dropout rate and held a workshop on teenage pregnancy.

Office of Adolescent Pregnancy Programs

The Office of Adolescent Pregnancy Programs (OAPP) was established to report directly to the Assistant Secretary for Health of HEW, in consultation and coordination with the Deputy Assistant Secretary for Population Affairs. Its responsibility is to administer the new grants program, under Title VI of the legislation; and carry out the coordination, technical assistance, and evaluation activities called for by Title VII. Under Title VI direct assistance grants are given to community-based agencies after a competitive application process. Funds pay up to 70 percent of the costs for the first two years, with the federal portion diminishing thereafter. The grants cannot extend beyond five years, with re-applications required annually. They are awarded to projects providing comprehensive services for pregnant adolescents, adolescent parents, and, to a lesser extent, those adolescents at risk of pregnancy, with a special emphasis on school-age parents. All grantees must provide certain "core" services (primarily health-related) either directly or through a network of providers, and may provide "supplemental" services (to include child care, family counseling, transportation). Grantees are required to develop linkages with related programs, charge fees based on ability to pay, seek reimbursement from other third-party payers, and meet a number of other assurances. Although $50 million was authorized for the first year of the Office of Adolescent Pregnancy Programs, only $1 million was appropriated. Lulu Mae Nix was appointed as Director. Her background as director of a successful comprehensive statewide yet community-based program in Delaware was a welcome indication to many that the program would not have an exclusively medical orientation. In its first year, two hundred twelve proposals were reviewed, but funds were only sufficient to award four grants—for a total of $740,000, which went to centers in Middlebury, Vermont; Houston, Texas; Bronx, New York; and Worcester, Massachusetts. The Office held six regional technical assistance seminars to advise prospective grant applicants, and published an Information Bulletin. Congress authorized $17.5 million for grants in fiscal year 1980; however, the Office was a victim of budget cuts and received only $7.5 million, of which $5.7 million was for newly funded programs. Three hundred and eighty proposals were received, of which one-half were approved for funding. However, funds were only sufficient to fund twenty-three new programs with four continued from the previous year. In fiscal year 1981, although Congress approved $10 million in the continuing resolution of December 1980, the Office was required by the Carter administration to operate at the same level as the previous year ($7.5 million). For the fiscal year 1982 budget, the Office of Management and Budget originally recommended a zero level of funding for the Office; however, on appeal by the department, the Office was reinstated at the level of $10.4 million. (The Office is clearly vulnerable in a period of budget cuts.)

The second major responsibility of the Office, spelled out in Title VII, is to coordinate federal policies and programs related to prevention of initial and repeat adolescent pregnancies. This task involves both identifying obstacles to improved coordination and delivery of service, and providing technical assistance to grantees to facilitate improved coordination between programs. A separate provision of this title assigns between 1 and 3 percent of appropriated funds to evaluate the activities of the Office. Such an evaluation is to be conducted by an independent program unit of HEW. The Office of Planning and Evaluation awarded in late 1980 a competitive contract to the Urban Institute, Washington, D.C., to conduct this evaluation, primarily of the Title VI funded programs. This contract will focus on setting up a required reporting system of agencies' aggregate data and an optional individual case management system. Title VIII of the legislation requires that an independent study examine more broadly the effectiveness of existing health, education, and welfare programs relating to the problem of teenage pregnancy; and that it recommend more effective approaches to reducing or eliminating unwanted teenage pregnancies. This ambitious task will be tackled by John R. Beyster Associates, McLean, Virginia, which was awarded in late 1980 a competitive contract from OAPP. Its study undertakes to compile a national directory of comprehensive adolescent pregnancy programs, an analysis of an OAPP survey of over two thousand teenage pregnancy programs, and in-depth studies of five model programs.

Soon after the passage of this legislation, I attempted an assessment of its written provisions in terms of potential impact on families. I used as criteria several family impact principles developed during the course of conducting the Seminar's teenage pregnancy study, and built on the findings of the commissioned papers.[40] (See also Chapter 12.) A summary of this family impact analysis follows.

There are three minor provisions of the legislation that do specifically attempt to recognize the value of involving the family context of the teenage client. One provision requires that, "unemancipated minors should be encouraged to consult with their parents with respect to receiving the programs' services"; a second clause includes counseling for the extended family as one of the optional supplementary services that can be funded;

INTRODUCTION 37

and finally, grant applicants that "involve the community to be served including adolescents and families, in the planning and implementation of the project" are to be given priority. However, in other respects, the legislation and accompanying regulations, in my view, do not sufficiently take into account the broader ecological and family context surrounding teenage pregnancy and parenthood. Specifically:

- In its analysis of the nature and severity of the problem, the legislation makes no mention of the complex causes of teenage pregnancy. Thus, to the extent that it speaks at all to prevention, the underlying assumption is that providing teenagers themselves with information and contraceptive services is all that is needed.

- Although the need that teenage parents have for day care and employment and referral services is given some recognition, the greatest priority is still placed on the provision of health-related services (seven out of ten of the required "core" services).

- The legislation continues to view teenage pregnancy primarily as a female problem. However, it has been pointed out that in contrast to previous legislative language which spoke only of teenage *mothers*, the eligible person for services in this legislation can be a nonpregnant (or pregnant) adolescent, or an adolescent parent, thus opening the door to serving teenage males.

- With the exception of one priority being to establish programs in underserved rural areas, there is no mention of the need to tailor the design of programs to different kinds of family backgrounds—differences of race, religion, ethnicity, income, or geographical residence.

- Finally, and most important, in emphasizing the theme of comprehensive services throughout, the legislation fails to differentiate between those teenagers whose families are an actual or potential source of assistance, and those who are estranged from their families and whose needs may indeed be truly comprehensive. There are no incentives (or requirements) for programs to assess the family context of their minor clients, or to attempt to work in consultation with any of the teenager's family members. My assessment is that, without such an emphasis, programs funded under this grants program are likely to be less efficient and effective; and an opportunity will be missed to help support families' own efforts to help their adolescents.

However, the Office of Adolescent Pregnancy Programs has considerable flexibility in administering the act. It is encouraging to note that various innovative features of the four programs funded in the first year do indicate an interest in broader family issues: one program includes a mothers-of-mothers group to work out intergenerational conflicts over childrearing; another focuses on male involvement and preventive outreach to junior high school students; another recruits older adult women and men to act as big sisters and big brothers to provide role-model relationships for isolated teen parents.

In its first two years the Office was seriously understaffed, and thus has concentrated most of its activities on an unusually vigorous and imaginative technical assistance effort in setting up the grants program. By mid-1980, it had, however, also taken the first important steps regarding its mandate to improve coordination of federal programs. It established two federal inter/intra-agency coordinating committees, one relating to programs and services, and the other to research and evaluation; and a network of coordinating committees in each of the ten regional offices of HEW to facilitate coordination between regional, state, and local governments. The agendas for these committees are substantial.

Information presented in this volume underscores the importance of coordination. Vigorous leadership is needed to help make the present, haphazard patchwork of programs and policies work together. However, the history of governments is littered with well-meaning attempts at coordination that fizzle

INTRODUCTION 39

out. Strong support for the Office's coordinating efforts from the very highest levels of government in several federal agencies will be necessary if the Director and her staff are to achieve solid success.[41]

In short, although passage of the legislation and establishment of the Office raised many expectations, they were largely symbolic acts and not a measure of substantial new federal investment in this area. The actual dollar amounts being expended are pitifully small—a poignant lesson in the power of the congressional appropriations process to bring good intentions and rhetoric down to earth. But the creation, for the first time, of a federal governmental unit whose energies and skills will be solely devoted to working on the problems of adolescent pregnancy is a promising and welcome development.

Conclusions

There is a general agreement on the goals of public policy towards teenage pregnancy: to lower the present rates of teenage pregnancy and births, especially for school-age adolescents; to ensure that pregnant adolescents receive health care; and that adolescent parents have the kinds of resources and support necessary to become adequate parents and prevent long-term public dependency. Taken together, the chapters in this volume constitute a strong critique both of the means by which the government is presently attempting to achieve these goals, and of the new directions being recommended by others.

One of the unusual features of the family impact approach to policy analysis is its emphasis on the need to examine the details of policy implementation. Thus, the chapters in this volume focus on various governmental levels, components of policy and agency characteristics, including the training, attitudes and actions of the staff who work directly with teenage clients. I shall end this introductory chapter by highlighting a few of the major conclusions that emerge from the contributors' chapters.

Sex education is considered one of the primary tools to help adolescents avoid unwanted pregnancy. In reviewing the role of schools in providing sex education, Scales, in Chapter 6, points up a puzzling fact. Although the large majority of parents approve of sex education being taught in school, few programs exist and those that do rarely provide the kind of information that will help adolescents avoid pregnancy. Educational policymakers have been, for the most part, timid and fearful of establishing broader-based programs. Such ostrich-like behavior in the public sector mirrors that of parents, few of whom, as Fox discusses (Chapter 3), can deal explicitly with the topic in their own homes. Many concerned professionals, policy makers, and citizens advocate the logical solution: leadership is needed to institute more sex education in schools at an earlier age, to include information about birth control, and more family planning programs should be geared to adolescents. Yet these proposed solutions are often greeted with some uneasiness. They seem too "technological," and, above all, it is feared that they may undermine even further the role of parents who, most people agree, should retain a primary role in the sex education of their children. Moreover, they seem to be based on an assumption that many would question: namely, that the public must come to terms with the fact that teenagers—even young teenagers—are going to be sexually active.[42] Scales suggests that viable models exist for overcoming the various barriers to sex education programs and building a supportive partnership between schools, parents, and other community leaders, (especially from churches and synagogues). The central dilemma of school sex education remains a difficult one: how to help parents overcome their distrust of the values that these programs may teach; and how, in turn, to help educators learn to respect parents' own, often quite conservative, values.

Family planning programs have definitely contributed to lowering the rates of unwanted pregnancies and in large segments of the population they receive broad acceptance. Yet, several contributors (Fox, Furstenberg and his co-authors, and Steinfels) suggest that these programs might be more effective with adolescents if the movement as a whole re-evaluated its assumptions that, one, birth control was the responsibility of the teenage girls alone, and, two, parental knowledge of their daughter's sexual activity, and clinic visits, was irrelevant, unnecessary, and even harmful to her using contraceptives successfully. The contributors agree that ways of involving family members more fully in such programs need to be tried, although they differ as to the best way to achieve this goal. One of the most controversial routes to family involvement, that of requiring parental notification, is discussed by Steinfels in the light of the general, and often confusing, framework of children's rights, parental autonomy, and family privacy. Other methods, involving training of counselors and changing administrative practices and funding mechanisms, are reviewed in Chapter 11 by Furstenberg and his co-authors.

Currently, most advocates and experts emphasize teenage parents' extensive need for services above and beyond health care, thus advocating more "comprehensive" community-based programs. When measured against such a criterion as comprehensiveness, current policy (and funding) is woefully inadequate. Yet, as the history of recent legislation illustrates, we are in an era when economic resources are limited and even diminishing, and we cannot expect any substantial new funding for social, ameliorative programs in the immediate future. This counseling of realism should not lead to inaction and cynicism, but rather to careful thinking and planning. We need to ensure maximum leverage from the use of existing funds, and this goal is best achieved when government resources supplement, and do not compete with, each other or with nongovernmental sources of assistance.

The chapters that follow amply document the many existing sources of formal and informal assistance and support for young parents. The challenge is twofold. First, we should ensure that programs already funded give priority to teenage parents, and develop the necessary interagency agreements to allow cooperation and outreach services to contact the young parents who need services. Second, and equally important, programs need to be redesigned to complement and support the resources and expertise of the teenagers' families, not duplicate or undermine them. And in all of this, policy needs to understand and respect the diverse values and traditions of different kinds of families.

This is no easy task; but the following chapters develop some of the themes further, and make them concrete through specific recommendations. In the final chapter, I define several family impact principles that can be used to assess or guide policy, discuss the sensitive issue of parental notification, and summarize and expand on some of the recommendations and suggestions made in earlier chapters regarding government policy, agency administration and practice, professional training, and research. It must be emphasized however, that while the contributors' writings have greatly influenced my thinking on this topic, the conclusions and recommendations in this and the final chapter are my responsibility alone.

While the scope of this book is broad and covers a variety of disciplines, no single volume can do justice to the complexity of the topic. Many issues have been omitted or are only lightly touched on. One particular omission needs explanation. There is only cursory reference to the health aspects of adolescent pregnancy and the notable efforts and achievements of health care programs. I chose to de-emphasize health issues and programs, in large part because they have received the greatest attention by professionals and policymakers to date. Furthermore, it is increasingly recognized that the health risks of adolescent pregnancy are not, except for the very youngest ages, primarily a function of age. Rather they are associated with poverty and lack of access to health care. Now that more pregnant adolescents have access to good medical care, substantial progress has been made—and it needs to be continued—in diminishing the negative health consequences of teenage pregnancy.

Clearly, the focus and framing of the particular questions for these chapters in family impact terms involves a bias that

INTRODUCTION

may not be shared by others. However, people's values and assumptions do evolve and change, sometimes in response to new evidence or through a redefinition of problems. Perhaps, this presentation of factual knowledge about adolescent sex and pregnancy in a family context, and of critical questions about present policy, will reshape some of the assumptions and beliefs of those who have not, until now, shared the family perspective. And for those who do share a commitment to the family perspective, I hope this book suggests ways to translate such commitment into practice.

One final personal note. As study director and editor of this volume, I should describe my own values and biases, which have influenced the design of this study and its recommendations. Trained as a social worker and family therapist, I became interested in teenage pregnancy when working with families who had experienced an adolescent daughter's pregnancy. From them, I learned directly of the anger, disappointment and hurt and observed their struggles, coping, acceptance, and even joy as they lived through the crisis of adolescent pregnancy. These experiences led to my professional interest in undertaking the Seminar's study. But I also have a personal interest: as a parent of three children, two of them adolescents, I found myself early on in the study identifying with parents everywhere whose anxieties, needs, views, and problems were so rarely mentioned in the literature I read, or at the meetings and conferences I attended.[43] (I wondered too how grandparents, siblings, and other family members felt.) I was surprised that professionals, who were deeply committed to improving services to adolescents, would often appear to regard parents as insignificant, or worse, as adversaries and talk as though it were their role to protect or rescue adolescents from their families. I think I now understand better both how and why this impression is conveyed, and that there are, indeed, some instances in which such attitudes are justified. It is my hope, however, that in attempting to correct the imbalance and ensure that the family perspective is better appreciated, this book has not tipped the scales too far in the other direction. It is the argument of this book that the needs, interests and rights of teenagers—and their children—are best protected within the context of their families and not in a world apart.

NOTES

1. Two other kinds of families may be affected by teenage pregnancy: foster families who offer temporary care to the pregnant teenager and/or her baby; and adoptive families whose chances of being able to adopt a healthy infant decline as more and more teenagers decide to keep their babies.
2. The state of the law regarding the rights of minors is in considerable confusion and flux. A recently published report provides a state-by-state comprehensive summary of much state law on the topic, and is a valuable reference. It explains how landmark Supreme Court decisions are often not consistently followed through in changes in state law. The report is called *Legal Status of Adolescents* (1980), and was developed under a grant from Office of the Secretary of DHEW, by Scientific Analysis Corporation, San Francisco, and the Regional Institute of Social Welfare Research, Inc. in Athens, Georgia. It is available from the Scientific Analysis Corporation, 2408 Lombard Street, San Francisco, CA 94123.
3. The National Association of Broadcasters' (NAB) voluntary code that regulates the "tastefulness" and sensitivity of television advertising permits television advertisements of feminine hygiene products, such as tampons and douches, if very carefully worded, and aired at certain hours. However, it has not yet permitted advertisements of contraceptives. The code may be changed soon; the NAB is presently funding a major opinion survey to ascertain public reaction to this policy, including information on sex and sexuality in public affairs programs, and public service announcements.
4. Parents who expect that their teenagers will be taught the biological facts of sex in their ninth- or tenth-grade biology class may be disappointed. For example, one widely used text, which seems otherwise comprehensive, glosses over the complex facts of human sexual intercourse with the single phrase, "in land animals . . . systems have evolved which further ensure the meeting of eggs and sperm"; it makes no reference to why the sperm should be at all interested in meeting the egg or how this is achieved. See Biological Sciences Curriculum Study Co., *Biological science: Molecules to man*, 3d ed. (Boston: Houghton Mifflin, 1976), p. 270.
5. Marjorie Tifford (College Park, Md.), "Deferred motherhood," Letters to the Editor, *Washington Post*, Jan. 25, 1980.
6. Catherine S. Chilman, *Adolescent sexuality in a changing American society: So-*

cial and psychological perspectives (HEW pub. no. [NIH] 79-146; Washington, D.C.: G.P.O., 1979), p. 300.

7. Jerome Kagan and Robert Cole, eds., *Twelve to sixteen: Early adolescence* (New York: Norton, 1971), Intro. Kagan, p. vii. This book presents a variety of perspectives on adolescence. Two other recent volumes on adolescence should be mentioned, although they make only passing reference to teenage pregnancy: Sigmund E. Dragastin, and Glen H. Elder, Jr., eds., *Adolescence in the life cycle: Psychological change and social context* (New York: Wiley, 1975); and Joan Lipsitz, *Growing up forgotten: A review of research and programs concerning adolescence* (Lexington, Mass.: D. C. Heath, 1977).

8. J. M. Tanner, "Sequence, tempo, and individual variation in growth and development of boys and girls ages 12-16," in Kagan and Coles, *Twelve to sixteen*, p. 8.

9. Erik H. Erikson, *Childhood and society* (New York: Norton, 1950, 1963; also, London, England: Penguin, 1965).

10. There is good research evidence to support this view: Kantner and Zelnik report that lack of knowledge about contraception or about where to get it appears to be of minor importance in the reasons why teenagers do not use contraceptives. A major reason cited by those finding themselves unintentionally pregnant is that they had not expected to have intercourse. See John F. Kantner and Melvin Zelnik, "Reasons for non-use of contraception by sexually active women aged 15-19," *Family Planning Perspectives* 2, no. 5 (Sept./Oct. 1979): 290. A somewhat different but not inconsistent view is argued by Kristen Luker, who claims that teenagers weigh the costs and benefits, but decide that the immediate disadvantages of using contraceptives outweigh the far more remote and uncertain disadvantages of pregnancy. See her *Taking chances: Abortion and the decision not to contracept* (Berkeley, Calif.: University of California Press, 1977).

11. See Gail Sheehy, *Passages: Predictable crises of adult life* (New York: Dutton, 1976); and Daniel J. Levinson, *Seasons of a man's life* (New York: Knopf, 1978).

12. Reuben Hill, "Methodological issues in family development research," *Family Process* 3 (March 1964); 186-206.

13. Jay Haley, *Uncommon therapy: The psychiatric techniques of Milton H. Erickson, M.D.* (New York: Norton, 1973), p. 41.

14. Haley, *Uncommon therapy*, pp. 60-63, 265-296.

15. John H. Gagnon and Cathy S. Greenblatt, *Life designs: Individuals, marriages, and families* (Glenview, Ill.: Scott Foresman, 1978), p. 79.

16. Frank F. Furstenberg, Richard Lincoln, and Jane Mencken, eds., *Teenage sexuality, pregnancy, and childbearing* (Philadelphia: University of Pennsylvania Press, 1981). This book consists of a collection of articles previously published in the journal, *Family Planning Perspectives*. See the editors' *Overview* chapter for a review of data and research on the topic.

17. Since going to press, John F. Kantner and Melvin Zelnik have published the preliminary findings of their 1979 survey of teenagers living in metropolitan

areas of the United States. This survey's results confirm the recent trends noted in their two previous surveys in 1971 and 1976: the proportion of teenage women having sexual intercourse continues to increase, especially among whites; and although contraceptive use is becoming more widespread, pregnancy and abortion rates are also increasing. John F. Kantner and Melvin Zelnik, "Sexual activity, contraceptive use, and pregnancy among metropolitan-area teenagers; 1971–1979," *Family Planning Perspectives* 12, no. 5 (Sept./Oct. 1980): 230–237.

18. Chilman, *Adolescent sexuality*, pp. 25–31.

19. For example, see Susan Ross, *The youth values project*, a report of a survey conducted by teenagers themselves on a cross-section sample of one thousand in New York City. The project was supported by the Population Institute of Washington, D.C., and the State Communities Aid Association, New York City. The report is available from Susan Ross, c/o The Experiment, Kipling Road, Brattleboro, VT 05301.

20. See Kristin Moore et al., *Teenage motherhood: Social and economic consequences* (Washington, D.C.: Urban Institute, 1979); and Catherine Chilman, *Adolescent sexuality*, pp. 223–246.

21. Wendy Baldwin and Virginia S. Cain, "The children of teenage parents," *Family Planning Perspectives* 12, no. 1 (Jan./Feb. 1980): 34–43.

22. Maris A. Vinovskis, "Adolescent pregnancy: Some historical considerations," *Journal of Family History* (in press).

23. Stanford Research Institute International (SRI), *An analysis of government expenditures consequent on teenage childbirth* (Menlo Park, Calif.: SRI, 1979).

24. Leontine Young, *Out of wedlock: A study of the problems of the unmarried mother and her child* (New York: McGraw Hill, 1954), p. 1.

25. In *Adolescent sexuality*, Chilman mentions Young's book as an example of the extensive clinical literature of the time when scholars wrote about the "presumed psychological problems of unmarried mothers . . . propounding that they have deep psychological disturbances" (pp. 215–216).

26. Young, *Out of wedlock*, p. 122.

27. Lucille J. Grow, *Early childrearing by young mothers: A research study* (New York: Child Welfare League of America, 1979), p. 1.

28. Young, *Out of wedlock*, p. 95.

29. Carl Degler, *At odds: Women and the family in America from the revolution to the present* (New York: Oxford University Press, 1980). In chap. 6, "Under stress: Families of Afro-Americans and immigrants," Degler cites interesting evidence in the early nineteenth century of an earlier age of first births amongst blacks. He suggests as an explanation not only a difference in cultural attitude, but that slave owners offered positive economic and other incentives to young black women to bear children (see p. 118).

30. Joyce A. Ladner, *Tomorrow's tomorrow: The black woman* (New York: Doubleday and Anchor Books, 1971, 1972), pp. 232, 233.

31. Family Planning Perspectives, "Anniversaries," *Family Planning Perspectives* 11, no. 1 (Jan./Feb. 1979): 2.

32. It is interesting to compare the British teenage contraceptive experience here: two recent British studies report that although levels of teenage sexual activity are similar to the United States, British teenagers are more successful contraceptors. The younger teenagers particularly use barrier methods, especially condoms, more than their American counterparts, whereas the older teens are more likely to shift to using prescription methods. These studies were reported on in recent issues of *Family Planning Perspectives*: see 11, no. 6 (Nov./Dec. 1979): 372; and 12, no. 2 (Mar./Apr. 1980): 108.

33. Harriet Pilpel and Nancy F. Wechsler, "Birth control, teenagers, and the law," *Family Planning Perspectives* 1, no. 1 (Spring 1969): 2-48; and "Birth control, teenagers, and the law," *Family Planning Perspectives* 3, no. 4 (July 1971): 37-45.

34. See Institute of Judicial Administration, American Bar Association Juvenile Justice Standards Project, *Rights of minors* (Cambridge, Mass.: Ballinger, 1980), pp. 50-85.

35. American Civil Liberties Union, press release regarding its position on the *Bellotti v. Baird* Supreme Court Decision, July 2, 1979.

36. Alan Guttmacher Institute, *11 million teenagers: What can be done about the epidemic of adolescent pregnancies in the United States*. (New York: Planned Parenthood Federation, 1976).

37. This opposition continues: at a meeting in Washington D.C. in June 1980, entitled the "American Family Forum," (attended by conservative, right wing organizations and individuals) in a workshop on Planned Parenthood and teenage pregnancy, Planned Parenthood was vehemently attacked by panelists as "doing the work of Satan" and "waging a war against the poor."

38. I am indebted to Maris Vinovskis who shared with me a draft of his article, "Adolescent pregnancy," which raised this point in a very interesting discussion about the regrettable lack of a historical perspective on the issue as it was being discussed in Congress.

39. See Vinovskis, "Adolescent pregnancy."

40. A more detailed family impact assessment of the new legislation, and a copy of the act itself (P.L. 95-626, Titles VI, VII and VIII) are included in our preliminary report, *Teenage pregnancy and family impact: New perspectives on policy* (Washington, D.C.: Family Impact Seminar, 1979).

41. Since going to press in March 1981, Marjory Mecklenburg, President of American Citizens Concerned for Life (ACCL), was appointed Director of the Office of Adolescent Pregnancy Problems. ACCL is a moderate pro-life organization which is dedicated to social justice and supports sex education, family planning, adoption, and other abortion alternatives.

42. A perusal of the issues of *Family Planning Perspectives* will find several instances of the assumption that policy must accept that teenagers will be sexually

active. For example, Phillip Cutright writes, "it is the control of the unwanted pregnancies—not the control of premarital sex—that is the problem. The former, but not the latter, can be affected by public and private programs" ("Illegitimacy: Myths, causes and cures," *Family Planning Perspectives* 3, no. 1 [Jan. 1971]: 25–48).

43. There are very few books designed to help parents communicate with their adolescents about teenage sex and pregnancy. A recent, comprehensive one takes the position that parents are an essential source of sexual knowledge and guidance for their children. It has an interesting discussion about how to help teenagers resist the many pressures in our society on them to engage in sexual intercourse, and it is sensitive to parents' own feelings and values. See Howard R. and Martha E. Lewis, *The parent's guide to teenage sex and pregnancy* (New York: St. Martin's Press, 1980).

2

Teenage Women in the United States: Sex, Contraception, Pregnancy, Fertility, and Maternal and Infant Health

Audrey E. Jones and Paul J. Placek

Teen Childbearing: Trends and Comparative Overview

During the last decade, birth rates for younger American teenagers have increased while rates for older teenagers have dropped. Despite these compensating trends among teens, teenage births are forming a larger proportion of all U.S. births.

A 1966–1975 trend report on teenage childbearing indicated that births to teenage mothers represented 19 percent of 3,144,198 births in 1975, compared with 17 percent of 3,606,274 births in 1966. Table 1 indicates that of the 594,880 births to mothers under twenty years of age in 1975; 354,968 were to mothers eighteen to nineteen years old; 227,270 were to mothers fifteen to seventeen years old; and 12,642 were to mothers ten to fourteen years old.[1] (Throughout this chapter, such phrases as "ten to fourteen" are used inclusively—that is, to mean "through the fourteenth year.")

Figure 1 plots the long range view of teenage childbearing in the United States by presenting central birth rates for whites and all other colors for the period 1917–1977. (Central birth rates are age-specific birth rates for single years of age, i.e., the annual

TABLE 1
TOTAL LIVE BIRTHS FOR WOMEN, 10–19 YEARS OF AGE, BY AGE OF MOTHER AND RACE, 1966–1975

Age of Mother and Race	1975	1974	1973	1972	1971	1970	1969	1968	1967	1966
10–14 years										
Total	12,642	12,529	12,861	12,082	11,578	11,752	10,468	9,504	8,593	8,128
White	5,073	5,053	4,907	4,573	4,130	4,320	3,684	3,114	2,761	2,666
All other	7,569	7,476	7,954	7,509	7,448	7,432	6,784	6,390	5,832	5,462
Black	7,315	7,291	7,778	7,363	7,264	7,274	6,650	6,312	5,742	5,370
15–17 years										
Total	227,270	234,177	238,403	236,641	226,298	223,590	201,770	192,970	188,234	186,704
White	148,344	152,257	153,416	150,897	143,806	143,646	128,156	121,166	118,035	119,800
All other	78,926	81,920	84,987	85,744	82,492	79,944	73,614	71,804	70,199	66,904
Black	74,946	77,947	81,158	82,217	79,238	76,882	71,020	69,594	68,133	64,922
18–19 years										
Total	354,968	361,272	365,693	379,639	401,644	421,118	402,884	398,342	408,211	434,722
White	261,785	267,895	271,417	283,089	302,920	319,962	306,118	305,336	317,204	345,312
All other	93,183	93,377	94,276	96,550	98,724	101,156	96,766	93,006	91,007	89,410
Black	86,098	86,483	87,615	90,132	92,446	94,944	90,918	87,986	86,410	84,818

Source: Stephanie J. Ventura, "Teenage childbearing: United States, 1966–1975," *Monthly Vital Statistics Report*, vol. 26, no. 5; supp., National Center for Health Statistics, Hyattsville, Md., Sept. 1977.

number of births to teen mothers at a given age per 1,000 females at that age.) As Figure 1 indicates, older teens and nonwhite teens had higher birth rates for the sixty-year period. After World War II, white increases eclipsed nonwhite increases, but during the 1960s, decreases for older white teens were more rapid than for nonwhite teens. Since the beginning of the 1970s, these central birth rates fell for nonwhite teens, but increased for the younger white teens. These central birth rates indicate the level of childbearing each year for females at each age. For example, about 100 out of every 1,000 nineteen-year-old white women had live births in 1930; and after fluctuating four decades, that rate was virtually the same in the early 1970s.[2] By way of comparison, white and all other women of the prime childbearing ages of twenty to twenty-nine had central birth rates in the 150 to 200 range in 1970. Historically, for 1917–1977, rate variations for older teens have followed a pattern similar to that for the twenty- to twenty-nine-year-old women.

Age at menarche may also account for some variation in age and color. During the last five decades there has been a decline in the age of menarche in the United States. One of the major factors contributing to this decline is improved health and nutrition.[3] Even though the age at menarche declined for white and black females, the percentage of black females who begin menarche between ten and fifteen is much higher than that of white females of the same ages.[4]

According to the Alan Guttmacher Institute's (AGI) publication, *11 Million Teenagers*, the United States has higher rates of adolescent childbearing than more than a dozen developed countries and several less developed countries, such as the Philippines, Tunisia, and East Malaysia. For example, the number of births per 1,000 women, age fifteen to nineteen, is only five in Japan, sixteen in the USSR, and thirty-six in Canada, compared to over fifty in the United States (see Figure 2).[5]

FIGURE 1
CENTRAL BIRTH RATES FOR WOMEN AGED FOURTEEN TO NINETEEN, BY COLOR: UNITED STATES, 1917–1977

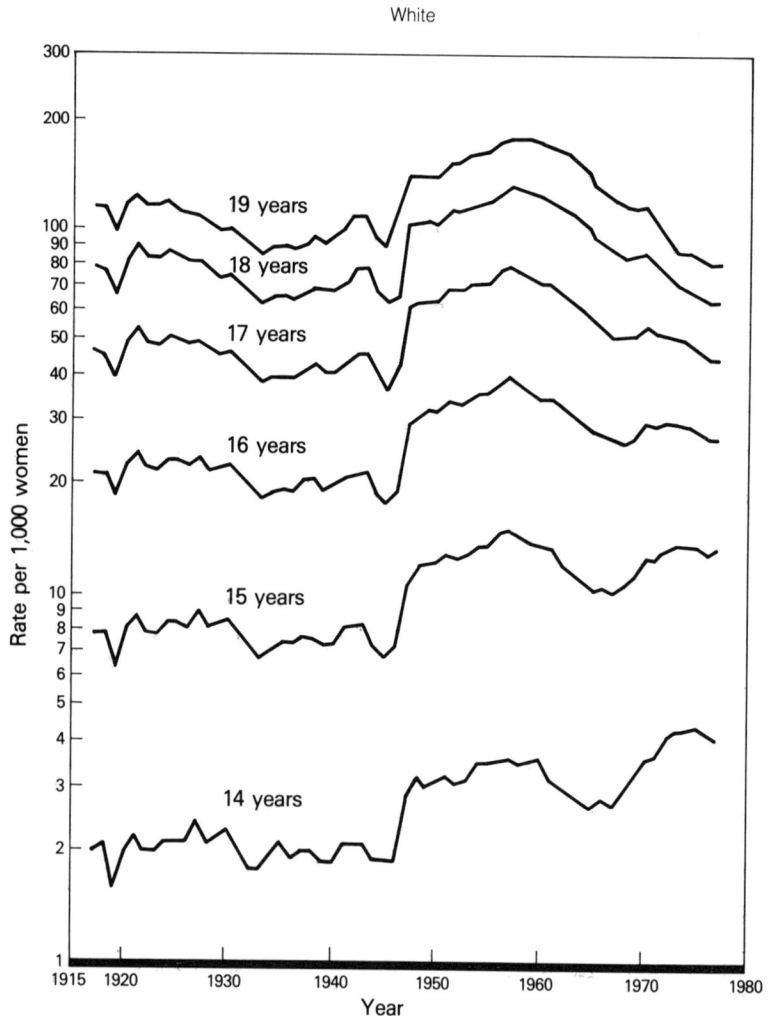

Source: Robert L. Heuser, "Sixty years of teenage childbearing in the United States, 1917–77," paper presented at the meeting of the Southern Regional Demographic Group, Myrtle Beach, S.C., Oct. 1979.

All Other

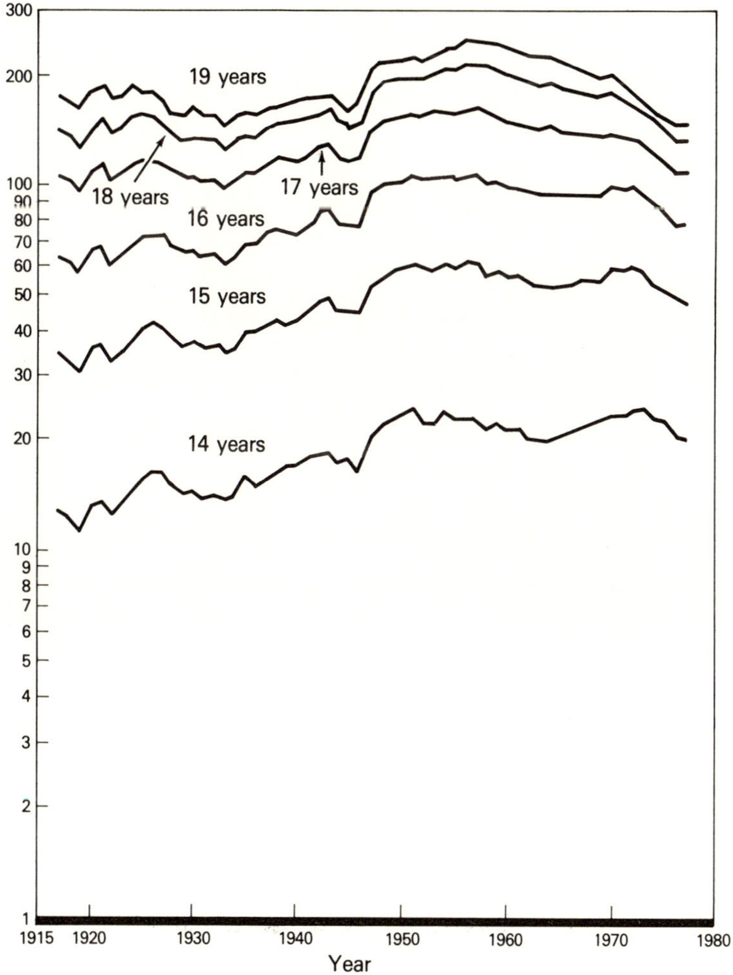

300
200
100
90
80
70
60
50
40
30
20
10
9
8
7
6
5
4
3
2
1
19 years
18 years
17 years
16 years
15 years
14 years
1915
1920
1930
1940
1950
1960
1970
1980
Year

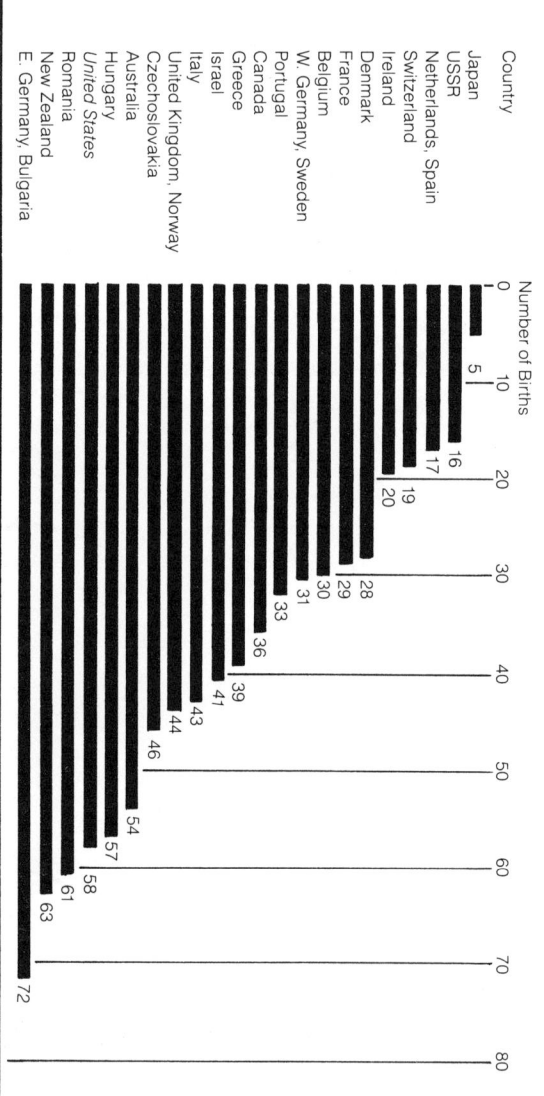

FIGURE 2
NUMBER OF BIRTHS PER 1,000 FEMALES AGED FIFTEEN TO NINETEEN, SELECTED COUNTRIES, 1970s

Source: AGI, 11 million teenagers: What can be done about the epidemic of adolescent pregnancies in the United States (New York: Alan Guttmacher Institute, 1976).

Sexual Activity

Most information on sexual activity comes from Zelnik and Kantner's work based on two national probability sample surveys of women, fifteen to nineteen years of age, in 1971 and 1976.[6] The authors found an increase in the percentage of never-married teenagers who have experienced sexual intercourse. In 1976, 31 percent of white and 63 percent of black females in that age group had engaged in premarital intercourse; this represents a significant increase over the 1971 rates of 21 percent for whites, and 51 percent for blacks (see Table 2). The percentage increase during that time (1971–1976) was twice as great for whites as for blacks (44 percent versus 23 percent). Despite the larger increase for whites, by 1976, the percentage of white females having experienced intercourse was still less than black females at all age levels.[7]

Among sexually active teens, Zelnik and Kantner found that both black and white teenagers' sexual activity is generally irregular and infrequent: 48 percent had not had sexual intercourse at all in the four weeks preceding the interview; 25 percent had sexual intercourse only once or twice; 12 percent had sexual intercourse only three to five times; and only 15 percent had sexual intercourse six or more times in the four week period. They found that eighteen- to nineteen-year-old women have a higher frequency of sexual activity than fifteen- to seventeen-year-old women; that white sexually active teens within each age group have a higher frequency of sexual activity than black teens; and that although the number of partners has increased, by 1976, half of the sexually experienced teens had only one partner.[8] The earlier initiation of sexual intercourse may be a partial explanation for the increase in birth rates for younger teens, but contraceptive use has concurrently increased among American teenagers.

TABLE 2
PERCENT OF NEVER-MARRIED WOMEN AGED 15–19 WHO HAVE EVER HAD INTERCOURSE, BY AGE AND RACE, 1976 AND 1971

Age	Study Year and Race														
	1976						1971						% increase 1971–1976		
	All		White		Black		All		White		Black		All	White	Black
	%	N	%	N	%	N	%	N	%	N	%	N			
15–19	**34.9**	**1,886**	**30.8**	**1,232**	**62.7**	**654**	**26.8**	**2,633**	**21.4**	**2,633**	**51.2**	**1,339**	**30.2**	**43.9**	**22.5**
15	18.0		13.8	276	38.4	133	13.8		10.9	642	30.5	344	30.4	26.6	25.9
16	25.4		22.6	301	52.6	135	21.2		16.9	662	46.2	320	19.8	33.7	13.9
17	40.9		36.1	277	68.4	139	26.6		21.8	646	58.8	296	53.8	65.6	16.3
18	45.2		43.6	220	74.1	143	36.8		32.3	396	62.7	228	22.8	35.0	18.2
19	55.2		48.7	158	83.6	104	46.8		39.4	287	76.2	151	17.9	23.6	9.7

Source: Melvin Zelnik and John F. Kantner, "Sexual and contraceptive experience of young unmarried women in the United States, 1976 and 1971," *Family Planning Perspectives* 9, no. 2 (March/April 1977).

Note: Base excludes those for whom no information was obtained on intercourse; this amounted in 1971 to 1.2 percent of the never-married blacks and 1.3 percent of the whites; and, in 1976, to 0.9 percent of the blacks and 0.7 percent of the whites. Percentages for whites and blacks are computed from unweighted data (Ns in tables); percentages for total sample are computed from weighted data and thus may sometimes appear to be inconsistent with figures by race. Figures for 1971 differ from earlier published reports because they exclude women living in group quarters. Except where indicated, the base excludes women who did not respond to the question analyzed in the table.

Contraceptive Use

The Zelnik-Kantner study indicated a definite improvement from 1971 to 1976 in contraceptive use among both black and white *unmarried*, sexually active teenage women. Still, by 1976, only 30 percent reported that they "always" used contraception; 45 percent reported that they "sometimes" used it; and 26 percent reported that they had "never" used it. Also, 64 percent reported that they had used a contraceptive at their last sexual intercourse. Younger sexually active teens are more likely to report they have "never" used contraception. Still, the majority of white teens at each age and black teens, age sixteen or more, had used contraception the "last time" they had intercourse.[9]

Figure 3 indicates the choice of contraceptive methods used by never-married teenage women at the time of their last intercourse: 31 percent, pill; 2 percent, intrauterine device (IUD); 13 percent, condom; 11 percent, withdrawal; 2 percent, douche; 5 percent, other methods; and 37 percent, none. Although the most popular method for both white and black fifteen- to seventeen-year-olds is the pill, they are still less likely to use the pill, and more likely to use the condom and withdrawal than older teenaged women.[10]

Using the Zelnik-Kantner data, Zabin found that most teens do not seek out contraceptive assistance until they have been sexually active for about a year, and that half of their first premarital pregnancies occur during the first six months after they begin intercourse.[11]

The use of contraceptives by *married* teenage women is available from the National Survey of Family Growth (NSFG). This survey of currently married women, fifteen to forty-four years of age, indicated that, in 1973, only 57 percent of married women, age fifteen to nineteen, were using contraception. Of married teens not using contraception, 36 percent were pregnant, postpartum, or seeking pregnancy; less than 1 percent were sterile; and 7 percent were other nonusers. The married teens'

FIGURE 3
PERCENT OF SEXUALLY EXPERIENCED NEVER-MARRIED WOMEN AGED FIFTEEN TO NINETEEN, ACCORDING TO METHOD USED AT LAST INTERCOURSE, 1976 AND 1971

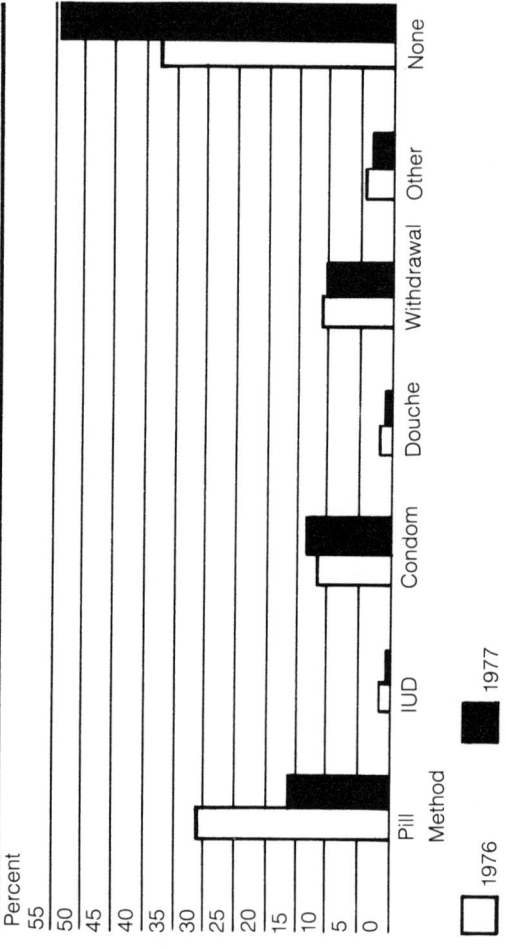

Source: Melvin Zelnik, John F. Kantner, "Sexual and contraceptive experience of young unmarried women in the United States, 1976 and 1971," *Family Planning Perspectives* 9, no. 2 (March/April 1977).

choice of contraceptive methods was as follows: 77 percent, pill; 5 percent, IUD; less than 1 percent, female sterilization; less than 1 percent, male sterilization; 1 percent, diaphragm; 8 percent, condom; 3 percent, foam; 1 percent, rhythm; 1 percent, withdrawal; less than 1 percent, douche; and 2 percent, other methods.[12] The 1976 NSFG indicated declines in the percentage who were pregnant, postpartum, or seeking pregnancy, but the distribution of method choices appears not to have changed substantially.[13]

Pregnancy Outcomes

Fecundity is defined as the biological ability to become pregnant, but the only proof of fecundity is fertility. Fecundity is high among young adult women, but declines with age.

AGI estimated that of ten million fifteen- to nineteen-year-old females in the United States in 1974, about one million became pregnant, the majority while single.[14] Furthermore, AGI estimated that approximately thirty thousand girls younger than fifteen years of age get pregnant annually. Natality statistics (Table 1) indicate 12,529 live births to females age ten to fourteen, in 1974 (5,053 to white women; 7,476 to all other women).[15] It is evident, therefore, that many pregnancies did not end in live births, but either terminated in stillbirths (late fetal deaths), miscarriages (early fetal deaths), and abortions, or were pregnancies not yet terminated.

Since the 1976 Zelnik-Kantner study included the ever-married as well as the never-married, it is possible to estimate pregnancy outcomes for all fifteen- to nineteen-year-old women, not just single women. Zelnik and Kantner reported that 57 percent of first pregnancies to teens resulted in live births, 1 percent in stillbirths, 10 percent in miscarriages, 18 percent in abortions; and 15 percent were currently pregnant. Black teenagers were more likely to have a live birth and less likely to have an abortion or miscarriage than white teenagers (see Table 3).[16]

TABLE 3
PERCENT DISTRIBUTION OF ALL FIRST PREGNANCIES TO WOMEN AGE 15–19 AT INTERVIEW, ACCORDING TO PREGNANCY OUTCOME AND RACE, 1976 AND 1971

Outcome	1976			1971		
	Total (N = 419)	White (N = 233)	Black (N = 186)	Total (N = 614)	White (N = 265)	Black (N = 349)
All	100.0	100.0	100.0	100.0	100.0	100.0
Live birth	56.8	50.1	76.0	62.8	58.9	71.9
Stillbirth	0.7	0.6	1.0	0.7	0.8	0.4
Miscarriage	9.9	11.7	4.9	7.5	7.8	6.8
Abortion	17.9	21.7	6.7	8.5	10.3	4.3
Currently pregnant	14.7	15.9	11.4	20.5	22.2	16.6

Source: Melvin Zelnik and John F. Kantner, "First pregnancies to women age 15–19: 1976 and 1971," Family Planning Perspectives 10, no. 1 (Jan./Feb. 1978): 16.

Legal Abortions

The AGI survey of abortion providers estimates that about 1,180,000 legal abortions were performed in the United States in 1976; 1 percent (or 15,820) were to females under 15; 31 percent (or 362,680) were to women age fifteen to nineteen; and the remainder were to women age twenty or more. The abortion rate in 1976 was 24.5 abortions per 1,000 women, fifteen to forty-four; for fifteen- to seventeen-year-old women, the rate was 24.4 (equal to the national average); and for eighteen- to nineteen-year-old women, the rate was 49.5 (twice the national average). AGI suggests that there is a large unmet need for additional abortion services, since four-fifths of all counties had no abortion facilities available; 70 percent of all non-Catholic, short-term general hospitals reported performing no abortions; and 8 percent of terminations were outside of the woman's state of residence. AGI asserts that a significant number of teenagers were unable to obtain legal abortions, with the result being additional unwanted births, out-of-wedlock births, and self-induced or illegal abortions.[17] The Center for Disease Control

(CDC) also collects and analyzes statistics on abortions voluntarily reported by the states. In 1977, approximately 30 percent of reported abortions in thirty-six states and the District of Columbia were to women age nineteen or younger. Thirty-two states reported abortions by single year of age for teens, over 55 percent of these abortions were to females eighteen and nineteen years of age.[18] Due to the Hyde Amendment, Medicaid-financed abortions have declined dramatically.

Miscarriage

Miscarriage is a term for early fetal death, that is, less than twenty weeks of gestation. AGI estimates that, in 1974, about 14 percent of the one million teenage pregnancies (or about 140,000 resulted in early fetal death or miscarriage.[19] The Zelnik-Kantner estimate would indicate about 100,000 miscarriages annually to teens.[20]

Stillbirths

Stillbirths, or fetal deaths of twenty weeks or more of gestation, totalled 33,053 in 1977. Of these, 216 were to females under fifteen years of age; and 6,177 were to women, age fifteen to nineteen. Fetal death ratios (the number of stillbirths per 1,000 live births) for females under fifteen, and between fifteen and nineteen were 18.9 and 11.0, respectively. Only women over thirty-five had higher fetal death ratios than teenage women. Among teen mothers who have second or higher order pregnancies, the risk of fetal loss increases significantly.[21]

Live Births

Since the early 1950s, the birth rates for the fifteen- to nineteen-year-old age group have decreased, with the exception of a small increase during the mid-1950s. Even though the birth rates generally decreased, the number of births to this age group increased a relatively small amount. The birth rates for the under-fifteen-year-old age group remained the same until a small increase occurred in the 1970s. Unlike the relatively small increase for the fifteen to nineteen group, however, the number of births to mothers under fifteen years of age has doubled since the early 1950s.[22]

Legitimate, legitimated by marriage, and out-of-wedlock births to teenagers in 1977 numbered 570,609. About one-fifth (or 120,176) of all births to teens were second, or higher order, births. Live births to females under fifteen numbered 11,455 (3 percent were second, or higher order, births); live births to females between fifteen and seventeen numbered 213,788 (12 percent were second, or higher order, births); and live births to females between eighteen and nineteen numbered 345,366 (28 percent were second, or higher order, births). This means that 225,243 births were to teens of school age, that is, age seventeen or under. Also, 249,800 (or 44 percent) of all teen births were out of wedlock in 1977; and women under twenty accounted for nearly half of all the 515,700 out-of-wedlock births in the United States. The illegitimacy ratio (the ratio of births to unmarried women compared with total births) was much higher for black women than for white women; for example, 33 percent of births to seventeen-year-old white women, but 87 percent of births to seventeen-year-old black women were out of wedlock in 1977.[23]

Data on live births are based on natality statistics collected through the vital registration system, in which birth data by age, race, and birth order are collected from fifty-two state and independent registration systems. Wedlock status information in 1977 was available from only thirty-nine states and the District of Columbia, making it necessary to estimate out-of-wedlock births for the remaining registration systems. However, births legitimated by marriage cannot be studied using registration data alone, since a date of marriage is not available as an item of information on the birth certificate. Therefore, special studies are necessary to study marriage-to-birth intervals. Placek analysed data from the 1964–1966 and 1972 National Natality Surveys (NNS).[24] The NNS studies only legitimate births, but legitimated births can also be measured, since date of birth is obtained from the birth certificate; and date of marriage, from the questionnaire mailed to the mother. Births occurring seven months or less after marriage are presumed to have been conceived out of wedlock but legitimated by marriage. The 1972 NNS data indicated that of first births to white mothers, age fifteen to nineteen, one-fourth were out of wedlock; one-fourth were legitimated by marriage; and the remaining half were legitimate, and occurred eight months or more after marriage. Of live first births to teenage mothers of all other colors, three-fourths were out of wedlock; one-tenth were legitimated by marriage; and one-seventh were legitimate, and occurred eight months or more after marriage.[25]

Although birth rates are higher among black teenagers, in terms of absolute numbers of babies born, births to white teenagers under eighteen far outnumber births to blacks of the same age. In 1977, for example, 142,894 babies were born to whites under eighteen, compared to 77,764 babies born to blacks in the same age group. However, there are more births to blacks under fifteen (6,582) than to whites under fifteen (4,671).[26]

Christopher Tietze has attempted to estimate how many of today's fourteen-year-olds would experience one or more pregnancies before they reach the age of twenty, assuming that current rates of sexual activity and contraceptive use and abortion for teenaged women continue. Tietze estimates that about 21 percent of all women would experience at least one birth; 15 percent would obtain at least one legal abortion, and 6 percent would have at least one miscarriage or stillbirth. Thus, 34–39 percent of today's fourteen-year-olds would experience at least one pregnancy before age twenty; and 20–22 percent would experience a pregnancy by the age of eighteen. Tietze also suggests that if the use of contraceptives increases, these estimates may be lowered.[27]

Number and Timing Failures

Number and timing failures, or unwanted and mistimed births, are very common among all age groups, but especially common among teenage mothers. The 1968, 1969, and 1972 NNSs collected information on this topic, with 1972 indicating fewer number and timing failures for teenagers than in previous years. Still, of all legitimate live births to women under twenty in 1972, 5 percent were unwanted (pregnancy not wanted then or at any time in the future); 34 percent were timing failures (pregnancy wanted later, but not then); and 61 percent were wanted then. Teenage mothers of all other colors were more likely to have unwanted births and timing failures than teenage mothers who were white.[28]

The Zelnik-Kantner analysis of teenage women in 1976 also studied intended and unintended pregnancies among the fifteen- to nineteen-year-olds. Table 4 indicates that only 29 per-

TABLE 4
PERCENTAGE DISTRIBUTION OF PREMARITALLY PREGNANT YOUNG WOMEN, BY WHETHER CONTRACEPTION WAS USED AT TIME OF CONCEPTION, ACCORDING TO RACE

Pregnancy Intent and Use at Time of Conception	Total (N = 316)	White (N = 151)	Black (N = 165)
Intended pregnancy	28.8	28.3	29.8
Did not intend	71.2	71.7	70.2
Used medical method	7.4	8.5	4.9
Used nonmedical method	13.7	17.0	6.0
Did not use	78.9	74.5	89.0
Total	100.0	100.0	100.0

Source: Melvin Zelnik and John F. Kantner, "Contraception and premarital pregnancy among teenagers," *Family Planning Perspectives* 10, no. 3 (May/June 1978):140.

cent of premaritally pregnant young women intended the pregnancy, while 71 percent did not. Of those who did not intend the pregnancy, only 7 percent used a medical contraceptive method; 14 percent, a nonmedical contraceptive method; and 79 percent, no method of contraception at all.[29]

Adoption is a choice that a small and diminishing number of teenagers are making regarding the disposition of their pregnancy. The AGI teen report refers to a 1971 study that found that among those teenagers who gave birth out of wedlock, 87 percent kept the child; 5 percent sent the baby to live with others; and 8 percent placed the baby for adoption.[30] If we speculatively apply this 8 percent figure to the more than two hundred thousand out-of-wedlock births to teens each year, it appears that perhaps sixteen thousand are placed for adoption. In 1973, nonwhite infants comprised only 13 percent of all adopted babies.[31] Many believe that the legalization of abortion has reduced the number of children available for adoption, since pregnant teens are deciding to keep their babies or to have abortions.

Maternal and Infant Health

Young mothers and their infants often have more health problems than older mothers and their infants. Teen mothers are less likely to have health insurance and obtain prenatal care, and they are more likely to have complications of pregnancy, forceps deliveries, low-birth-weight infants, and infants with low Apgar scores. Most of the elaboration of this statement will be based on a number of papers based on the 1972 National Natality Survey (NNS), a one-in-five hundred nationwide sample survey of legitimate live births linked with a followback mail survey of the mothers, physicians, and hospitals associated with those births.

Findings from the 1972 NNS indicate that when teenage mothers are compared with mothers who are twenty and over, the teenagers are only half as likely to have health insurance to cover prenatal care, hospital bills, or doctor bills. For example, only 17 percent of mothers under eighteen, and 26 percent of mothers, age eighteen to nineteen, had health insurance that covered one-fourth or more of the prenatal care bill, as compared to older mothers, 52–59 percent of whom were covered. When the color of the mother is considered, teenage mothers of all other colors are even less likely to be covered by insurance than are white teenage mothers.[32] Apparently, the lack of health insurance for prenatal care results in fewer prenatal care visits: national natality statistics indicate that teenage mothers are about twice as likely as older mothers to have no prenatal care visits.[33]

NNS data from 1972 indicate that teenage mothers are as likely as older mothers to have underlying medical conditions existing during their pregnancies (such as diabetes or asthma). However, this same analysis indicated that 16 percent of mothers under eighteen, and 20 percent of mothers between eighteen and nineteen had one or more complications of pregnancy (urinary infection, hypertension, toxemia, preeclampsia, eclampsia, anemia, rubella, embolism, obesity, and others), compared to 16 percent of mothers in their early twenties and 15 percent of mothers age twenty-five to twenty-nine. Furthermore, 21 percent of mothers under twenty had one or more complications of labor (inadequate pelvis, transverse lie, multiple birth, abnormal position of placenta or cord, premature rupture of membranes, unusual bleeding, prolonged labor, anesthesia reaction, placenta abruption, and others), compared to 20 percent of mothers age twenty to twenty-four, and 20 percent of mothers age twenty-five to twenty-nine. Thus, teenage mothers have at least as high a rate of complications of pregnancy and labor as older mothers.[34]

Poor maternal and infant health have been found to be associated with higher levels of fertility, and there is substantial evidence that women who begin childbearing in their teens will have higher fertility than women who begin childbearing in their twenties. A parallel analysis of the 1972 NNS and the 1973

NSFG indicated that married women whose first birth occurred before age eighteen had 3,393 and 3,755 total births expected, respectively, compared to only 2,854 and 2,527 total births expected for women whose first birth occurred when they were twenty-five to twenty-nine, respectively.[35] Thus, early childbearing is associated with higher completed fertility, which is, in turn, associated with poor maternal and infant health, especially at the time when the higher order births occur.

Type of delivery has also been found to be related to age of mother. Teenage mothers who delivered legitimate live births in hospitals in 1972 were less likely to have spontaneous deliveries (associated with better maternal and infant health), and more likely to have forceps deliveries (associated with birth injuries) than mothers age twenty and over. Among women under eighteen, 47 percent had spontaneous deliveries, 46 percent had forceps deliveries, 6 percent had Caesarean section deliveries, 1 percent had breech deliveries, and less than 1 percent had other types of deliveries; the corresponding percentages for mothers age twenty-five to twenty-nine were 55 percent, 36 percent, 7 percent, 2 percent, and 1 percent, respectively.[36]

One could hypothesize that infants born to teenage mothers might be healthier due to the idea that younger women are generally healthier than older women. Unfortunately, such is not the case. Natality data from forty-two reporting states and the District of Columbia for 1975 indicate that 21 percent of mothers under fifteen, and 11 percent of mothers between fifteen and nineteen received late or no prenatal care, as compared with only 6 percent for all mothers. The same data indicate that 10 percent of infants of mothers under twenty were low birth weight (2,500 grams or less; 5 lbs. 8 ozs. or less), as compared with 7 percent low birth weight for mothers in their twenties. Of teenage mothers with no prenatal care, 26 percent had low birth weight infants.[37] Furthermore, a study of Apgar scores (an index of infant health ranging from 0 to 10, and based on the infant's heart rate, respiratory effort, muscle tone, reflex irritability, and skin color) of 1972 NNS infants indicated that teenage mothers had the lowest percentage of infants with one- and five-minute Apgar scores in the satisfactory (8 to 10) range.[38]

In sum, teenage mothers, in contrast to older mothers, are much less likely to have health insurance or to obtain less prenatal care; are slightly more likely to have complications of pregnancy and labor, and to expect higher-than-average completed fertility (which is associated with poorer maternal and infant health and higher rates of postpartum sterilization); are less likely to have spontaneous deliveries, and are more likely to have forceps deliveries. Infants born to teenage mothers are more likely to be of low birth weight than infants born to older mothers; and are more likely to have low one- and five-minute Apgar scores.

Venereal Disease. CDC tabulates reported information on sexually transmitted diseases, although much disease is unreported. Focusing on females only, in 1978, fifteen- to nineteen-year-old women had the second highest rates of primary and secondary syphilis and gonorrhea; only females twenty to twenty-four had higher rates than the teens. In 1978, 153,227 teenage females were reported to have contracted gonorrhea; and 1,316 were reported to have contracted syphilis. Even though the rates for females between ten and fourteen are low, the rates for the incidence of gonorrhea among them have more than doubled since 1956; they also doubled for fifteen- to nineteen-year-old females in the same period.[39]

Data Gaps, Limitations, and Needed Future Studies

The first gap concerns unmarried fertility: natality and fertility surveys have often excluded it. Natality followback surveys in 1963–1969 and 1972 excluded out-of-wedlock births. It is possible that the infants born out of wedlock and their young mothers experienced more severe health problems, but these problems go unmeasured, due to the sensitivity of studying out-of-wedlock births in some states. However, the 1980 NNS will include medical information on out-of-wedlock births. Even as an item of information on the certificate of live birth, marital status of the mother is now included by only thirty-nine states and the District of Columbia. The NSFG focused its 1973 and 1976 cycles on currently or previously married women, and single women with children; the next cycle will include a nationally representative sample of women, age fifteen to forty-four, including single women.

A second major gap in the data is the lack of inclusion of males in fertility studies. Fatherhood probably has a relatively major impact on the lives of young men, just as motherhood does on young women. Consequently, a nationally representative survey of males, age seventeen to twenty-one, is currently being undertaken by Zelnik and Kantner.[40]

A third major gap in available data is the lack of detailed ethnic background information, including Hispanics. Typically, Hispanics have been included in the "white" group, which was then contrasted with "all others" or "blacks." Data on Hispanics are now available through the National Survey of Family Growth (NSFG) (Cycle 1 and 2 only). Also, the 1980 NNS will include more detailed ethnicity data on mothers and fathers than have ever been collected on previous followback surveys.

A fourth major problem involves the paucity of small-area studies that are comparable with national studies. Because most national studies, such as the NNS or NSFG, cannot be broken down to the state or county level of analysis, more localized fertility studies of teens would enrich our understanding, and fill an important part of the data gap.

Fifth, a variety of age group categories have been used in different studies of teenage women. The most desirable categorization is by single years of age, if available; however, the under-fifteen and fifteen-to-nineteen age categories are fairly standard; and increasingly, the latter is broken down into fifteen to seventeen, and eighteen to nineteen.

Most of the data limitations identified here are recognized and being dealt with squarely in current and planned research, in part, due to increased attention to the problems of adolescent childbearing.

NOTES

1. Stephanie J. Ventura, "Teenage childbearing: United States, 1966-1975," *Monthly Vital Statistics Report* 26, no. 5 (supp.), National Center for Health Statistics, Hyattsville, Md., Sept. 1977.
2. Robert L. Heuser, "Sixty years of teenage childbearing in the United States, 1917-1977," paper presented at the meeting of the Southern Regional Demographic Group, Myrtle Beach, S.C., Oct. 1979.
3. Phillips Cutright, "Illegitimacy in the United States: 1920-1968," *Demographic and social aspects of population growth*, ed. Charles F. Westoff and Robert Parke, Jr. (Washington, D.C., GPO, 1972).
4. Brian MacMahon, "Age at menarche: United States," *Vital and Health Statistics*, ser. 11, no. 133, National Center for Health Statistics, Rockville, Md., Nov. 1973.
5. Alan Guttmacher Institute (AGI), *11 million teenagers: What can be done about the epidemic of adolescent pregnancies in the United States* (New York: Alan Guttmacher Institute, 1976).
6. *Editor's note:* Since going to press, Melvin Zelnik and John F. Kantner have published the preliminary findings of their 1979 survey of teenage women living in metropolitan areas of the United States. This survey's results confirm the recent trends noted in the authors' previous surveys in 1971 and 1976; the proportion of teenage women having sexual intercourse continues to increase especially among whites; and although contraceptive use is becoming more widespread, pregnancy and abortion rates have also increased. Melvin Zelnik and John F. Kantner, "Sexual activity, contraceptive use, and pregnancy among metropolitan area teenagers; 1971-1979," *Family Planning Perspectives* 12, no. 5 (Sept./Oct. 1980): 230-237.
7. Melvin Zelnik and John F. Kantner, "Sexual and contraceptive experience of young unmarried women in the United States, 1976 and 1971," *Family Planning Perspectives* 9, no. 2 (March/April 1977): 55-71.
8. Zelnik and Kantner, "Sexual and contraceptive experience," pp. 60-61.
9. Zelnik and Kantner, "Sexual and contraceptive experience," p. 62.
10. Zelnik and Kantner, "Sexual and contraceptive experience," pp. 63-67.
11. Laurie Schwab Zabin, John F. Kantner, and Melvin Zelnik, "The risk of ad-

olescent pregnancy in the first months of intercourse," *Family Planning Perspectives* 11, no. 4 (July/Aug. 1979): 215–222.

12. Kathleen Ford, "Contraceptive utilization among currently married women fourteen to forty-four years of age: United States, 1973," *Monthly Vital Statistics Report*, 25, no. 7, supp., National Center for Health Statistics, Hyattsville, Md., Oct. 1976.

13. Kathleen Ford, "Recent changes in contraceptive practice among American couples: Results from the 1976 National Survey of Family Growth," paper presented at the meeting of the Population Association of America, Atlanta, April 1978.

14. AGI, *11 million teenagers*, p. 10.

15. Ventura, "Teenage childbearing," p. 9.

16. Melvin Zelnik and John F. Kantner, "First pregnancies to women aged fifteen to nineteen: 1976 and 1971," *Family Planning Perspectives* 10, no. 1 (Jan./Feb. 1978): 11–20.

17. Jacqueline Darroch Forrest, Christopher Tietze, and Ellen Sullivan, Abortion in the United States, 1976–1977, *Family Planning Perspectives* 10, no. 5 (Sept./Oct. 1978): 271–279.

18. Center for Disease Control, *Abortion surveillance—United States*, 1977 (Atlanta: Public Health Service, HEW, 1979).

19. AGI, *11 million teenagers*, p. 10.

20. Zelnik and Kantner, "First pregnancies," pp. 13–15.

21. National Center for Health Statistics, Mortality Statistics Branch, Division of Vital Statistics, unpub. tabulations for 1977 (HEW Washington, D.C.: The Center, 1979).

22. Heuser, "Sixty years," p. 3.

23. National Center for Health Statistics, "Final natality statistics, 1977," *Monthly Vital Statistics Report* 27, no. 11, p. 10, supp. (1979).

24. Paul J. Placek, "Trends in legitimate, legitimated by marriage, and illegitimate first births: United States, 1964–1966, and 1972," paper presented at the meeting of the American Statistical Association, San Diego, Calif., Aug. 1978.

25. Placek, "Trends," p. 3.

26. National Center for Health Statistics, "Final natality."

27. Christopher Tietze, "Teenage pregnancies: Looking ahead to 1984," *Family Planning Perspectives* 10, no. 4 (July/Aug. 1978): 205–207.

28. Robert H. Weller and Robert L. Heuser, "Wanted and unwanted childbearing in the United States: 1968, 1969, and 1972 National Natality Surveys," *Vital and Health Statistics*, ser. 21, no. 32, National Center for Health Statistics, Hyattsville, Md., Sept. 1978.

29. Melvin Zelnik and John F. Kantner, "Contraceptive patterns and premarital pregnancy among women aged fifteen to nineteen in 1976," *Family Planning Perspectives* 10, no. 3 (May/June 1978): 135–142.

30. AGI, *11 million teenagers*, p. 11.

31. Wendy H. Baldwin, "Adolescent pregnancy and childbearing—growing concerns for Americans," *Population Bulletin* 32, no. 2 (1976): 10–12.

32. Paul J. Placek, unpub. tabulations presented at National Institute of Child Health and Development/Belmont Conference, Baltimore, MD, May 1975; Marcie L. Cynamon and Paul J. Placek, "Insurance coverage for prenatal care, hospital stay, and physician care: United States, 1964–1966, and 1972 National Natality Surveys," paper presented at the American Public Health Association, New York, Nov. 1979.

33. Selma Taffel, "Prenatal care: United States, 1969–1975," *Vital and Health Statistics*, ser. 21, no. 33, National Center for Health Statistics, Hyattsville, Md., 1978.

34. Paul J. Placek, "Underlying medical conditions, complications of pregnancy, and complications of labor to mothers of legitimate live hospital births in the United States," paper presented at the meeting of the Population Association of America, Atlanta, April 1978.

35. Gordon Scott Bonham and Paul J. Placek, "The relationship of maternal health, infant health, and socio-demographic factors to fertility," *Public Health Reports* 93, no. 3 (May/June 1978): 283–291.

36. Paul J. Placek, "Type of delivery associated with social and demographic, maternal health, infant health, and health insurance factors: Findings from the 1972 National Natality Survey," paper presented at the meeting of the American Statistical Association, Chicago, Aug. 1977.

37. Paul J. Placek, "Maternal and infant health factors associated with low infant birthweight: Findings from the 1972 national natality survey," *Epidemiology of Prematurity*, ed. D. M. Reed and F. J. Stanley (Baltimore: Urban and Schwarnzberg, 1977); see also Taffel, pp. 20–21.

38. Paul J. Placek, "The relationship of social and demographic maternal health, and infant health factors to one and five minute Apgar scores: Findings from the 1972 National Natality Survey," paper presented at the meeting of the American Public Health Association, Miami Beach, Oct. 1976.

39. Center for Disease Control, *Sexually transmitted disease statistical letter* (Atlanta: Public Health Service, HEW, 1978).

40. *Editor's note*: Preliminary results of the Kantner and Zelnik survey of adolescent males ages seventeen to twenty-one living in metropolitan areas were published just as this chapter went to press. The survey findings indicate that the percentage of school-age males who are sexually active is only a little higher than that of females of the same age: In 1979 55.7 percent of seventeen-year-old males as compared with 48.5 percent of seventeen-year-old females reported that they had ever had sexual intercourse. John F. Kantner and Melvin Zelnik, "Sexual activity, contraceptive use and pregnancy among metropolitan-area teenagers: 1971–1979," *Family Planning Perspectives* 12, no. 5 (Sept./Oct. 1980): 230–237.

3

The Family's Role in Adolescent Sexual Behavior

Greer Litton Fox

Introduction

The purpose of this chapter is to consider the part the family of origin—mother, father, siblings, other relatives—plays in adolescent sexual behavior. It attempts to answer the questions that follow. What do we know about the facts, values, and attitudes about sex that parents teach or indirectly communicate to their children? What seems to distinguish these families who communicate more directly with their children from those who do not? What effects does such communication have on the children's attitudes and behavior? Finally, what specific attempts do parents make, if any, to guide and control their teenagers' sexual behavior?

In defining the family's role and functioning, I adopted a broad view of families that was to include three distinct but overlapping aspects of family life. First, various objective sociocultural and economic characteristics of families—the education and income level of the parents; their religious, racial, and ethnic background—can affect the attitudes, expectations, values, and behavior of teenagers. Second, each family system has established patterns of relating—patterns that govern the distribution of power and authority within a family, the setting of rules, the enforcing of certain sanctions, and the setting of boundaries. Such patterns may be characterized as authoritarian or permissive, paternal or maternal, highly structured or disorganized, rigid or flexible. A third aspect is the quality of affective relationships among family members—such as the marital relationship or mother-daughter relationship—and may include the amount and quality of communication, the closeness or distance of the relationship, and the balance between affection and hostility. The various studies reviewed below investigate or touch on all these various attributes of family roles and functioning.

I took a more restrictive approach to the inclusion of research materials concerned with sexuality. Spanier[1] suggests five aspects that are involved in sexual development: development of a gender identity; development of gender roles; development of sex object preference; acquisition of sexual skills, knowledge, and values; and development of sexual attitudes or a disposition to behave. For the most part I concentrated on the role of the family in the latter two aspects of sexual development, the development of sexual scripts and sexual attitudes. In addition, I looked for evidence of family impact on sexual behavior, including contraception and pregnancy resolution.

It seems important at the outset to emphasize the dramatic discrepancy in the amount of good research on adolescent male sexuality, as compared to that on adolescent female sexuality. There is a dearth of research on the sexual socialization process for young men; on the roles they play in decisions to have sex or to use contraception; on their involvement in pregnancy resolution decision-making; and on the extent of their participation in the actual parenting and support of the newborn child. Fortunately, a national survey of the sexual behavior of young men, which is currently underway, will correct some of the gaps in our knowledge of adolescent men. The study, conducted by Kantner and Zelnik, is designed to be comparable to their previous studies of the sex, contraception, pregnancy, and childbearing behavior of young women, which have been of enormous value in charting the dimensions of sexual activity among older teenage women. In the meantime, however, the present review necessarily reflects the current research emphases and biases of the field. The obvious omission of young men from much of the discussion that follows should serve to underline the need for more research on young men, thus far the "silent partners" in adolescent sexual behavior and childbearing.

The Role of the Family in Sexual Socialization

Sex-role Learning

The importance of the family in the eventual sexual behavior of its teenage members stems, in large part, from its centrality as a socialization structure for the adult life course. Parents serve as initial sources of sex-role learning for their daughters and sons. It is from their parents, for example, that sons and daughters begin to observe ways of negotiating the familial and marital social order of wife-mothers and husband-fathers. Indeed, for daughters, the absence or loss of a father, as well as conflict within an intact parental marital relationship, have all been found to carry over into a daughter's ability to establish intimate ties with men of her own generation.[2] The work of Lipman-Blumen, among others, has established the central importance of the mother's values, attitudes, and behavior as both direct and indirect determinants of the sex-role attitudes and behaviors of daughters.[3] An impact of fathers on sex-role development of daughters has also been found, although the mechanisms through which a father's impact occurs are subject to debate.[4] Presumably, somewhat similar dynamics would hold with regard to the impact of same-sex and cross-sex parental influences on sons, although the research data are both less abundant and less conclusive on these points.[5]

Direct Transmission of Sexual Information

Long before the right and responsibility to initiate children into adult roles were parcelled out to agencies external to the family, the function of sexual socialization was handled within the context of the family and its primary community. Rites of passage marking the attainment of puberty, lusty customs celebrating the significance of the wedding night, the gathering of kin to watch through the event of childbirth are all examples of the structures and patterns used to transmit information about human sexuality and adulthood from generation to generation. Central to these patterns were the same-sex, parent-child units: mothers-daughters and fathers-sons. A question that must be addressed is: To what extent has the parent-child relationship retained its centrality in the transmission of sexual information to young people? And if this relationship is no longer so central—as seems to be the case—then why might this be so?

Before looking specifically at the research in this area, we should consider some of the limitations of sample survey research as a methodological approach to sexual socialization. Most survey research elicits respondent self-reports, generally retrospective reports at that; the question is usually some version of "from whom did you first learn about 'X'?" Sometimes respondents are asked, "What did your mother/father say to you about 'X'?" or "What did you say about 'X' to your son/daughter?" At best, what we are getting from such question formats is some measure of direct verbal transmission of information or values. It is easy to challenge the validity of data gathered in this way; for instance, the retrospective report is subject to recall error (selective reinterpretation, memory lapse, and so forth); moreover, the message that is sent may not be the one received, and vice versa; parents' and children's reports of the same instance of communication may vary tremendously.[6] Perhaps most serious is the fact that such communication about sex and sexual values is unspoken, indirect, and nonverbal. It is not captured by asking who said what to whom when. Moreover, the process of sexual socialization is a long-term one, beginning for each child in her or his earliest days within the family. The research produced from cross-sectional designs with questions like "who's talking to you now about what" misses the richness of a transmission process that stretches back through some fifteen years of a daughter or son's life.

While keeping in mind some of the limitations of the research picture, let's turn now to some recent studies in this area. Constance Lindemann in her sensible book, *Birth Control and Unmarried Young Women*, reflects much of the conventional professional wisdom on the matter of parents as resources to teenage children:[7]

> A girl cannot readily ask her parents about birth control. They are usually ambivalent about, if not downright opposed to, premarital sex. Even in families that have a permissive attitude toward premarital sex, parents are not able to help their daughters plan for birth control in concrete terms. When it comes to what to do, where to go, and which method to use, the family doesn't tell and the girls don't ask (p. 29).

Much literature in family sociology suggests that parents and children do not communicate directly or positively about sex, sexual values, contraception, and so forth.[8] Indeed, some go so far as to claim that parents and children cannot communicate about sexuality within a familial context.[9]

In Figure 4, I have summarized the findings from fifteen studies on the initial or most important source of sexual information, as reported by young people. Indicated in the figure are the sources of information young respondents have rank-ordered first, second, and third, in terms of their importance. Since our interest is in the role of parents, available data for each parent are indicated in parentheses below the top-ranked choices.

There are three important points to be made from Figure 4. First, it is clear that the role of parents as formal sex educators of their children is minor, at best, although this differs somewhat by sex of parent and child, and by topic. In only one of the stud-

FIGURE 4
PARENTS AS SOURCES OF SEX EDUCATION FOR TEENS IN RELATION TO THREE MOST FREQUENTLY CITED SOURCES

Authors	Study Population	Topic	Rank Order of Most Often Mentioned Sources	
			Source	Percentage Reporting

Elias (1978)*	"My study of high school students"	"Sex education"	Same-sex peers
			Opposite-sex peers
			Teachers
			Males
			  Mother
			  Father
			Females
			  Mother
			  Father
				(no percentages reported)
				
				10
				26
				
				65
				2

Finkel and Finkel (1975)†	421 male high school students	"Sexual intercourse and reproduction"	Male friends Professionals i.e., doctors, teachers Female friends Father Brother Mother	37 23 18 9 8 5
Fox (1976)‡	690 male and female college students	Birth control	*Males* Books, reading Same-sex friends Girlfriend Father Mother Brother	90 84 51 23 17 13

Gebhard (1977)[§]	Kinsey sample—college males and females	"Sex"	*Females*
			Books, reading 89
			Same-sex friends 84
			Boyfriend 52
			Mother 43
			Father 8
			Sister 25
			Males
			Male friends 61
			Mixed 20
			Mass media 10
			Father 3
			Mother 2
	114 male and female college students	"Sex"	*Females*
			Female friends 39
			Mixed 24
			Mass media 14
			Mother 13
			Father 1
			Males
			Male friends 42
			Mixed 30
			Mother 10
			Father 2
Goldfarb et al. (1977)[†]	639 pregnant teens	"Sex education"	Family 44
			Peers 44
			School 12
	114 never-pregnant teens	"Sex education"	Family 47
			Peers 38
			School 15

Authors	Study Population	Topic	Rank Order of Most Often Mentioned Sources	
			Source	Percentage Reporting
Ktsanes (1977)[‖]	116 teen clinic clients	Birth control	Mother Sister or other relative Friend	38 31 20
Lewis (1973)[#]	419 male and female college students	"Sex"	*Males* Parents *Females* Parents	8 43
Libby et al. (1974)[**]	250 parents	Sex education	Peers Mothers "Others" Fathers	46 28 13 9
Manley, as reported in Goodman and Goodman (1976)	1,000 male and female teens	"Sex"	*Males* Peers Media Parents *Females* Peers Parents Media	54 16 15 42 32 16
Shipman (1968)[††]	400 male and female college students	Sex education	*Males* Parents *Females* Parents	5 14

Study	Sample	Topic	Source	%
Spanier (1977)‡‡	1,177 male and female college students	"Sex"	*Males*	
			Male friends	81
			Reading	67
			Father	30
			Mother	24
			Females	
			Female friends	70
			Reading	67
			Mother	62
			Father	12
Thornburg (1970)‖	88 female college students	Summary of 11 topics concerning sex	Girlfriends	35
			Mother	23
			Books	17
			Father	1
Thornburg (1972)‖	381 female college students	Summary of 11 topics concerning sex	Peers	38
			Books	21
			Mother	19
			Father	2
Warren and Pierre (1973)**	266 male and female college students	"Sex knowledge"	Friends	33
			Books	27
			Parents	19
Weiss et al. (1974)§§	374 male and female teens	Family planning	Mother	59
			Father	38
			Peers	18

* Mode of presentation: major source of information, except for parents ("ever discuss sex with").
† Mode of presentation: source of information.
‡ Mode of presentation: "ever used as source of information or advice." Percentages total more than 100 since more than one source could be indicated.

§ Mode of presentation: main source of early sex education.
‖ Mode of presentation: first source of information.
Mode of presentation: percentage receiving most of their sex education from a parent.
** Mode of presentation: most important source.
†† Mode of presentation: percentage receiving "adequate sex education from parents."
‡‡ Mode of presentation: source of a good deal of information at the beginning of high school.
§§ Mode of presentation: ever discuss with.

Percentages total more than 100 since more than one could be indicated.

Sources: James E. Elias, Adolescents and sex," *The Humanist* (March/April 1978): 29–31; Madelon and David Finkel, "Sexual and contraceptive knowledge attitudes, and behavior of male adolescents," *Family Planning Perspectives* 7, no. 6 (1975): 256–260; G. L. Fox, "A comparison of characteristics of the first coital episode by timing of sexual initiation among a sample of sexually-active single men and women," unpub. paper, 1976; Paul H. Gebhard, "The acquisition of basic sex information," *Journal of Sex Research* 13, no. 3 (1977): 148–169; Joyce L. Goldfarb, David M. Mumford, David A. Schum, Peggy B. Smith, Charles Flowers, and Carolyn Schum, "An attempt to detect 'pregnancy susceptibility' in indigent adolescent girls," *Journal of Youth and Adolescence* 6, no. 2 (1977): 127–144. Barry Goodman and Normal Goodman, "Effects of parent orientation meetings on parent-child communication about sexuality and family life," *The Family Coordinator* 25, no. 3 (1976): 285–290; Virginia K. Ktsanes, *Assessment of contraception by teenagers,* final report, National Institute of Child Health and Human Development (contract no. 1HD-52833), Jan. 1977; Robert A. Lewis, "Parents and peers: Socialization agents in the coital behavior of young adults," *Journal of Sex Research* 9, no. 2 (1973): 156–170; Roger W. Libby, Alan C. Acock, and David C. Payne, "Configurations of parental preferences concerning sources of sex education for adolescents," *Adolescence* 9, no. 33 (1974): 73–80; E. J. Roberts and J. Gagnon, *Family Life and Sexual Learning,* vol. 1 (Cambridge. Mass.: Population Education, 1978); G. Shipman, "The psychodynamics of sex education," *The Family Coordinator* 17, no. 1 (1968): 3–12; Graham B. Spanier, "Sources of sex information and premarital sexual behavior," *Journal of Sex Research* 13, no. 2 (1977): 73–88; Hershel D. Thornburg, "Age and first sources of sex information as reported by eighty-eight college women," *Journal of School Health* 40 (1970): 156–158; Hershel D. Thornburg, "A comparative study of sex information sources," *Journal of School Health* 42, no. 2 (1972): 88–91; Carrie Lee Warren and Richard St. Pierre, "Sources and accuracy of college students' sex knowledge," *Journal of School Health* 43, no. 9 (1973): 588–590; Eugene Weiss, F. Gerald Kline, Everett M. Rogers, Michael E. Cohen, and Jennifer A. Dodge, "Communication and population socialization among youth: Communication behavior and family planning information," paper presented at the annual meeting of the Population Association of America, New York City, 1974.

THE FAMILY'S ROLE

ies did parents emerge as the predominant source of sex education; and even in this study, less than half of the teens nominated "the family" as their major source of sex education.[10] As might be expected, the mother is consistently the parent more involved with daughters. Perhaps unexpectedly, sons indicate mothers as major sources about as often (and sometimes more so) as fathers. Indeed, and this is the second major point from Figure 3-1, the most notable aspect about the father is his almost complete absence as a source of sex education for his children. A less stringent indicator of parental involvement than being a "major source" of sex information is merely having discussed sex with one's children at least once. Two studies in Figure 4 show teens' reports of ever having discussed sex and family planning with fathers: Elias suggests that only one in four boys, and one in fifty girls have ever talked about sex with fathers.[11] Weiss reports 38 percent of the teens in his study as having ever talked about birth control with fathers.[12] The high degree of noninvolvement of fathers indicated by the studies in Figure 3-1 is consistent with accounts of low levels of male involvement in other aspects of child rearing.[13]

A third point to be made from the studies summarized in Figure 3-1 is that the caliber of research in this area is not especially impressive. With two or three exceptions the studies are based on rather woeful collections of questionnaires handed out to classroom gatherings of college students. Moreover, the studies tend to be descriptive rather than analytic. In only a few cases did the researchers push beyond the simple, although important, question of, From whom did you learn? to, How did you learn? or, How did your parents teach you? or, What kinds of people learn from family members as opposed to peers? or, What difference does the source of information make to one's sexual behavior? Answers to these questions are necessary if we are to understand much of the complexity of the family's role in sexual socialization. Additional studies are reviewed below in an attempt to find at least partial answers to each of these questions.

Mothers and Daughters

Given the importance of the mother-daughter relationship as the key familial context within which sexual information is transmitted (as indicated in Figure 4), it was somewhat surprising to find only three studies that look specifically at the process of sexual communication within this relationship. One of these, reported by Bloch, investigated the sex education practices of a random sample of 124 mothers of seventh-grade girls in two communities in California.[14] The modal age of daughters was twelve; only 35 percent of the daughters had passed menarche at the time the mothers were interviewed. Bloch asked for detailed answers to questions about what mothers had said to daughters about menstruation, about the male role in reproduction, and about birth control. Even using a liberal scoring system for their responses, which would have the effect of biasing her results toward greater communication, Bloch found that 20 percent had never told their daughters anything about menstruation; 50 percent had not discussed the father's role in reproduction; and 68 percent had not talked to them about any aspect of birth control or fertility regulation. When she shifted focus to the women who had said at least something to their daughters about one or more of these topics, then rated the adequacy of what had been said in terms of the level of sex education that "a mother might reasonably be expected to have achieved with a twelve-year-old daughter" (p. 11), the results were even more distressing: only 26 percent had achieved adequate levels in menstruation education; only 12 percent adequately discussed the male role in reproduction; and only 10 percent provided adequate birth control education. When all three areas were considered simultaneously, it turned out that 18 percent of the daughters had never been told anything about any of the three topics; and only 7 percent had received adequate instruction, appropriate to their age, from their mothers. As Bloch herself concludes, "The data from this study seem to support findings from prior studies which have consistently indicated that children get little sex education in the home" (p. 11).

A second study is that of Rothenberg, who analyzed a stratified random sample of 163 Cincinnati, Ohio, mothers, and also two of their children between ten and eighteen.[15] Rothenberg asked whether, and to which children, the mother had given reading material about sexual relations, explained the act of sexual intercourse, and talked to children about birth control. Among her findings were the following:

> Only about one-third of the mothers provided reading material, some 45 percent of the mothers explained intercourse, but nearly 3/5 talked about birth control to at least one child. Most mothers were consistent, in that they communicated with neither child or both children, but when communication was with only one child, it was usually the older one (p. 3).

Because Rothenberg's sample included both male and female children and covered an age range from ten to eighteen, it is possible to examine mothers' communication patterns with younger as compared to older children, and with sons as compared to daughters. She found that mothers reported that the age of the child made little difference in explaining coitus, but that giving reading material and discussing birth control occurred more often with the older children—that is, children over fourteen. The sex of the child made little difference in the likelihood of receiving reading material about sex from their mothers. However, more than twice as many daughters as sons were told about intercourse (58 percent, versus 28 percent) while more than one and a half as many daughters as sons were told about birth control (49 percent, versus 30 percent). When asked directly, more mothers reported that discussion of sex was easier with daughters than with sons. The greater amount of discussion with daughters may also reflect an awareness of the greater severity of consequences of sexual activity for daughters than sons.

The third study that examines patterns of communication about sex within the context of the mother-daughter relationship is one that I am currently engaged in.[16] Our sample consists of 449 mother-daughter pairs drawn systematically from among fourteen- to fifteen-year-old public school students in Detroit; 56 percent of the sample is black; 48 percent of the mothers are currently married to and living with the daughter's father; and 33 percent of the daughters are sexually active. Mothers and daughters were asked separately about the nature and extent of their discussions about menstruation, dating and boyfriends, sexual morality, conception, sexual intercourse, and birth control. The independent reports of mothers and daughters were highly consistent, and suggest that nearly all mothers and daughters have discussed all six topics at some point in the girl's life-time. "Menstruation" and "dating and boyfriends" are the topics that most of the mother-daughter pairs report ever having discussed, while "sexual intercourse" and "birth control" have been discussed by the fewest respondents (although even here over 70 percent of both mothers and daughters report that they have talked at least once about sex and birth control). When asked at what age a topic was first introduced, the mothers and daughters agreed that menstruation and conception are introduced when the daughter is around ten or eleven, while the other four topics generally are first discussed when she is thirteen or fourteen.

To assess the frequency of discussions about sex between mothers and daughters we asked them to say how often they had talked with each other about the six sex-related topics during the six months preceding the interview. The consistency in their responses is worth noting: although interviewed simultaneously but separately, mothers and daughters differed surprisingly little both in the order and magnitude of their responses. Dating and boyfriends is the topic discussed most often with some regularity (61 percent of the daughters and 67 percent of the mothers report having discussed this five times or more in the six months preceding the survey). This is followed by discussions of menstruation and morality, discussed frequently by about one-half of the sample; next are sexual intercourse and birth control, discussed frequently by about one-third of the sample. The least frequently and regularly discussed topic is conception; apparently, once the basic points are made, little additional elaboration or discussion is called for on this topic.

Determinants of Direct Communication

In order to begin to understand communication patterns we need to move beyond prevalent data of the sort reported above, and to begin to specify the conditions under which communication is likely to occur. What distinguishes the families in which interaction between mothers and daughters (or sons) on the topic of sexual matters occurs, from those families in which children never receive instruction or assistance from their parents? The homogeneity of most samples used in studies of sexual socialization (see, for example, those in Figure 1) makes the search for differentials almost futile.

Rothenberg has reported some data, however, that provide a few clues. Looking at family socioeconomic characteristics she finds that:

> Greater percentages of whites, high school graduates, and mothers in families with incomes over $10,000 provided reading material about sex to their children. Conversely, though the differences are smaller, greater percentages of black, lower income, and less educated mothers discussed birth control with their children. Although neither race nor income was related to whether mothers explained intercourse, those with more education were slightly more likely to have done so.[17]

Among our Detroit sample we found that mothers who are black, mothers without a high school diploma, mothers who are not currently married to the daughter's father, and mothers from lower income families tend to talk more frequently (that is, at least five times in the six months preceding the interview) about sexual intercourse and birth control than other members in the sample.

Besides race, income, and education, family composition—that is, whether the family type is a female-headed household or a husband-wife household—appears related to discussion about sex. Akpom and his co-authors report data from their study of 303 white Michigan teenage clients of a family planning agency that suggest daughters of female heads reported significantly more often than daughters of male heads that they had discussed contraception with parents (63 percent, versus 42 percent); that they felt parents would understand if the daughters tried to discuss contraception with them (63 percent, versus 43 percent); and of those currently using contraception, that their parents were aware of the daughter's use of contraception (48 percent, versus 18 percent).[18] These findings lead the authors to suggest that communication about contraception appears easier when the household head is female.

This result and another from the Rothenberg study, which is that mothers who themselves had premarital sex were considerably more likely to discuss birth control with their children, are consistent with Reiss's "autonomy theory of heterosexual permissiveness"; this theory predicts greater permissiveness about sexual matters among those least involved in, or tied to, a traditional marital and family form.[19] An alternative explanation, which is not necessarily inconsistent with Reiss's autonomy theory, is that the divorced, separated, or single mother may share considerably more role similarity with her teenaged daughter, vis à vis men, than the mother in an intact marriage. In the former setting both mother and daughter could potentially, or actually, be simultaneously engaged in dating or love relationships. One could posit a greater degree of similarity in the female role (despite the generational difference between mother and daughter) in these relationships than between the female roles occupied by a dating daughter and a married mother. In addition to having a greater degree of common ground as a basis for communication, still another factor that may be operative in facilitating mother-daughter communication in female-headed households is the induction of the teenage daughter into the role of quasiadult confidante by the mother. There is some evidence to suggest that children in single-parent households take on adult roles, vis à vis their parent, somewhat earlier than children in intact households. (We will have data in the Mother-Daughter Communication Study that will allow us to put some of these speculations to empirical test.) At the same time, it must be kept in mind that the potential for mother-daughter communication in female-headed households as a category may be reduced by the generally lower socioeconomic status of female-headed households. Lower levels of education, in particular, which are characteristic of female-headed households, foster neither a high degree of verbal interaction nor a particularly empathetic, introspective, or self-disclosing style of communication. It seems clear that a great deal more information is needed to clarify the effect of family type on the mother-daughter relationship.

Another type of variable that we are investigating for its influence on mother-daughter communication in our Detroit data set is the mother's attitudes toward sex roles and birth control, and her knowledge of sex and contraception. Preliminary analyses of the frequency of mother-daughter communication about sexual morality, sexual intercourse, and birth control suggest that sex-role traditionality may be related to whether these topics were ever discussed between mothers and daughters. We found that the most traditionally oriented mothers were more likely never to have talked on all three topics; for example, 21 percent of the most traditional mothers, compared to 15 percent of the most nontraditional mothers, had never discussed sexual intercourse with their daughters.

Several unexpected findings were encountered about the relationship between talking about sex and attitudes towards birth control and knowledge of sex and contraceptives. Contrary to expectations, mothers who held unfavorable attitudes toward contraceptives and mothers who were not very knowledgeable about sex and contraceptives tended to have more frequent discussions with their daughters on two of the topics, sexual intercourse and morality. For example, 35 percent of the mothers with the most negative attitudes towards birth control, compared to 25 percent of the mothers with the most positive birth control attitudes, talked five or more times in the last six months about sexual intercourse. A similar inverse association was found between knowledge and talking about sexual intercourse. Again, less knowledgeable mothers were more likely to have talked recently and frequently about sexual intercourse (30 percent of the low-knowledge mothers, versus 21 percent of the high-knowledge mothers).

Turning to the third topic, birth control, however, we found that birth control attitudes are related in the expected direction. Mothers with positive birth control attitudes were more likely to discuss birth control with their daughters frequently in the last six months; and they were least likely never to have broached the subject. Similarly, in terms of level of knowledge about sex and contraceptives, knowledgeable mothers in our study were least likely never to have discussed birth control with their daughters. We can speculate that mother-daughter discussions on sexual intercourse and morality occur in a different context than discussions on birth control. Talking about sexual intercourse and talking about sexual morality may, in fact, involve negative, one-way messages from mother to daughter about what to do and what not to do (e.g., "nice girls don't . . ."), rather than positive, two-way discussions. Talking about birth control, however, is more likely to be constructive and helpful.

These differences in the nature of the three topics may partly account for the unexpected findings that positive attitudes and high knowledge are related to less talking about sexual intercourse and morality, on the one hand, and more talking about birth control, on the other. Clearly, a next step in our analyses of the Detroit data is to untangle the interrelationships among social-structural and attitudinal variables to understand how family background variables are translated into effects on sex-related communication between mothers and daughters.

Age of the child might be expected to influence the nature of parent-child sexual communication. Children of different ages in adolescence have need for different kinds of sexual information, profess different sexual values and attitudes, and differ in terms of their stage of cognitive development—and perhaps in their capacity for moral judgment. Yet, surprisingly, in neither of the two studies in which amount of parent-child interaction was discussed as a function of child age was age of child found to matter very much.[20] Roberts and Gagnon, however, found in their study of Cleveland parents that parents justified their not having discussed sex-related topics with their children on the grounds that their children were "too young" or "not ready" for such information.[21]

The clinical, therapeutic, and applied literatures point to a rather different set of conditions as conducive to communication between parents and adolescents. In this literature, the concern is with interaction styles and tones, and with actor attributes, rather than gross social characteristics and structural variables. This literature tends more toward didacticism than description or analysis; yet, it comprises a not insignificant portion of the extant material on family determinants of teen sexuality. Familiarity with this literature can be of use to more formal researchers by suggesting, for example, criteria by which communication structures and styles may be judged more or less effective, by suggesting elements to be used to build scale items or measures of components of the parent-child relationship, and the like. Thus, although the material in this genre is not formal research per se, it is certainly not without value of its own. Some of the earlier literature of this type addresses such questions as "the parents' share" and whether or not mothers should inform their teenage daughters on contraceptives,[22] and exhorts both parents and professionals to increase their involvement in the sexual socialization of teens. The following description of the good male parent educator is provided by Gadpaille.[23]

> Essentially, a man must respect himself as a man so as to provide a basis for his son's self-respect. Such self-esteem would allow him to inform himself as fully as possible and to express his own attitudes consistently and without being dogmatic. At the same time he would respect his son's growing individuality so as to want to teach him how to think and to prepare him for independent decision-making, even when those decisions differ from his own.

It is perhaps worth noting that this description is similar to that of Baumrind in describing the parenting style of the parents of children designated "social agents," that is, high in social responsibility, social activity, and individuality.[24]

Gadpaille and Hodgman, who also address the father-son relationship, both suggest that the most important functions of fathers vis à vis sex education of sons are: (1) to reassure sons of their (the sons') normality regarding sexual interests, activities, and size and configuration of genitalia; (2) to model appropriate behavior in male-female relationships as exemplified in the father's day-to-day treatment of and interaction with the wife-mother; and (3) to discuss sexual attitudes and values with sons. Garfield and Morgenthau have written a comparable paper on mother-daughter communication.[25] In their paper, they emphasize the necessity for openness, accuracy, responsiveness, initiative, sensitivity, and integrity on the part of mothers for effective communication.

THE FAMILY'S ROLE 93

The authors of the papers just mentioned ask no more of parents than teens themselves want. Couch reports on a teen conference in which teens were asked to describe those from whom they would like to receive sex education.[26] According to Couch, while teens almost unanimously desired to receive sex education first and primarily from parents, they voiced the following complaints about parents: that parents were themselves uninformed; that they implied condemnation of a youth's behavior if she or he sought information; that parents acted shy, embarrassed, and ashamed to talk about sex; that parents were too often evasive and uncomfortable; and finally that parents seemed unable to cope with the reality that their children were really growing up (p. 261). Couch summarized their position as follows: "The composite qualities desired in a sex educator were that she or he be a young person, open-minded, warm, empathetic, with a flexible personality, skill in teaching, experienced, and specially educated for this rather complex subject" (p. 259). This last idea, special training in sex education for parents, is one that has been voiced not just by teens but by professionals as well, and is discussed at length by Peter Scales in this book (Chapter 6).

Impact of Communication on Behavior

We have considered certain parental attributes and family characteristics that are either felt to be or have been found to be of importance in distinguishing families in which there is communication about sex from those where there is none. A next question is to ask what impact—if any—having received sexual instruction from parents or other family members has on the sexual attitudes and behavior of teens.

Jessor and Jessor, in their study of the transition of youth from virginity to nonvirginity, found that parental values, support, and degree of connectedness with the youth distinguish between teenagers who remain virgins and those who become nonvirgins.[27] The more consistent the parental-youth values and the closer the ties to home, the less the likelihood of becoming sexually experienced.

Lewis provides data from a nonrandom questionnaire survey of 410 college students at two universities that address the question of the relationship between source and extent of sex education and premarital coital experience.[28] Lewis found that only 8 percent of males, compared to 43 percent of females, had received most of their sex education from a parent. Using gamma as a measure of association, Lewis found that receiving sex education from someone other than a parent was associated for both males and females with having experienced premarital coitus, with having had more than one sexual partner, and with a younger age of sexual initiation. Conversely, "where parents were the main source of sex education, the children tended to follow more traditional (chastity) norms in their premarital sexual relationship" (p. 162). When the number of sexual topics discussed by parents was considered, Lewis found that the greater the number of topics, the less likely were both male and female students to have had coital experience or to have had more than one partner. Lewis summarizes this portion of his data as follows: "rather than stimulate coital experimentation, sex information given primarily by parents seems to contribute to more restrictive premarital sexual behavior" (p. 163).

In an analysis similar to that of Lewis, but with a considerably more adequate sample and analytic procedure, Spanier explores the influence of different sources of sex information on premarital sexual behavior among a national probability sample of 1177 college students; he, again, found that those women students whose mothers were their major source of sexual information were somewhat less likely to be sexually experienced.[29] Spanier was also able to examine the effects of fathers, brothers, sisters, and other relatives, respectively, as sources of sex information on the index of sexual experience; he found that none of them had any appreciable effect on the subsequent sexual behavior of either male or female students (pp. 81–83). Perhaps it is worth emphasizing here that Spanier's analysis is virtually the only published report of the influence of one sibling, as a source of sex instruction, on the sexual behavior of another.

In a separate analysis, Spanier goes on to compare the relative influence of formal (classroom instruction) and informal (including parents) sources of sexual socialization on subsequent sexual behavior.[30] He finds that while informal sources of sex education have significantly more impact on premarital sexual behavior than formal sources, "there are indications that pressures and experiences confronting young people in a given dating or peer group situation take precedence over all past sexual socialization influences" (p. 40). This suggests that while parents, specifically the mother (see above), have some influence on their children's sexual behavior, their influence is outweighed—at least for college-age children not living in the home setting—by more immediate situational factors. A similar finding is reported by Lewis in the study described earlier.

Furstenberg reports on communication about contraception between mothers and daughters in his study of 404 pregnant teens and their mothers in Baltimore.[31] His study sample is predominantly black; and 40 percent of the families represented are female-headed. Close to 60 percent of the mothers interviewed reported that they had frequently attempted to talk to their daughters about sex; and nearly all (92 percent) reported discussing sex occasionally with their daughters. Birth control was reported to have been discussed by 61 percent of the mothers and 45 percent of the daughters. Although Furstenberg questions the accuracy and directness of the information transmitted by mothers to daughters, nevertheless, he finds that even limited instruction had an impact on the daughter's use of contraception. In families in which birth control was discussed, 52 percent of the daughters had used contraception at some time, compared to 23 percent when birth control had never been discussed by mothers and daughters.

Other researchers have found similar effects of mother-daughter communication on behavior. For instance, in our Detroit study we found that the frequency of mother-daughter discussion of sexual intercourse and birth control was positively and significantly related (p ≤.01 as measured by Pearson's r) to the daughter's knowledge, attitudes, and use of contraceptives. In his comparison of successful contraceptors with women seeking abortion, Miller found that the two groups differed significantly with respect to information about sexual intercourse: "Approximately 40 percent of the successful contraceptor group indicated their mothers as the first important source of information on this subject, whereas only 12 percent of the therapeutic abortion group indicated their mother."[32] Goldfarb and her coauthors found that receiving early education about menstruation and sex from one's family could be used along with a set of additional variables to predict accurately what they termed "pregnancy susceptibility" among adolescents.[33] That is, those who do not receive instruction from sources within the family are more susceptible to pregnancy.

Ager and his co-authors, in their study of dropouts from a teen contraceptive program, report preliminary data that suggest that mothers are an important influence both on teens' enrolling in the program and on their continuing in it.[34] Furthermore, those teens who report parental influence as being strongest tend to be those who either are not sexually experienced or who use effective contraception. Those for whom parental influence is weaker tend to use ineffective methods or no methods at all.

Ktsanes, in a study of 116 teenage family planning clinic attenders in Louisiana, attempted to discover how the girls had made the decision to come to the clinic.[35] Three-fifths of the respondents talked directly to someone in their immediate family, predominantly the mothers, about whether to come. Only four girls said that no one in their family knew that they were coming to the clinic. When asked about family reactions, 88 percent reported family members approved or supported them in their use of birth control or encouraged their clinic attendance. Ktsanes attributes the good contraceptive practice records of the study participants, in part, to their perceptions of the supportiveness of their families, and especially their mothers, for their practice of contraception. Brody and his co-authors interviewed 150 working-class women from Kingston, Jamaica, about their initial sources of sex information, their relationships with their mother, and their subsequent sexual and fertility behavior.[36] Although the women ranged from sixteen to forty-seven years of age, the median age was 25.5; and 83 percent were thirty or younger. The investigators found that more than three-fourths of the women had never received any information about sexual relations from their parents or surrogates, and almost one-half had no adequate instruction about sex or reproduction from anyone prior to menarche. Close to two-thirds of the women expressed resentment toward their mothers for their failure to give them any sex instruction. In a correlational analysis of their data, the authors found that women who received sex education from their mothers were older at first coitus, had fewer sex partners (and for women with two or more pregnancies, fewer impregnators), and fewer children by the time of their participation in the study than women who had not had such sexual instruction. More impregnators and more children (but not age at first coitus or first pregnancy) were correlated with expressions of resentment about lack of information from or communication with the mother about sex. Thus, this small study suggests that the nature of one's early sexual instruction may have long-lasting effects that manifest themselves in one's adult sexual and reproductive behavior.

Let me summarize the research evidence about parent-child communication cited thus far. First, there is not much detailed published research specifically on this topic, but the state of affairs should change rather soon. Second, it would appear that there is not a lot of direct communication about sex within the home. In the studies reviewed thus far, parents were never cited by a majority of respondents as their first or major source of sex instruction. Clearly, not many children receive much direct instruction about sexuality, or sexual intercourse, or fertility regulation from their parents. Furthermore, to the extent that intentional sex instruction occurs at all in American families, it would appear that it is due to the efforts of the female parent. Mothers are clearly the more involved parent. Perhaps because of this, daughters tend to fare better than sons in receiving sexual instruction within the family. The mother-daughter dyad is the only familial relationship of much significance in the direct transmission of sex education within the context of the family. However, it bears repeating that even for daughters, the mother is not often mentioned as an important source of sex information.

Of those children who do receive sex education from their parents (that is, from their mothers), the impact is often marked. The research reviewed above seems to suggest that communication, however minimal or inaccurate, is associated with the following patterns of sexual behavior: (1) parental communication about sex may forestall or postpone a child's sexual activity; and (2) among those daughters who are sexually active, parental communication appears related to more effective contraceptive practice on the part of the child.

Scientific prudence makes me want to underline the fact that the cause and effect relationship between communication, on the one hand, and sexual and contraceptive behavior, on the other, is not at all clear or well-established. It is plausible that many children wait to talk to their parents until after they become sexually active or have a pregnancy scare, or until after they start using contraception; and only then do they talk to their mothers about it. Whatever the sequence, however, it appears that daughters whose mothers have talked to them about sex and contraception are more often regular and effective contraceptors. It may well be that such discussion is important not so much for the factual information imparted as because such discussion can make explicit the daughter's sexual behavior, and can encourage the daughter's awareness and acceptance of her own sexuality, which is often a prelude to taking contraceptive responsibility for oneself.[37] Trying to understand why parental communication has the effects on children's sexual behavior that it does is an important problem that needs considerably more research attention.

Indirect Familial Sexual Socialization

Thus far we have considered patterns of open or direct communication and instruction about sex within the family. Such forms of sexual socialization are only one way in which families transmit sexual values, attitudes, and information from one generation to another, or within the same generation. Equally, and perhaps even more important are the less conscious ways in which sexual instruction is conveyed. For example, it is obvious that mothers and daughters are linked through their common female sexuality. The events of menarche, menstruation, conception, gestation, birth, and menopause provide a universal experiential link among women, most especially among the women of one familial unit. Indeed, mothers and their daughters are bound together in a time-lagged mutuality of shared sexual experience, a bond that is nonetheless potent for all its unspokenness. Moreover, as mentioned in earlier sections of this paper, parents are important in modeling appropriate sexual behavior vis à vis each other. Most of the sexual behavior we consider "normal" in this culture is enacted within a heterosexual dyad. Role theory suggests that in order to enact properly one's own role, one must learn the elements of both roles in a complementary role set. This suggests that the cross-sex, parent-child relationship may be just as important as the same-sex, parent-child relationship in learning, rehearsing, and in reinforcement of behavior in the paired roles of the complementary male-female role set.[38]

Apart from the influence of parents on children's sexuality through their enactment of sex roles in sexual behavior (and about which there is a large literature that includes Freudian and neo–Freudian analyses), there is only limited empirical research linking "family" variables with children's sexual attitudes and behavior. Part of the explanation for this surely lies in the difficulty of measuring "sexual climate" within the home. The handling of nudity necessitated by sharing bathroom facilities, the concealment of menstrual equipment, the responses to "dirty words" at the dinner table, the explanation of athletic supporters sent through the family laundry, the reactions to "living" lingerie advertisements on television during family viewing—in response to a thousand similar mundane and picayune incidents in daily living, sexual information and orientations are transmitted within the family; but I know of no researchers who have tried to measure family sexual climate at this level, and have published their findings. Even though family sexual climate failed to show up in the literature I reviewed for this paper, other aspects of family patterns have been analyzed for their influence on children's sexual attitudes and behavior.

Family Interaction

Lewis investigated the effect that level of family conflict had on the premarital sexual experience of sons and daughters.[39] He found weak or no relationships between measures of familial interpersonal conflict and sexual activity among males. Among females, however, there was an indication that unhappiness in the parental home and not feeling close to the mother were associated with a greater incidence of coital activity, with earlier age of initiation of sexual activity, and with having two or more sexual partners.

Consistent with Lewis's findings are those of Barglow and his co-authors.[40] In a clinical study of seventy-eight adolescent unwed mothers they found "an intensely ambivalent mother-adolescent bond . . . to be a relevant etiological factor in the pregnancy of a group of girls eleven to sixteen years old" (p. 672). Abernethy, in proposing a screening technique to identify those girls at high risk of becoming premaritally pregnant, highlights similar factors when she suggests that the following family variables identify high-risk daughters: (1) not liking the mother and finding her inadequate as a mother; (2) preferring the father to the mother, and having "an intimate, exclusive, quasi-sexual father-daughter relationship" (p. 663); and (3) hostility in the parental marriage that is accompanied by the daughter's failure to side with the mother against the father.[41]

In our Detroit study we found the quality of the mother-daughter relationship, as assessed by the daughter in a series of descriptive statements, to be a stronger predictor of the daughter's sexual status as a virgin or nonvirgin than many other factors, including race, daughter's age, family socioeconomic status, sex of the household head, and parental supervision of the daughter's social activities. Moreover, the quality of the mother-daughter relationship was strongly and positively related to the amount of discussion about sex-related topics between mothers and daughters prior to the daughter's twelfth year, and at her current age. Apparently, communication about sensitive topics like sex is less difficult in the middle teenage years if it follows and builds upon a more general pattern of trust and open communication in the mother-daughter relationship.

One of the most competently handled studies of the impact of marital discord on daughters' sexual behavior was that of Uddenberg, who conducted interviews in Sweden with 101 mothers and their daughters pregnant with a first child.[42] Uddenberg found that although daughters from harmonious and discordant homes differed neither with respect to age at first pregnancy nor educational level, daughters from discordant homes more often described their pregnancies as inconvenient and undesired. They reported a higher number of sexual partners, and were more likely to report unsatisfactory relationships with their male partners than daughters from harmonious homes.

Family Values

A cluster of studies have investigated various effects of parental religious and moral values on children's sexual behavior.[43] Jessor and Jessor found evidence that the mother's ideology (as assessed through her attitudes toward deviant behavior, her traditionality, and her religiosity) was strongly related to an index of children's problem behaviors, which included sexual activity.[44] They found that the more traditional the mother, the more conventional the child's behavior. Similarly, mother-child affectionate interaction and mother's exercise of control and regulation of child behavior were correlated with the problem behavior index; for example, the more affectionate and regulative the maternal behavior, the more conforming was the child. Again the mother was found to have a much stronger effect than the father.

Furstenberg, in his study of pregnant teens, suggests that the mother's sexual standards had a direct effect on the daughter's use of contraception.[45] He found that "women whose mothers strongly disapproved of premarital sexual relations were far less likely to have had experience with birth control than adolescents from more permissive families."

Two studies of college students' attitudes towards sex compared with their parents found a perceptual gap between generations, in that parents were far more likely to believe that their college-age children shared their values and attitudes about premarital sex than was the case in the students' own reports.[46] These findings are of interest because they offer a possible explanation for the negligible amount of talking about sex in American families; that is, to the extent that parents believe (wrongly) that their children share their "conservative" attitudes about premarital sex, they may feel little need to discuss sexual attitudes, values, behavior, and information with their growing children.

Family Structure

Earlier in this chapter it was pointed out that various sociocultural and structural factors appear to influence the degree of communication about sex; in particular, female heads of household are more likely to communicate with their daughters about sex and birth control. It is interesting to compare the influence of these kinds of family characteristics on sexual behavior itself. Roebuck and McGee examined the impact of family decision-making structures on premarital sexual attitudes and behavior in a sample of 242 black female high school students in rural Mississippi.[47] Families were classified as "matriarchal," "egalitarian," or "patriarchal" on the basis of the presence or absence of a husband-father, and according to daughters' responses as to which parent was the major decision maker in the family. The authors found that daughters in mother-led homes had the most permissive attitudes, while daughters in father-led homes had the least permissive attitudes. When sexual experience was considered, they found that close to 50 percent of daughters from mother-led and egalitarian homes were sexually experienced, as compared to 30 percent from father-led homes.

Barglow and his co-authors also found that family structure (that is, whether a household was headed by a female or was a husband-wife household) was related to adolescent premarital pregnancy; girls from households headed by females were more likely to be pregnant.[48] Their findings are consistent with those of Kantner and Zelnik, who report, from their national probability sample survey of fifteen- to nineteen-year-olds, higher proportions of daughters from families headed by females as having some sexual experience, in comparison with daughters in father-present homes.[49] We found a similar relationship between daughters' sexual intercourse experience and parental marital status in our Detroit sample of fourteen- and fifteen-year-olds. Goldfarb and her co-authors, in their paper on "pregnancy susceptibility," found that growing up in a large family of orientation, and having unmarried sisters with children of their own were predictive of premarital pregnancy among adolescents.[50] The Akpoms's study of 303 white Michigan teenage family planning clients also reported earlier initiation of sexual activity among daughters from female-headed families.[51]

Finally, there is evidence to suggest that such parental and familial characteristics as socioeconomic status and the work status of the mother distinguish among daughters, in terms of their sexual and contraceptive behavior. Kantner and Zelnik find that, in general, for both blacks and whites there is an inverse association between parental socioeconomic status and a daughter's sexual experience.[52] An exception to this relationship is the educational level of the parent or guardian. In black families the more education the father has, and to a lesser extent the mother, the less likely his daughter is to be sexually experienced. However, this is not so in white families, where, at the college level or above, the reverse is true: the more education either parent has, the more likely the daughter is to be sexually experienced. Relative to contraceptive use, Kantner and Zelnik find a positive association with parental socioeconomic status, with the education of the female parent/guardian particularly important in this regard.[53]

The work status of the female parent has been infrequently investigated for its relation to the daughter's sexual and contraceptive behavior. In a comparison of pregnant teens with their nonpregnant classmates in his Baltimore study, Furstenberg found that mothers of the nonpregnant teens are slightly more likely to be in the labor force than mothers of the pregnant teens (66 percent, versus 60 percent).[54] In unreported data from my own study of women students at a midwestern university, daughters of mothers working outside the home were more likely to be sexually experienced than daughters of mothers who did not work outside the home (62 percent, versus 54 percent); and the former were more likely than the latter to have used a contraceptive at their most recent coital episode (64 percent, versus 50 percent). Without more information about the conditions under which mothers worked outside the home, their occupational status, or their contributions to family income, as well as more information from a larger pool of studies, it is difficult to interpret the meaning of the relationship between the mother's work status and the daughter's sexual and contraceptive behavior.

Let me conclude this section on the indirect or unintentional effects of parents on children's sexual behavior by underlining the evidence that points to the critical importance of the mother-daughter relationship. The absence of a solid bond between mothers and daughters was found in several studies of sexually active and pregnant adolescents. The importance of the mother found in the studies reviewed here provides independent corroboration of the similar conclusion reached in the section on direct parent-child communication.

What is also evident from these studies, but did not emerge so clearly in the previous section, is the importance of the father-mother relationship to a daughter's sexual behavior. Whether measured in terms of harmony or conflict, power structure, or simply the presence or absence of the husband-father, the tenor of the parental relationship carries over into a daughter's sexual behavior. There are several possible explanations of why this may be so. It may be a function of social learning of adult male-female interaction patterns; of the additional moral authority that a father could add to the value positions and behavior regulations posited by the mother; of the additional social resources that an adult male could bring to a family unit; or of some combination of these.

Perhaps the surest conclusion that can be drawn from this section is that, in fact, we know very little about how teenagers are affected by the individual members of their families and by the interactions among them. The problem is partly methodological, and partly has to do with the fact that some of the right questions have yet to be asked. Needed is more research that is specifically designed to assess the impact of family-level variables on sexual initiation, activity, contraception, and pregnancy. Sibling relationships, for example, are felt to be of considerable importance; yet, we know very little about them, as a thorough literature review has demonstrated; and we know perhaps even less about siblings' effects on sexual behavior.[55] Until we have studies that will allow for the simultaneous examination of many factors thought to be relevant, we will be constrained to build explanations of behavior out of unconnected and noncumulative research that is, of necessity, inconclusive.

The Role of the Family in Social Control

To sociologists, social control is simply socialization's "other face." Both work in conjunction to ensure the normative order. Thus, there are theoretical reasons for considering the family's role in the social control of sexual behavior, as well as its role in sexual socialization.

The most effective form of social control is the internalization of the values and norms of appropriate behavior that encourages an individual to want to do what he must do. This is generally accomplished through socialization. There are, however, other mechanisms through which control is engineered. These include monitoring behavior and keeping it under surveillance, so that tendencies toward inappropriate behavior can be altered at once. An additional mechanism of control is to punish the manifestation of inappropriate behavior, through physical, psychological, or social sanction.

With regard to the sexual behavior of their children, once families have taught them "to know right," they are then expected to "keep them in line" and make sure they "do right." What evidence exists of the family's attempts to regulate the sexual behavior of its younger members? As in the other sections of this paper, I found little empirical research on this issue. There were some interesting, though nonempirical, papers that touched on social control of teenage children's sexual behavior that are reported below. First, however, let us consider the admittedly limited empirical evidence on parental control.

Jessor and Jessor, cited earlier, found that the mother's efforts to regulate or sanction children's behavior—in terms of setting family curfew, use of leisure time, doing homework, and the like—were related negatively and significantly to an index of problem behavior (including sex) for both male and female children: "The greater the controls exercised by the mother, the less the child's participation in the different areas measured by the problem index."[56]

In a previous paper on the social control of women, I suggested that internalization of the concept, "nice girl," was a potent method of constraining women's behavior to conform to rather strict guidelines of propriety.[57] Although the concept of "nice," versus "not nice," has long been used by parents as a means to govern the sexual behavior of their daughters, I suggested that it is counterproductive for generating a sense of self-responsible sexuality among young women. As it pertains to contraceptive use among young women, the "nice girl" construct was described as follows:

> Because one of the most effective ways to maintain chastity in public while deviating in private is through regular use of contraception, one might expect that the "nice girl" construct would encourage contraceptive use among young women. However, it has just the opposite effect. Regular use of contraception requires preparedness and preplanning, acknowledgement prior to coitus of the probability of coitus, and a willingness to take responsibility for sexual behavior. But the only excuses a young woman may give for sexual intercourse prior to marriage and still claim some vestige of niceness to herself are coercion (rape) and, more important here, to be so uncontrollably in love as to be virtually swept away by the spontaneous and unrestrainable passions of the particular moment. Obviously, to be prepared for coitus with contraceptives would give lie to the rationale that each act of intercourse was unanticipated and unplanned, merely a temporary and transitory lapse of virtue. In short, in order to be responsible to her "virtue" or "niceness," the nice girl construct requires that a woman be irresponsible sexually with regard to contraceptive use (pp. 815–816).

Two other formulations that, like the "nice girl" construct, have yet to be tested empirically, but, when taken together, pose an interesting contrast in the roles of the mother in the social control of her teenaged daughter's behavior are those of Bernard and Reiss.[58] In *Women, Wives and Mothers,* Jessie Bernard suggests that one of the most worrisome and problematical aspects of the "middle motherhood" stage is the renegotiation of the maternal role relationship with adolescent sons and daughters. Relative to the mother-daughter relationship, Bernard suggests that, until recently, mothers were held responsible for the sexual purity of their daughters. However, in the face of the often radical changes in sexual behavior among young women of the seventies, Bernard suggests that mothers have given up trying to prevent sexual experimentation by their daughters, and have adopted what I would call an "ostrich response"; that is, they no longer feel responsible for the virginity of daughters, go to great lengths to protect themselves from knowledge of their daughters' sexual behavior, and hope only that the daughters will refrain from becoming pregnant out of wedlock.

Bernard's thesis contrasts sharply with that of Reiss and Miller, which suggests that, as their daughters reach puberty, women become measurably less permissive in their attitudes about premarital sexual behavior.[59] Reiss and Miller attribute this to the mother's heightened sense of responsibility for the sexual behavior of their daughters. Thus, following Reiss and Miller, we might expect mothers to be likely to take a more active rather than a less active role in their daughters' transition from sexual innocence to awareness, and to be likely to take steps to decrease the opportunities for sexual experimentation by their daughters. It also seems probable that the formulations of both Bernard and Reiss and Miller capture some of the realities of the mother-daughter relationship, but that each is describing a different aspect of the mother's role in the process of the daughter's transition.

It would appear that, although teenagers complain often and loudly about parental restrictions and rules, although the family is generally expected to continue to safeguard and protect its children by monitoring their behavior, and although parents appear to worry endlessly about how, in fact, to do this, there is little research on this family function. The papers reviewed in this section clearly raise several questions that need further investigation.

Family Involvement in Pregnancy Resolution

For many parents, the first direct involvement in the sexual behavior of their daughters comes with the discovery of the daughter's pregnancy. Furstenberg, for example, notes that three-fourths of the mothers of the pregnant teens he studied expressed shock and surprise at learning of their daughter's pregnancy.[60] In this section I want to review briefly a few papers that look at the part that parents (most typically the mother) play in pregnancy resolution.

Rosen's study of problem pregnancy decision making suggests that teens seeking abortions rarely consult with their parents, while those who carry their pregnancies to term nearly always do.[61] Those who obtain abortions reported their parents as not influential in their decision; when parents were reported as influential, the woman was more likely to decide to keep her baby than when they were not influential.

Once the decision is made to bring the pregnancy to term, we find several studies—in particular, Smith—that confirm that parents, upon learning of a daughter's pregnancy, express anger and disappointment, then move through stages of a gradual accommodation; frequently there is a growing closeness, especially between mother and daughter.[62] Furstenberg's chapter (which follows) provides some vivid clinical examples of this process of family accommodation, and evidence that confirms the findings of Young and her co-authors, who describe how influential a mother is, both in helping the teenage mother make basic decisions, and providing practical assistance.[63] Of equal relevance, especially to the family planning demonstration project described in Chapter 11, are the three studies that show how critical parental support and values are to teenage mothers' use of contraceptives after their first birth.[64]

Sources of Strain for Families in Responding to Adolescent Sexuality

Sources within Family Systems

In this final section, I will explore some possible, and admittedly partial explanations for why sexuality, specifically adolescent sexuality, appears to be so difficult an area for families. Some of the difficulty lies in the internal dynamics that are inherent in the life stages of families with adolescents.

One of the strengths of the family as a social organization is its multigenerational character. The fact that within the family each member moves through time in concert with others who are at different stages of life distinguishes the family as a social body within which change is experienced. Persons of differing ages are exposed to one another, as each attempts to grapple with her or his own age-differentiated developmental tasks. Thus, parents are able to watch their daughters and sons struggle with the events and tasks of childhood and youth, developmental tasks similar to those faced by the parents themselves at that age, but which are enacted in a temporal context that has been altered by a generation of time. Similarly, children, while experiencing their lives as children, are able to telescope the experience of time and preview their adult roles by observing how their parents, as adults, deal with the same events that they, the children, experience as children. The family, in brief, provides an experiential laboratory for transcending the temporal dimension of human life through involvement in the continual changes in the lives of loved ones.

But while this is a source of strength, it is also a source of strain for the family unit. It is often the case for parent-adolescent units within the family that the development of the child as an adolescent is occurring simultaneously with the tasks and challenges of mid-life development for the parent; moreover, the separate developmental agendas of the parent and adolescent are, in many ways, in conflict; and within both roles, but more particularly that of the parent, there are serious internal inconsistencies in the demands of the role set. Finally, the developmental tasks of both parents and children have been exacerbated by cultural shifts in the norms governing sex roles and sexual behavior. Let me say a bit more about each of these sources of strain, because I think they may offer some clues about the difficulty of direct communication about sex between parents and adolescent children.

The daughter's or son's developmental agenda in adolescence includes the development of autonomy and separation, that is, gaining distance from and resolving feelings about one's family. The task is accompanied by erratic and unpredictable pulls toward, and pushes away from, the family; by an intense need for closeness and an equally intense feeling of being smothered by the family; and by a simultaneous need to gain independence from, yet retain one's dependence upon, the family. Seeking out and turning to peers become important activities during adolescence, and contribute to the separation from one's family. A second task is the establishment or consolidation of one's identity, the defining of one's own self. The difficulty of coming to terms with the "who am I?" question has been especially intensified for young women, but also for young men, by the current unsettled nature of sex-role prescriptions. A third developmental task of adolescence is the establishment of appropriate attachments to people outside the realm of one's family. This is consistent with the process of separation from one's family; and both are often facilitated by the participation of the son or daughter in dating, going steady, and falling in love. A final developmental task of adolescence is self mastery, that is, gaining mastery over one's own impulses, and developing the ability to anticipate future consequences of present actions. The preoccupation of adolescents with themselves, their own needs, and the demands they make on their families are great, and occasionally, overwhelming, but no more so than the tasks confronting them during this phase of their lives.

The parents' developmental agenda during their children's adolescence are equally exacting. The recent research of Levinson on adult men, popularized and extended to include women by Sheehy, has focused considerable attention on the process of development throughout adulthood.[65] Let me offer a view of the mother's developmental agenda from the perspective of the mother-daughter relationship.

As the parent of a maturing daughter, the mother must serve both as a protector of the daughter-as-child and a guide for the daughter-as-woman. Learning to manage the conflict between these two aspects of the mother's role is one of the major developmental tasks of this period, and one for which there are few clear guidelines. It is hard work to discern when to let go and when not to yield; when to share information and when not to; when to allow a child to find her own way and to live out the consequences of her own decisions, and when, instead, to take charge and make decisions in her behalf. It takes untold amounts of psychic energy to be attentive enough to the needs of a child to know which action among the alternatives is the better one for her. And it often takes a lot of time. Moreover, renegotiation of the mother-daughter relationship is painful; it is often far simpler to allow existing patterns of parent-child interaction to continue unaltered by changing realities in the life of the child. Thus, in many families, we find that children choose to protect their parents from knowledge about themselves and their peers on the quite reasonable grounds that the parents cannot cope with knowing that their children know what they know; and parents are sometimes eager for this protection.

A second task on the mother's developmental agenda is to come to terms with her own stage of adulthood. This is termed the mid-life crisis by some, and includes several "crises." One is the *crisis of being*, that is, finding meaning beyond one's role as mother, or alternatively, finding ways to extend the role as mother. Another is the *crisis of doing*, which, for many women, is a crisis of implementation, that is, of making decisions about entry or return to the labor force, resumption of education, or career changes, and the like. The *crisis of aging* also pervades this phase of female adulthood; for many women, the perceived loss of culturally valued youth, with its uncontrived beauty, at the very same time that their daughters are sensing and exercising their own youthful attractiveness, is a bitter experience, one that some writers suspect of fostering an unintentional hostility and one-sided competition between a mother and her daughter.[66] In sum, part of what women who are mothers of adolescents must deal with is the conflict between their role as a parent and their own selfhood; both demand time, energy, and concern.

In any social system, the growth and development of one member of an interdependent whole calls for the expenditure of social resources above and beyond the relatively constant resource expenditures necessary for meeting daily needs. Resources are needed to compensate for, and accommodate to, the change, and to readjust and realign the relationships among the interdependent members. The simultaneous (and often divergent) development of two or more members increases the problems of adjustment many times. Families differ in their elasticity for managing the structural strain that results from the concurrent development of parents and adolescent children. Families differ in their store of available social resources, and in their ability to mobilize those resources at the right time and in the appropriate way. The modal pattern appears to be one of "muddling through." Most teenagers survive adolescence; most women and men survive their children's adolescence, and also negotiate their own mid-life crises; and most families survive—although there are certainly enough studies of family happiness to suggest that the period is neither an easy one nor a terribly satisfying one for most people. (It is easy to overdraw a picture of adolescence as a traumatic phase in the family life cycle. The inconsistencies in the empirical and theoretical literature on adolescence as a time of tempest or calm are reviewed, and a synthesis attempted via the "focal" theory of adolescent development, in a brief article by J. Coleman.[67])

Some families, however, simply lack the resources to manage the structural problems inherent in concurrent growth. Teenage pregnancy may well be an indicator, or symptom, of such a resource shortage. Indeed, two of the more popular motivational explanations for teenage pregnancy are couched in terms of family system deficits: namely, that teens have babies in order to have someone to love, to relate to, to care for, to compensate for their family's lack of attention to them. The other version is that teens have babies in order to break away, establish their own independence, and force a renegotiation of their relationship with their parents. Both of these versions imply that when the family lacks the social resources needed to attend to the needs of the teen, the teen will seek to meet them herself through a pregnancy. One of the challenges for all of us concerned with adolescents should be to discover ways to regenerate and supplement the social resources of families.

Sources of Strain from the Social-Cultural Context

While some of the explanation for a family's role in the sexual behavior of adolescence can be couched in terms of internal family system dynamics, it is also necessary to take into account the fact that families exist in a cultural context. Above and beyond subcultural differences of race, religion, and ethnicity (which are addressed elsewhere in this book), families are affected by patterns of cultural values and shifts in those values, most particularly those that relate to sexuality, on the one hand, and parent-child relationships, on the other.

In the mid-sixties, in his studies of standards for premarital sexual behavior, Reiss detected a shift away from abstinence codes (in both sex-equal and sexist double-standard forms) toward a contingency code that permitted permissiveness on the condition of affection between partners.[68] Virtually every study conducted since then on the same topic has found the permissiveness-with-affection standard to have gained adherence at the expense of abstinence codes.[69] Among the many consequences of such a shift in values is that it has complicated the task of parents as sex educators, in part because the system of ethics that underlies a contingency standard is more complex than one that underlies an absolute standard. It is far easier to teach children that a behavior is inappropriate under all circumstances than to attempt to specify not only the defining condition of the appropriate circumstances (i.e., "affection"), but also how to detect when, in fact, the condition is "real," not ersatz or ephemeral. Moreover, the fact that the value shift is not complete across the population as a whole means that there is less consensus on the appropriate moral postures for parents, or on what the outcomes of parental sexual socialization and control efforts should be. Put as a blunt question, should a goal of parental socialization be to prevent premarital sexual activity entirely among their sons and daughters, or merely to forestall it until an "appropriate age?" Should it be to prevent sexual activity or merely conception? Should it be to prevent sexual activity or merely the enjoyment of sexual activity? Rephrasing these questions in the positive (i.e., "A goal of parental socialization should be to encourage children toward responsible sexual behavior, which may or may not include coitus; if it does, it is to be engaged in joyfully with a loved and loving, contraceptively protected partner") may be less jarring to our sensitivities, but it does little to reduce the confusion about the desired outcomes of parental socialization. In the face of such confusion, it should not be surprising that many parents have sidestepped the matter entirely.

Not only does there seem to be a lack of consensus on what to teach one's children about sex, but two sociologists have suggested that our general cultural understanding of sexuality lies at the heart of the difficulty of parent-child communication about sex. In their enormously important book on the science of human sexuality, Gagnon and Simon have written lucidly on the ways we think about sexuality, and of the impact that sexual ideology has on the full scope of our lives. Against the Freudian view of sexuality—as a potent biological drive, or instinctual force, that is only incompletely and temporarily restrained by the civilizing forces of socialization and social control, but which threatens constantly to break through and disrupt our social conventions—they present an alternative view of sexuality as a process of learning "sexual scripts," that is, learning how to organize, code, and attribute sexual meaning to thoughts, acts, situations, and actors.

Gagnon and Simon's work in this area is important for two reasons. First, it puts into perspective several conventional and interrelated explanations of why sexual socialization is a source of difficulty within the context of the family, and why parent-child communication about sex is so rare. Shipman discusses several of these in detail; for example, the incest taboo has been viewed as strong enough to prohibit even verbal communication about sex, because open communication about sex within the family was felt to be a form of symbolic incest.[70] Udry also talks of a need to neutralize, or "desexualize" family relationships for the sake of comfort and survival.[71] In such a situation, sex is too explosive a topic for internal family communication.

Another explanation discussed by Shipman is the idea that human beings have an instinctual need for privacy, which is manifested in the establishment of boundaries between parents and children in dealing with sex. The tendency of adults to deny childhood sexuality and the refusal of children to accept the sexual nature of their parents are also offered as reasons why parents and children cannot communicate about sex. Beiser, in a classic Freudian analysis, accounts for antagonism between mothers and adolescent daughters in terms of the covert sexual rivalry between them: "A relatively normal woman with a good marital relationship may not be aware that she sees her daughter as a painful reminder to her husband and herself of her own youthful beauty that is now fading. It is a rare woman who can sincerely welcome her daughter into puberty."[72]

These explanations make sense only if one understands sexuality as a natural force, or biological drive, that presses constantly for expression. Sexuality, understood in this way, indeed poses a threat to such an intimate group as the family, and would require that steps be taken to keep it from spilling over into, and disrupting the life of, the family. One way to keep it in check would be to deny its existence by not talking about it.

On the other hand, these explanations fail to be credible if sexuality is seen as a product of social learning, in the way that Gagnon and Simon have suggested. It is precisely by conceptualizing sexual development in such a fashion that we are able to look at the way parents teach their children about sex. Gagnon and Simon hold that parents rarely initiate sexual instruction, but rather react to a child's questions about, or expression of, behavior that the parents, but not necessarily the children, interpret as sexual. The authors further suggest that parents apply very different strategies for teaching about sexual behavior than they use in teaching other kinds of behaviors. They describe a pattern of typical response that parents make: (1) parents impute "sexual capacities, or qualities in children that the children may not have had but that result in—however imperfectly—children learning to act as if they had such capacities or qualities"; and (2) parents respond to a child's behavior (which the parent interprets as having sexual meaning) by "describing the behavior as sexual and saying that it is wrong, . . . mislabel[ing] the behavior, describing it as something it may not be, or . . . nonlabel[ing] the behavior by ignoring or providing a judgment without a specific label."[73] Gagnon and Simon assert first, that applying judgment without naming the behavior is the most frequent parental response; second, that such moral judgments and evaluations are rarely reassessed or revised by either the parent or child as the child passes into or through adolescence; and third, "the young are trained, more often informally than formally, in the sexual vocabulary without associating it with sexual activity, [which allows] the words to develop a complexity of meanings and associations long before they are ultimately applied to the realm of sexual behavior" (p. 38). Among the many tangled consequences of this pattern of sexual socialization, Gagnon and Simon suggest, are a child's turning to peers for sexual information—which is, however, filtered through the value orientations and attitudes toward sex fostered by the parents; the development of guilt and anxiety about sexual behavior; and the "capacity and need to keep sexuality secret, especially from those one loves" (p. 42).

Why is it that parents teach sexuality in this way? As sexual pedagogy, the parents' methods are fully compatible with an understanding of sexuality as an instinctual drive, as was described earlier. In other words, that parents handle sexuality with their children in the way that they do is not so much a function of the need to "desexualize family relationships" by limiting even the discussion of sex, as it is a function of the *belief* that that is necessary.

A final cultural pattern that I will but mention here, since others have dealt with it in great detail quite recently, has to do with age-grading in our society.[74] Specifically, the structural patterns that maintain segregation across generations keep parents and children apart, and limit the amount of time and opportunity for shared activity and interaction. Adolescent children and parents who exist in barely overlapping spheres will not communicate very often about anything, including sex.

Exacerbating the problem of age-grading is the rather low valuation attached to the adult parenting role. In comparing the differential permeability of work roles and family roles, Pleck observed that for men, but not for women, family roles were open to intrusion and disruption by the demands of a job, but not vice versa.[75] I suspect that the sex differential here is narrowing, so that women are increasingly under the same pressures as men not to let their families' needs intervene in their work lives. Far from being rewarded for placing the highest priority on their responsibilities to their spouses and children (except insofar as this responsibility is defined as providing for their economic well-being), parents are prevented from doing so by the organization of work. As more and more women continue to enter and remain in the labor force, and as the conditions under which they work become more and more like those of men, there will be fewer and fewer adult parents who have the reservoirs of time, patience, and flexibility of schedule that adolescent children need.

Bronfenbrenner has already predicted some of the consequences of rearing children under conditions of relative isolation from parents and other adults.[76] Therefore, we should not be surprised that some of the consequences are making themselves manifest, as in patterns of adolescent sexuality and childbearing.

A final source of strain for families in dealing with the sexual behavior of teens may well be the interrelationship between families and external agencies in the handling of sex education and related services for teens. An inventory of such agencies would include: the formal educational system; the church or religious system; the formal medical system; the broadening network of less formally organized clinics offering specialized medical services to teenage clientele; and the social service system. How are responsibilities for the sexual socialization of children divided up and parceled out among families and agencies? One of the underlying criteria for the current division of labor is the age of the child. It is generally the practice that the family is responsible for little children, say sixth grade and under, while external agencies have access only to children, middle-school-age and older. A second criterion is content. The family is generally assigned the responsibility for instilling sexual values, while the other agencies handle "the facts"—biological, physiological, health-related, and so forth.

I would suggest that this division of labor has not been the product either of a rational consideration of alternatives or of a well-conceived policy planning, but rather is an ad hoc system that has grown out of the perception on the part of various professional interest groups (educators, social workers, clerics, physicians) of needs for their skills and services. One of the unintended consequences of this division of labor is that it appears to pit "the family" against "the world," and reinforces an artificial, and in my view, harmful dichotomy between the sacred and the profane in matters of sexuality. It casts families in the role of protectors of innocent children, and portrays external agencies as the major corruptors of teenage children. It makes families and agencies into competitors when mutual supportiveness, rather than competition, is sorely needed. I am not wholly convinced that a re-thinking and intentional restructuring of the division of labor between family and external service providers could come up with a better system, but it is certainly the case that we could hardly do worse.

A second issue in the family-agency interrelationship is the matter of confidentiality in the provision of services to teens. Certainly, it is too large an issue to be dealt with in a brief paragraph; nevertheless, as a family sociologist I would like to make a few observations. It is simply not clear how to balance the right and responsibility of parents to know about, and participate in, decisions their daughters make to seek contraceptive or abortion assistance against the agency obligation and desire to serve teens effectively. Agency personnel apparently believe that parental involvement, most particularly parental notification as a prerequisite for service delivery, will have a chilling effect on a teen's help-seeking behavior. A recent national study by Urban and Rural Systems Associates (URSA) on ways to improve family planning services to teens emphasized strongly the vital importance of assuring confidentiality in order to gain teens' acceptance of services.[77] Unless teens know for sure that their parents will not find out, the study said, they will refuse to come to clinics for contraceptive assistance.

The Ktsanes study cited earlier, however, suggests otherwise: in this study of clinic attenders, 60 percent had talked to their mothers or another family member about coming to the clinic prior to the initial visit; moreover, nearly all of the teens reported having told their families they were receiving contraceptive assistance after coming to the clinic; and only 5 percent of the teens reported that confidentiality was of concern to them. Torres reports similar data from a pilot study of 1,442 young clinic attenders from fifty-three clinics across the country.[78] Her findings are consistent with those of Ktsanes. Torres found that parents of 55 percent of the young women were aware of their daughters' clinic attendance. Of those women whose parents did not know, 10 percent said that a parental notification policy would not have deterred their coming to the clinic for assistance. Thirty-six percent of the young women guessed that a parental notification policy would have kept them from coming to the clinic; of this group, the majority guessed that they would obtain a nonprescription method of contraception when having sex. Only one out of eight girls in the study indicated explicitly that they would have sex without using contraception if the clinic had a parental notification policy.

Unfortunately, none of these studies is methodologically strong enough to provide a definitive answer about the effect of parental notification policies on the contraceptive help-seeking behavior of teens. In the first place, it is not good enough to sample only clinics or clinic users, as the above three studies have done. Moreover, both the URSA and Torres samples are poorly drawn; and the Ktsanes study pertains only to Louisiana, and thus is of questionable generalizability to the United States as a whole. One needs to understand the perceived barriers to clinic use by those who are not clinic attendees; in other words, the population of interest has not yet been studied, although some promising research projects are underway that may provide information on girls who are contraceptively at risk but who are not clinic attendees.[79]

It may be for many teens at risk that parental notification policies are only a minor barrier, when considered alongside the difficulties of accessibility due to inadequate urban transportation systems, the psychological reluctance to admit the need for contraception, or simple inertia. On the other hand, parental notification could also emerge as a highly significant factor in clinic nonuse. At this point, we simply do not know which is the case for the majority of teens.

In the face of inadequate knowledge, if the goal is to reach the largest number of teens, it would appear safest to assume that parental notification policies (and certainly those requiring parental consent for service delivery) are a barrier to help-seeking. However, recognition of some of the hidden costs of an open, no-notification policy is also essential. Maintaining confidentiality may be necessary for many teens; a no-notification policy allows for a swift response to teens' immediate needs, which may forestall the even more serious problems that come with pregnancy. At the same time, bypassing the family robs both parents and teens of a critical opportunity to renegotiate their relationships. Furthermore, this bypass constitutes one more way in which we are systematically undermining what has traditionally been the most effective support group, one's family.

A third issue in the family–external agency interface is related to the emergence of teenage pregnancy and its *sine qua non*, teenage sexuality, as major social concerns. Does the management of teenage sexuality (sex education, provision of services, pregnancy assistance, and so forth) need to be handled by experts who are specially trained to deal with such problems? This question has a corollary; and that is that parents of teens need special help and training in order to deal effectively with their children's sexuality. That these notions, in fact, may be accurate is not the point. The point is that the institutionalization of teenage sexuality as a major social problem—with an attendant array of experts, programs, policy initiatives, and so forth—carries with it at least two unintended consequences: first, by articulating the ineptitude of parents as sex educators of their children, we may encourage, not the desired parental help-seeking behavior, but rather, an even greater parental noninvolvement ("learned helplessness" may be appropriate theoretical construct here), as parents leave the entire field to "the experts."

The second consequence is also related to expertise. With the emergence of an identifiable corps of experts who are specially charged with (and possibly equipped for) handling the given problem, comes a widespread belief that "something is being done" about the problem, and a concomitant contraction in the number of people (and agencies) who perceive a personal responsibility for responding to the problem. What is created, in effect, is a vicious circle in which the unintended consequences of our responses to a social problem themselves exacerbate the problem. Some of this can be avoided by seeking to hold the reification and mystification of expertise to a minimum in any programs or policies that are developed to deal with teenage sexuality.

Conclusions

It would be satisfying to be able to offer a series of policy recommendations that flow logically out of the existing research on the family's role in teenage sexuality; but the list would necessarily be based as much on what we do not know as on what we do know. Nevertheless, a few suggestions for future action can be made.

It seems fairly clear that more research on the role of the family in teenage sexuality is needed; but it needs to be informed by the questions that grow out of the programmatic needs of practitioners. Such research needs to be intelligently designed and competently executed. Some of it needs to be cross-generational; some should be longitudinal; and not all should be based on sample survey designs. Throughout this review, I have suggested questions that are worthy of further research. For instance, we need to know more about the role of *fathers*, vis-à-vis daughters and sons; fathers present an intriguing riddle, in that there is little empirical evidence of their direct involvement or impact in the sexual socialization and control of children, even though a considerable body of data suggests a strong indirect influence. Understandably, most of our research has been directed at teenage women; but we absolutely must begin to learn something about the sexual socialization and behavior of *young men*, and the part they play in sexual, contraceptive, and pregnancy resolution decisions.

More attention also needs to be addressed to the entire *family* unit, as well as to specific relational configurations within it, such as mother-daughter dyads, father-daughter, father-son, sister-sister, brother-sister, and so forth. While we already know something of the association of family size, composition, and socioeconomic characteristics with the sexual behavior of teens, the effect of intrafamilial interaction (communication skills, problem-solving strategies, decision-making and governance styles) on the transmission of sexual values and information, and on the availability of the family as a support system for teen members is less well charted in the current research literature.

A particularly important area for further research lies in the *interface of the family with formal service agencies that assist teens*: does formal involvement of the family in agency programs help or hinder the teen? How might agency personnel best serve the needs of the teen, in light of the larger familial context in which she/he is found? How can parents effectively join with the agency in meeting the needs of their teens? How can the needs of parents be recognized and dealt with by agency personnel? What components of programs engender the most enthusiasm and resistance from parents?

With regard to policies concerning teenage sexuality, the evidence from existing research suggests a rather simple cardinal principle: ways of involving the parent or parents of teens must be developed; implemented as a core component of the program; and evaluated, whether the specific program is primary prevention, sex education, contraceptive service provision, or pregnancy and post-partum assistance. Policies that ignore familial support, and undermine, rather than supplement, the efforts *and effectiveness* of parents are likely to yield programs that are wasteful, inefficient, and ineffective; and, what is more serious, are likely to do a considerable disservice to the teenagers about whom we are so concerned.

NOTES

1. Graham B. Spanier, "Formal and informal sex education as determinants of premarital sexual behavior," *Archives of Sexual Behavior* 5, no. 1 (1976): 39–67.

2. Mavis E. Hetherington, "Effects of father absence on personality development in adolescent daughters," *Developmental Psychology* 7, no. 3 (1972): 313–326; and Nils Uddenberg, "Mother-father and daughter male relationships: A comparison," *Archives of Sexual Behavior* 5, no. 1 (1976): 69–79.

3. Jean Lipman-Blumen, "How ideology shapes women's lives," *Scientific American* 226, no. 1 (1972): 34–42.

4. See, for example, Anne Doherty, "Influence of parental control on the development of feminine sex role and conscience," *Developmental Psychology* 2, no. 1 (1970): 157–158; Alfred B. Heilbrun, Jr., "Identification with father and sex-role development of the daughter," *Family Coordinator* 25, no. 4 (1976): 411–416; and David B. Lynn, "Fathers and sex-role development," *The Family Coordinator* 25, no. 4 (1976): 403–409.

5. Henry B. Biller, "Father absence and the personality development of the male child," *Developmental Psychology* 2, no. 2 (1970): 181–201; E. Herzog and C. Sudia, "Children in fatherless families," in *Review of child development research*, E. M. Hetherington and P. Ricciuti, eds., vol. 3 (Chicago: University of Chicago, 1974); David B. Lynn, *The father: His role in child development* (Belmont, Calif.: Wadsworth, 1974); and Donald E. Payne and Paul H. Mussen, "Parent-child relations and father identification among adolescent boys," *Journal of Abnormal and Social Psychology* 52, no. 3 (1956): 358–362.

6. Frank Furstenberg, *Unplanned parenthood: The social consequences of teenage childbearing* (New York: Free Press, 1976).

7. C. Lindemann, *Birth control and unmarried young women* (New York: Springer, 1974).

8. Robert R. Bell and Jack V. Buerkle, "The mother and daughter attitudes to premarital sexual behavior," *Marriage and Family Living* 23 (1961): 390–392; Stella Chess, Alexander Thomas, and Martha Cameron, "Sexual attitudes and behavior patterns in a middle-class adolescent population," *American Journal of Orthopsychiatry* 46, no. 4 (1976): 689–701; M. C. Dubbe, "What parents are not told may hurt: A study of communication between teenagers and parents," *Family Life Coordinator* 14 (April 1965): 51–118; L. A. Kirkendall and H. S. Cox, "Starting a sex education program," *Children* 14 (1967): 136–141; G. Shipman, "The psycho-

dynamics of sex education," *The Family Coordinator* 17, no. 1 (1968): 3–12; and Arlene S. Skolnick, *The intimate environment* (Boston: Little, Brown, 1973).
   9. D. R. Mace, "From the President: Some reflections on the American family," *Marriage and Family Living* 24 (1962): 109–113.
   10. Joyce L. Goldfarb, David M. Mumford, David A. Schum, Peggy B. Smith, Charles Flowers, and Carolyn Schum, "An attempt to detect 'pregnancy susceptibility' in indigent adolescent girls," *Journal of Youth and Adolescence* 6, no. 2 (1977): 127–144.
   11. James E. Elias, "Adolescents and sex," *The Humanist* 38 (March/April, 1978): 29–31.
   12. Eugene Weiss, F. Gerald Kline, Everett M. Rogers, Michael E. Cohen, and Jennifer A. Dodge, "Communication and population socialization among youth: Communication behavior and family planning information," paper presented at the annual meeting of the Population Association of America, New York City, 1974.
   13. Robert Fein, "Men and young children," in *Men and masculinity*, eds., J. H. Pleck and J. Sawyer (Englewood Cliffs, N.J.: Prentice-Hall, 1974); M. Polatnick, "Why men don't rear children: A power analysis," *Berkeley Journal of Sociology* 18 (1973–74): 45–86; and C. S. Stoll, *Female and male* (Dubuque, Iowa: William C. Brown, 1974).
   14. Doris Bloch, "Sex education practices of mothers," *Journal of Sex Education and Therapy* 7, no. 1 (1972): 7–12.
   15. Pearila Brickner Rothenberg, "Mother-child communication about sex and birth control," paper presented at the Population Association of America, Atlanta, April 1978.
   16. For more detailed reports of the findings discussed below, see G. L. Fox and J. K. Inazu, "Mother-daughter communication about sex," *Family Relations* 29 (1980): 347–352; and G. L. Fox and J. K. Inazu, "The effect of mother-daughter communication on daughter's sexual and contraceptive knowledge and behavior," paper presented at the annual meetings of the Population Association of America, Philadelphia, April 1979.
   17. Rothenberg, "Mother-child communication," p. 4.
   18. Amechi C. Akpom, Kathy L. Akpom, and Marianne Davis, "Prior sexual behavior of teenagers attending rap sessions for the first time," *Family Planning Perspectives* 8, no. 4 (July/Aug. 1976): 203–206.
   19. Rothenberg, "Mother-child communication," p. 7; and I. L. Reiss and B. Miller, *A theoretical analysis of heterosexual permissiveness*, technical report no. 11 (Minneapolis: Minnesota Family Study Center, 1974).
   20. Karin Schoof-Tams, Jurgen Schaegel, and Leonhard Walczak, "Differentiation of sexual morality between eleven and sixteen years," *Archives of Sexual Behavior* 5, no. 5 (1976): 353–370; and L. Kohlberg, "Moral development and the education of adolescents," in *Adolescent Readings in Behavior and Development*, ed. E. D. Evans (Hinsdale, Ill.: Dryden, 1970); Joseph Adelson, "The development of

ideology in adolescence," in *Adolescence in the life cycle,* eds. S. E. Dragastin and G. H. Elder, Jr. (New York: Wiley, 1975); and D. Elkind, "Recent research on cognitive development in adolescence," in *Adolescence in the life cycle,* eds. S. E. Dragastin and G. H. Elder, Jr. (New York: Wiley, 1975); Rothenberg, "Mother-child communication"; and John F. Kantner and Melvin Zelnik, "Sexual experience of young unmarried women in the United States," *Family Planning Perspectives* 4, no. 4 (Oct. 1972): 9–18.

21. E. J. Roberts and J. Gagnon, *Family life and sexual learning,* vol. 1 (Cambridge, Mass.: Population Education, 1978).

22. Hugo B. Beigel, "The parent's share," *Journal of Sex Research* 26, no. 1 (1966): 47–50; and Walter R. Stokes, "Should mothers inform their teenage daughters on contraceptives?" *Journal of Sex Research* 2, no. 1 (1966): 59.

23. W. J. Gadpaille, *Father's role in sex education of his son* (reprint available from American Association of Sex Educators and Counselors, n.d.).

24. D. Baumrind, "Early socialization and adolescent competence," in *Adolescence in the life cycle,* eds. S. E. Dragastin and G. H. Elder, Jr. (New York: Wiley, 1975).

25. Christopher H. Hodgman, "Talks between fathers and sons," *Medical Aspects of Human Sexuality* 9 (1975): 9–29; Mary G. Garfield and Joan E. Morgenthau, "Sex talks between mothers and daughters," *Medical Aspects of Human Sexuality* 10 (Nov. 1976): 6–18.

26. Gertrude B. Couch, "Youth looks at sex," *Adolescence* 2, no. 6 (1967): 255–266.

27. Shirley L. Jessor and Richard Jessor, "Transition from virginity to nonvirginity among youth: A social-psychological study over time," *Developmental Psychology* 11, no. 4 (1975): 473–484.

28. Robert A. Lewis, "Parents and peers: Socialization agents in the coital behavior of young adults," *Journal of Sex Research* 9, no. 2 (1973): 156–170.

29. Graham B. Spanier, "Sources of sex information and premarital sexual behavior," *Journal of Sex Research* 13, no. 2 (1977): 73–88.

30. Spanier, "Formal and informal sex education," pp. 39–67.

31. Furstenberg, *Unplanned parenthood: The social consequences of teenage childbearing* (New York: Free Press, 1976).

32. Warren B. Miller, "Sexual and contraceptive behavior in young unmarried women," *Primary Care* 3, no. 3 (1976): 427–453.

33. Goldfarb et al., "'Pregnancy susceptibility,'" pp. 127–144.

34. J. Ager, F. Shea, and S. Agronow, "Comparisons of participants and dropouts from a teen contraceptive program," paper presented at the 84th Annual Convention of the American Psychological Association, Washington, D.C., Aug. 1976.

35. Virginia K. Ktsanes, *Assessment of contraception by teenagers,* final report, National Institute of Child Health and Human Development, contract no.- 1HD-52833, Bethesda, Maryland: Jan. 1977.

36. Eugene B. Brody, Frank Ottey, and Janet Lagrandade, "Early sex education in relation to later coital and reproductive behavior: Evidence from Jamaican women," *American Journal of Psychiatry* 133, no. 8 (1976): 969–972.

37. G. L. Fox, "Sex-role attitudes as predictors of contraceptive use among unmarried university students," *Sex Roles* 3, no. 3 (June 1977): 265–283.

38. For a different explanation of the role of fathers in enhancing traditional sex role development in daughters see Heilbrun, "Identification with fathers," pp. 411–416.

39. Lewis, "Parents and peers," pp. 156–169.

40. P. Barglow, M. Bornstein, D. B. Exum, M. K. Wright, and H. M. Visotsky, "Some psychiatric aspects of illegitimate pregnancy in early adolescence," *American Journal of Orthopsychiatry* 38 (1968): 672–687.

41. Virginia Abernethy, "Illegitimate conception among teenagers," *American Journal of Public Health* 64, no. 7 (1974): 662–665.

42. Uddenberg, "Mother-father," pp. 69–79.

43. Kantner and Zelnik, "Sexual experience," pp. 16–17; H. S. Gill, "The influence of parental attitudes on child's reaction to sexual stimuli," *Family Process* 9, no. 1 (1970): 41–50; Roger W. Libby, "Parental attitudes toward content in high school sex education programs: Liberalism-traditionalism and demographic correlates," *The Family Coordinator* 20, no. 2 (1971): 127–136; and Ira L. Reiss, *The social context of premarital sexual permissiveness* (New York: Free Press, 1967). Robert H. Walsh, Mary Ferrell, William Tolone, and Ollie Pocs, "Gender, sex role equalitarianism, and sexuality in student and parent samples," paper presented at the annual meetings of the National Council on Family Relations, New York City, Oct. 1976.

44. Shirley L. Jessor and Richard Jessor, "Maternal ideology and adolescent problem behavior," *Developmental Psychology* 10, no. 2 (1974): 246–254.

45. Furstenberg, *Unplanned parenthood*.

46. Harvey R. Freeman, "The generation gap: Attitudes of students and of their parents," *Journal of Counseling Psychology* 19, no. 5 (1972): 441–447; and Joseph LoPiccolo, "Mothers and daughters: Perceived and real differences in sexual values," *Journal of Sex Research* 9, no. 2 (1973): 171–177.

47. Julian Roebuck and Marsha G. McGee, "Attitudes toward premarital sex and sexual behavior among black high school girls," *Journal of Sex Research* 13, no. 2 (1977): 104–114.

48. Barglow et al., "Some psychiatric aspects," pp. 672–687.

49. John F. Kantner and Melvin Zelnik, "Contraception and pregnancy: Experience of young unmarried women in the United States," *Family Planning Perspectives* 5, no. 1 (Winter 1973): 11–25.

50. Goldfarb et al., "'Pregnancy susceptibility,'" pp. 127–144.

51. Akpom et al., "Prior sexual behavior," pp. 203–206.

52. Kantner and Zelnik, "Sexual experience," pp. 9–18.

53. Kantner and Zelnik, "Contraception," pp. 11–25; see also their report in

Farida Shah, M. Zelnik, and J. Kantner, "Unprotected intercourse among unwed teenagers," *Family Planning Perspectives* 7, no. 1 (Jan./Feb. 1975): 39–44.

54. Furstenberg, *Unplanned parenthood*.

55. B. Sutton-Smith and B. G. Rosenberg, *The sibling* (New York: Holt, Rinehart and Winston, 1970).

56. Jessor and Jessor, "Maternal ideology," p. 250.

57. G. L. Fox, "Nice girl: Social control of women through a value construct," *Signs: Journal of Woman in Culture and Society* 2, no. 4 (Summer 1977): 805–817.

58. Jessie Bernard, *Women, wives, and mothers* (Chicago: Aldine, 1975).

59. Reiss and Miller, *A theoretical analysis*.

60. Furstenberg, *Unplanned parenthood*.

61. R. A. H. Rosen, "Pregnancy resolution decision-making among minors," paper presented at the annual meetings of the American Psychological Association, San Francisco, Aug. 1977.

62. Eleanor Wright Smith, "The role of the grandmother in adolescent pregnancy and parenting," *Journal of School Health* 45, no. 5 (1975): 278–283.

63. Alma T. Young, Barbara Berkman, and Helen Rehr, "Parental influence on pregnant adolescents," *Social Work* 20, no. 5 (1975): 387–391.

64. See Young et al., "Parental influence," pp. 387–391; William L. Graves and Barbara R. Bradshaw, "Early reconception and contraceptive use among black teenage girls after an illegitimate birth," *American Journal of Public Health* 65, no. 7 (1975): 738–740; and Georgiana M. Selstad, Jerome R. Evans, and Wayne H. Welcher, "Predicting contraceptive use in postabortion patients," *American Journal of Public Health* 65, no. 7 (1975): 708–713.

65. G. Sheehy, *Passages: Predictable crises of adult life* (New York: Dalton, 1974).

66. For a clinician's description of this pattern see Helen R. Beiser, "Sexual factors in antagonism between mothers and adolescent daughters," *Medical Aspects of Human Sexuality* 11 (1977): 32–42.

67. John C. Coleman, "Current contradictions in adolescent theory," *Journal of Youth and Adolescence* 7, no. 1 (1978): 1–11.

68. Ira L. Reiss, *Premarital sexual standards in America* (New York: Free Press, 1960), and Ira L. Reiss, *The social context of premarital sexual permissiveness* (New York: Free Press, 1967).

69. Kenneth L. Cannon and Richard Long, "Premarital sexual behavior in the sixties," *Journal of Marriage and the Family* 33, no. 1 (1971): 36–49.

70. Shipman, "Psychodynamics," pp. 3–12.

71. J. R. Udry, "Sex and family life," *Medical Aspects of Human Sexuality* 4 (1968): 100.

72. Beiser, "Sexual factors," p. 32.

73. J. H. Gagnon and W. Simon, *Sexual conduct: The social sources of human sexuality* (Chicago: Aldine, 1973), pp. 32, 42.

74. Urie Bronfenbrenner, *Two worlds of childhood* (New York: Russell Sage Foundation, 1970), and Kenneth Keniston and the Carnegie Council on Chil-

dren, *All our children: The American family under pressure* (New York and London: Harcourt, Brace, Jovanovich, 1977).

75. Joseph H. Pleck, "Work roles and family roles," paper presented at the annual meetings of the American Sociological Association, San Francisco, Aug. 1975.

76. Bronfenbrenner, *Two worlds*, pp. 116–119.

77. Urban and Rural Systems Associates (URSA), *Improving family planning services for teenagers*, final report, Contract HEW-OS-74-304 (Washington, D.C.: HEW, June 1976).

78. Aida Torres, "Does your mother know . . . ?" *Family Planning Perspectives* 10, no. 5 (Sept./Oct. 1978): 280–282.

79. Joel W. Ager and F. Shea, "Consequences of teen contraceptive program dropout," paper presented at the Workshop on Adolescent Pregnancy and Childbearing, Center for Population Research of the National Institute of Child Health and Human Development, Bethesda, Md., 1979; Alan Guttmacher Institute, "AGI parental notification study: Research protocol," unpublished paper, New York: Alan Guttmacher Institute, 1979; Betty Cogswell, "Adolescents' perspective on the health care systems: A determinant of fertility," paper presented at the Workshop on Adolescent Pregnancy and Childbearing, Center for Population Research of the National Institute of Child Health and Human Development, Bethesda, Md., 1979.

4

Implicating the Family: Teenage Parenthood and Kinship Involvement

Frank F. Furstenberg, Jr.

Introduction

During the past five years, a conjunction of moral, economic, and political forces has lifted teenage pregnancy from the relative obscurity of a private concern, and placed it in the arena of pressing public issues.[1] The erroneous assumption that teenage childbearing is new or unprecedented has led to a host of dubious theories about its causes, accompanied by some hastily assembled programs that promise more than they can deliver.[2]

No less disturbing than the absence of a historical perspective on the problem is the tendency to ignore the social context of early childbearing. All too little attention has been given to the complex, if implicit set of rules governing peer group activity in general, and teenage heterosexual relationships, in particular.[3] Finally, although many researchers acknowledge a professional interest in the sociology and social psychology of families, almost no studies have examined either the link between early childbearing and family organization, or the ramifications of teenage parenthood for family functioning.[4]

The question of why the family's involvement has been neglected cannot be addressed in detail here. I contend that the American ethos of individualism pervades our notions of how social problems come about, as well as how we go about dealing with them.[5] Researchers are trained to study individuals, not families; policies and programs are designed to serve individuals, not families. In the case of early childbearing, we prefer to act as though the adolescent mother is solely responsible, and accordingly, the services we design single her out for attention. I shall try to show in this paper that the practice of treating collective behavior exclusively at the individual level misshapes our policies and our programs; and in the conclusion, I will advocate an alternative approach to intervention.

Researchers are compelled to employ different strategies when their sight expands from the individual to the family. When we must take into account the perspectives of several actors at once, our understanding becomes far greater, if far more difficult to achieve. As I shall try to show, pregnancy is not greeted similarly by all family members at any one point; and its meanings for various parties change over time, as well. Consequently, the task of the analyst is complicated when the unit under study is the family, rather than a single individual. Early childbearing simultaneously produces burdens and benefits within the group. Pregnancy in adolescence has multiple meanings for different family members, especially at different stages of family development. Without this dialectical perspective, the onlooker is likely either to become confused or to be forced to ignore a certain portion of reality.

Sources of Data

My early research on teenage childbearing developed from a longitudinal study of adolescents that was conducted in Baltimore from 1966 to 1972. (A brief description of this study is presented later in this paper, and a detailed account of the methods can be found in my book, *Unplanned parenthood*.) I discovered that although an early pregnancy created distinct disadvantages for most adolescents, some adapted rather successfully to the challenge posed by premature parenthood. My data analysis revealed that the success of these young parents was linked, at least in part, to support provided by their families. Following the completion of my book on the consequences of teenage childbearing, I received additional funding to reexamine the Baltimore data explicitly for the purpose of identifying the family's involvement in what I had previously referred to as the "process of unplanned parenthood." In this reanalysis, I also investigated the conditions that govern the flow of support to the adolescent during the transition to parenthood, and examined the impact of family resources on the teenager's adaptation to motherhood. The final objective of this research was to detail how the pregnancy altered family functioning, and what implications it had for members of the family other than the teenage parent and her child.

The data I collected in Baltimore on the family's involvement were meager at best. In order to address the issue the Family Impact Seminar was interested in—the impact of teenage childbearing on the family—additional sources of information were needed. In 1978, collaborating with a team of clinicians at the Philadelphia Child Guidance Clinic, I assembled case studies of a small number of families with an adolescent member who had recently become pregnant or delivered a child. The families were not part of the clinic's client population, but were paid subjects in a pilot study exploring changes in family functioning following adolescent pregnancy and childbirth.[6]

The design of the pilot study called for interviews with twenty such families at the clinic. Our invitation was extended to the adolescent and to any family member living in the household, as well as to the father of the child. In the beginning, we insisted on seeing at least a core subsystem of the family: the adolescent, her parent(s), and sibling(s) closest to her in age. Eventually, this requirement was dropped due to the difficulty of recruiting all of these family members; and we settled for interviews with the young mother and at least one other family member. With the participants' knowledge and permission, the interviews were videotaped for later analysis.

The clinicians were given considerable license to proceed as they saw fit. However, we devised a protocol of content areas to guide their discussion, and as a means of gaining further information on family functioning, contrived one or two tasks for the family to perform. Initially, the therapists consciously tried to assemble information on each of the content areas outlined in the protocol. As they went on, some clinicians became bolder in pursuing their own course, with the result that the interviews were less comprehensive, but much richer in detail. To supplement the clinical sessions, a research assistant made a visit to each home. Although we originally intended to conduct a more structured, sociologically oriented interview, we eventually abandoned this strategy, seeking instead to follow leads provided in the clinical session. By questioning family members directly, we were often able to get them to elaborate on points made at the clinic, or to verify our impressions and interpretations.

It is easier in theory than in practice to study entire families. Even though the families were paid fifty dollars for their participation in the study, it was exceedingly difficult, during two months of field work, to fill our quota of ten black, five white, and five Hispanic families, with ten in prenatal situations and ten in post-partum situations. We avoided drawing our sample from the clinic's client population, fearing that our results would be biased if families were selected exclusively from this single source. Thus, in hopes of recruiting participants, we contacted a number of local agencies that provide services to adolescent parents. In the end, we felt extremely lucky (and overworked) to have interviewed fifteen families (nine black, three white, and three Hispanic) by the end of the two-month field work period.

The small number of cases precludes any formal content analysis; the main value of the materials we assembled is to provide an agenda of research questions about the impact of early childbearing on the family of origin, to explore in future studies. In this paper, I use the clinical data to illustrate more concretely some leads suggested by the reanalysis of the Baltimore study data.

The first section below summarizes the results of the secondary analysis of the Baltimore data. It provides a macroscopic overview by presenting demographic information on the residential careers of adolescent mothers following the birth of their first child. I shall show how the family of origin is inextricably involved in supporting the young mother and her child in the period immediately after the birth; and shall discuss implications of their participation for the mother, for the child, and to some extent, for the family members who provide assistance themselves. I then turn to the clinical data for a more microscopic view of the process of family support, identifying certain themes which surfaced in my examination of the case studies.

Changes in Household Structure: The Baltimore Study

The study in Baltimore evolved from an evaluation of one of the nation's first comprehensive care programs for adolescent parents. In the course of assessing the impact of this program, it became apparent that the results of the prenatal clinic and family planning service could not be understood without a broader consideration of the life course of the adolescent parent. To undertake such an investigation, it was necessary to look, as well, at the experiences of teenagers from similar backgrounds who had managed to avoid an early birth. Thus, in addition to conducting four periodic interviews with teenage parents, I also carried out two interviews in the later stages of the study, with a sample of classmates who did not become pregnant in their early teens.

Some 400 adolescents who registered for prenatal services at Sinai Hospital in Baltimore were first interviewed during pregnancy (in 1966–1967), and then again, one, three, and five years after delivery. This paper will largely be confined to data collected from the 320 women who were faithful participants in all four stages of interviewing. At the time of the initial contact, we also conducted home interviews with one of the expectant mother's parents, usually her mother; some of the information to which I will refer was obtained from those interviews.

The Baltimore sample was not selected to guarantee representativeness. It consisted predominantly of low-income blacks who became pregnant for the first time before their eighteenth birthday. Most came from the community surrounding the hospital where the prenatal program was based; although in the later stages of the study, a number of participants were referred to the program by schools and health clinics in other parts of the city. Comparable data drawn from health and vital statistics on the population of the City of Baltimore suggests that the participants in the study were reasonably representative of the general population of early childbearers in Baltimore. Subsequent research based both on more carefully selected local samples and national samples indicates that the results drawn from the Baltimore sample appear to be generalizable in most respects, particularly to families from the same socioeconomic group.[7] (Unfortunately, there are virtually no research studies on adolescent parenting experienced by families who have higher incomes or live in rural areas.)

Until the final interview, very little information was obtained about the family's involvement in childcare or its economic contributions to the young mother. However, the interviews do contain a record of the composition of the adolescent mother's household at each point in the study. When inspected longitudinally, the data on residential situations provide a useful way of mapping this feature of family support.

From the limited information available, it appears that mothers were much more likely to receive substantial amounts of familial and financial assistance when they remained with their relatives.[8] Moving out of the parental household, whether to marry or to establish an independent residence, not only reduced the subsidies provided by the family in the form of room and board, but also lessened the chances that a relative would be available to provide day care.

One popular stereotype of the adolescent mother portrays her as a social isolate, removed from parental or conjugal support; our data belie this image. Most mothers in our study stayed close to home, especially during the early years of the study. During their first pregnancy, when most of the women were in their early or middle teens, nearly 90 percent lived with a parent or a close relative. One year after delivery most young mothers (77 percent) were still living with parents or close relatives. Separation from the family of origin became more common in the ensuing years, but even five years after the birth of their child, nearly half (46 percent) remained with their parents or other kin. Only 26 percent of the young mothers were married.

By following a young mother's household situation through the different points in the study, we can introduce animation to the snapshots provided above. The pattern of residential careers reinforces the impression gained from the cross-sectional data, which is that the family of origin is the most significant refuge for the adolescent childbearer. The most common residential career, occurring more frequently than marriage or heading a single-parent household, was unbroken residence with the family of origin: 29 percent of the young mothers remained with their parents throughout the study. By contrast, 24 percent moved out at the inception of pregnancy in order to marry and remained married; and 15 percent left to establish an independent household, and remained in that situation. It is of some interest that the fourth most common residential sequence, followed by nearly 11 percent of the young mothers, was to return home after the dissolution of a marriage. Thus, one reason why so many young mothers are residing with their parents at the five-year follow-up is that a significant number of women come back to their families, refugees from broken marriages.

The Determinants of Family Support

A major objective of the reanalysis of the Baltimore data was to discover why some families provided support for adolescent mothers while others did not. Two general classes of conditions that shape a young mother's residential career were identified in the analysis. The first is related to the young mother's need for assistance, and is termed, accordingly, the "demand" factor. The second, relating to the family's capacity to respond, was labelled the "supply" factor. In the discussion that follows, I shall make reference to each set of conditions in turn.

One might anticipate that an adolescent's family would shoulder much more responsibility when she remained single than when she married. Detailed inspection of the data certainly bears out this expectation. Especially in the early years of the study, the women moved away from their families only when they married. Even then, they frequently remained in the household for a time after marriage. One year after delivery, 43 percent of the currently married mothers were living with kin; at the second follow-up, 31 percent of the married couples were living in households with other relatives. From comments in response to unstructured questions, I learned that a major deterrent to marriage was the possibility that it might require forfeiting family support. The decision to remain in the home after marriage may, of course, be dictated by economic considerations, but I suspect that it also reflects ambivalence about substituting a tenuous conjugal bond for a functioning family network. As will be shown later, these two types of support systems are more often competitive than complementary.[9]

Surprisingly, age was not an important determinant of residential careers. Apart from its connection to marital prospects, age was not strongly related to the young mother's continuing residence with her parents. By contrast, educational status clearly predicted residential arrangements. Young mothers who continued their education after becoming pregnant were significantly more likely to rely on their parents than those who dropped out of school. Furthermore, parents often had an explicit understanding with their offspring that they would supply childcare so long as the young mothers were attending school.

The quality of the relationship between the adolescent mother and her parents during pregnancy also foreshadowed subsequent residential choices. In households where the bond between parents and daughters was close, marriage was less likely to occur; and in the event that the young mothers remained single, they usually stayed with their parents. A series of items in the initial interviews, tapping the degree to which the adolescents openly relied on their parents for advice and assistance, was combined into a single index. This index predicted rather well a young mother's likelihood of remaining at home during the course of the study. Women who expressed a low level of dependency were almost twice as likely as those who were more dependent to move out after delivery, either to marry or to establish a household of their own.

By the time the interview with the family took place, usually in the second trimester of the pregnancy, most prospective grandmothers had already signaled their intention to help out after the child was born. The few who stated that they hoped the baby would be given up for adoption were, in fact, less likely to provide room and board or childcare assistance following the birth. Thus, the parents' willingness to supply assistance may explain at least a small part of their daughters' residential choices.

Given the inclination of all but a few parents to lend assistance, the capacity of their families to provide aid became a major factor in shaping the young mothers' residential careers. Contrary to what I had thought might be the case, adolescents were much more likely to remain in couple-headed households than in female-headed households. This pattern can be traced to several factors. First, young mothers in couple-headed households were more likely to return to and remain in school. The greater economic resources of the couple-headed families either were used to purchase childcare services or enabled the grandmother to remain at home while the young mother resumed her education.

Second, under certain conditions, the provision of public assistance facilitated movement to independent household headship, particularly when increased benefits were provided to women who established a separate household. Couple-headed households were far less likely to receive welfare payments, providing a lower incentive for the young mother to move out.

Finally, since space was more abundant in two-parent households, there was less pressure to leave the parental home. Although the data collected were not fine-grained enough to permit examination of crowding as a cause of separation from parents, it is clear that young mothers were more likely to move out when a second pregnancy occurred. Repeat pregnancy occurred more frequently in female-headed families, which were already pressed for space and strained for resources.

Consequences of Family Support

Up to this point, I have touched on some of the circumstances that led to the departure of adolescent mothers from the parental household. However, most adolescents and their offspring stayed in the household for at least several years after the birth of a child. By this time most had completed or dropped out of school, had married the father of the child or had abandoned plans to do so, and were employed or had gained stable support from public assistance. Their children were in school, or at least old enough to be cared for outside the home. In short, the family had tided the young mother over during the difficult period of transition to parenthood.

As we have seen, some young mothers benefitted from greater amounts of family assistance than others. Does the provision of such support, particularly when it is abundant and long-lasting, improve the life chances of the young mother and her child? The weaknesses of our data preclude a definitive answer, but there are strong hints that young mothers who received significant amounts of aid were more likely to be in an economically favorable position at the conclusion of the study than those who did not. Adolescents who remained with their parents were more likely to advance educationally and economically than their peers who left home before or immediately after their child was born. Most participants in the Baltimore study stayed home because they were being provided with childcare assistance by a parent, sibling, or other relative. Losing that advantage often forced them to terminate their education, or, if they were working, to quit their jobs.

Most mothers were willing to accept childcare from a day care center but lacked either the money or the know-how to make such an arrangement for their offspring; a minority were unwilling to rely on people outside their family for child care. When asked to designate the most suitable custodian, the great majority indicated a preference for a relative, inside or outside the home. The early interviews did not show precisely how childcare responsibilities were being divided among family members when the adolescents remained at home. However, the last two interviews revealed that the young mothers who lived at home received more help from family members than those who were not residing with relatives. At the five-year follow-up, for example, 35 percent of the adolescents stated that a parent or close relative either took most of the responsibility for childcare or shared it equally with them, while 20 percent of those who lived alone received regular childcare from a parent or close relative.

How did collaborative childcare arrangements affect the well-being of the mother and her offspring? Based on the mothers' self-reports and on observations by interviewers in the home, we found no sizable differences between the full-time mothers and the women who collaborated with a relative. For example, the mothers who received substantial help in raising their children were only slightly more likely to express positive views about their offspring, and were a little less likely to report the presence of behavior problems (e.g., bedwetting, talking back, or throwing temper tantrums).

The information obtained from the children themselves provided a somewhat stronger indication of the benefits of collaborative care. On a test of cognitive performance, the Pre-School Inventory, children of unmarried mothers achieved higher scores when their parents were not their full-time caretakers. As we have already shown, the provision of childcare assistance was more likely to occur when the young mother remained with her parents. Thus, unless there was continuity of collaborative childcare, moving out may have resulted in some cognitive decrement for the child.

Perhaps the quality of care was higher when the mother received supervision from an experienced relative or when she was simply relieved of full-time responsibility. Possibly, children received more stimulation when they had multiple caretakers. Or, conceivably, the mothers who remained in the home (or their families generally) were more upwardly mobile. Finally, moving out of the home may have deprived the child of a familiar caretaker, creating certain emotional and developmental difficulties.

Even though we do not have the means at hand to explore these differing interpretations, we can say with some confidence that, on the basis of our data, family assistance confers certain benefits to both mother and child in the initial years. How long-lasting they are cannot be ascertained from the Baltimore data.

The findings presented up to now provide a bird's eye view of the impact of early childbearing on the family. We have learned, from data on the women's residential arrangements and from selected interview items, that most families become heavily involved when a pregnancy occurs, because they are called upon both to render aid to the adolescent mother and to assume child-rearing responsibilities. In short, most adolescent mothers do not stop being their parents' children, in the sense of requiring and receiving care and support when they, themselves, become parents. As a corollary, most of the parents are not relieved of child-rearing duties when their daughters become parents.

The data collected at the Child Guidance Clinic of Philadelphia afford a more intimate view of how the family responds when a pregnancy occurs to a teenage member. Earlier, I described the data collection procedures used to assemble the case studies. I must reiterate that what follows is not a formal analysis of the interview material. Instead, I have attempted to identify common responses to critical events or tasks that arise when a pregnancy occurs, and to illustrate these prototypical responses with portions drawn from the interviews.

The areas still to be covered can be classified into four categories: the part the family plays in the process by which the adolescent becomes pregnant, the family's role in the disposition of the pregnancy, the participation of the family in caring for and supporting the mother and child, and the implications of providing assistance for the well-being of various family members.

Becoming Pregnant

A characteristic of the families in my Baltimore study was an inability to communicate directly about sexual matters. Their elliptical communication was a response to the difficulties parents experienced in providing direct sexual socialization. Mother and daughter made an implicit pact not to discuss sex, and their oblique communication heightened the chances of pregnancy when the adolescent began to have intercourse. Moreover, the likelihood of the adolescent's using contraception was strongly related to the degree to which her sexual activity was openly acknowledged and accepted by her parents. Greer Litton Fox in Chapter 3, reviewing the meager survey data on sexual socialization, strongly indicates that patterns of sexual communication within the family are related both to the age at onset of sexual activity, and to the practice of birth control among sexually active teenagers.

To understand the nature and influence of communication between family members, we must study their interactions and communications directly through clinical interviews. The Child Guidance Clinic interviews have convinced me that intensive studies of ongoing interaction within families are needed to augment what can be learned from surveys. The major limitation of surveys is their insensitivity to the process and style of communication, and their inability to pick up subtle ambiguities in family communication patterns. Let me take an illustration from an interview with a sixteen-year-old pregnant adolescent and her mother, herself a single parent. Mother and daughter are explaining to the interviewer how the pregnancy occurred:

> Daughter: Well, I had started having sex in December, and when I started, well, the week after, I came to my mother and I was going to ask her to have me put on birth control. But then she said, well, let's wait and see if a period comes up. December had passed, it was around the 27th or something, and we had made an appointment because she wanted the doctor to give me a checkup. It was too late to get on birth control.
> Mother: (a minute later in the interview, recalling her discussion with her daughter around the time the daughter started to have sexual relations) I was trying to get my heart up to talk to her.
> *How did that go?*
> Mother: Well, when I confronted her about her sex life, I knew she liked the guy, and I told her to demand respect from her boyfriend. He should respect her and her morals, and if they choose to get involved, to think about the repercussions because your mother is living proof. She has no husband. . . . I gave her that to look at and I chose birth control. She is against birth con-

trol, she reads so much in the books. You know, what it does to health and cancer. (Interviewer asks if she considered other forms of birth control like the coil.) She did not want to consider that. And, I myself do not know of any other. I told her he could go in and talk to the drugstore man, and get something for himself. And I heard no more until she thought she was pregnant.

Although this is a family in which the mother and daughter are at some pains to communicate with one another, their mode and manner of conversation can be seen as effectively blocking the flow of information. In some respects mother and daughter appear to be talking past each other; from another point of view they seem to be collaborating. Either perspective suggests that the two were negotiating a way of dealing with the daughter's sexual status that would accommodate both of their respective (and not necessarily compatible) beliefs about the desirability of sexual relations and the advisability of using various methods of birth control.

Our clinical interviews provided many examples of the ambiguity, tentativeness, and obliqueness of parental communication towards their adolescents' sexual behavior. In many of the family situations there was considerably less discussion than in the family quoted here. In only one or two was there really open communication between mother and daughter. Our clinical data thus confirmed the impressions from surveys that adolescents are receiving confused messages on sexual matters.

Further research is needed to explore the individual meanings attached to sexual topics by various family members (not just mothers and daughters), the ways that families arrive at shared meanings, and the strategies they employ to avoid reaching a common understanding. Both the content and techniques of sexual socialization, as Fox observes, are incompletely understood.

But even our limited information points to some important

implications for sex education and family planning programs. Family planning programs have generally operated on the assumption that it is important to reach the sexually active adolescent; but they rarely attempt to make contact with the parents, at the risk of violating the adolescent's confidentiality and privacy. Yet, what we are now learning about the influence of family members on their adolescents' sexual behavior would strongly suggest that programs that attempt to educate or treat the young adolescent at the exclusion of the family run the risk of being neutralized, if not sabotaged, by the adolescent's family. The lesson for practitioners is that programs of sex education and birth control must take into account the entire family and not just the individual child or adolescent.

A more active policy of extending services to families of sexually active teenagers need not require mandatory notification of the parents, a practice that is probably counterproductive and ineffective. Indeed, it is not always necessary to involve families directly in order to penetrate the veil of secrecy that exists in many families at the time teenagers become sexually active. Programs can increase the level of communication within the family without insisting that parents be provided with specific accounts of their adolescent's level of sexual experience.

In collaboration with Roberta Herceg-Baron, I have designed a program that will reach out to the families of adolescents seeking contraceptive assistance in an effort to build kinship support for the teenager's use of birth control. In Chapter 11, we describe the development of this experiment, which is in its early stages, and share our initial observations.

The Disposition of the Pregnancy

With few exceptions, most notably studies by Rains and by Luker, there is little research on the family's involvement in the disposition of the pregnancy.[10] A detailed phenomenological account of what happens when an adolescent discovers she is pregnant would greatly advance our understanding of the meaning of the pregnancy to the teenager, and how her definition of the situation influences her strategy for dealing with it. At what point does she tell her family, and how does their response to the news affect her course of action?

In many of the families we interviewed, the initial reaction to the pregnancy was one of shock and dismay. But when asked whether they had considered an alternative to having the child, most of the early childbearers replied that they had rejected abortion for moral reasons. ("A baby shouldn't have to pay for his mother's mistake." "It's wrong to kill.") Of course, our sample was confined to those who had decided to have the child. Despite the deep reservations many had about abortion, some interesting exceptions appeared. One family had arranged for an abortion, only to back out at the last minute, when the mother made it clear to her pregnant daughter that if she wanted the child, a way would be found to support it. A couple of other parents acknowledged that they might have urged their daughters to obtain an abortion, had they learned about the pregnancy sooner. It was not uncommon, within our small sample, for the parents to find out late in the second or even in the third trimester. Sometimes, the parents had considerable influence on the outcome; in other cases, the decision was presented to the family as a *fait accompli*, usually because the adolescent, after consulting with the father of the child and/or a physician, had decided to proceed with the pregnancy. The clinical data illustrate just how critical it is to examine the interplay between the adolescent and her family at the time of conception:

> *Tell me a little bit about what it was like when Sandra got pregnant, for the family?*
> Mother: Well, to me, it was—I could not accept it. I blamed it on myself because she wanted to be a mommy. I had to let her do as she wanted to do. . . .
> [Interviewer then asks at what point the mother talked

to her daughter after noticing that she was probably pregnant.] I had tried to, but she hadn't talked to me. Then she came out and told.

What happened then?

Mother: Nothing really, I asked her what her plans were, if she was going to get married or what. And she said, no. She was not going to get married, she was going to have this baby and that was it . . .

When you discussed it with Sandra, did she propose that there were other options, or did you propose to her that there might be other options?

Mother: I was told by a psychiatrist to leave things alone, leave her to solve the problem herself. If she wanted to have the baby, keep it. So, I should go along with it. I should not make any decisions for her.

Many of the parents in our study portrayed themselves as bystanders. Some bitterly observed that although they had little to say in the decision of whether the pregnancy would be brought to term, they were forced to assume a full measure of responsibility for the child after birth. Many families, if given the opportunity, would no doubt have endorsed the adolescent's decision to have the child, but they were generally not considered to be interested parties in the decision. It is an intriguing and highly debatable question about who should have a say in the disposition of the pregnancy. What is clear is that the family is often only consulted after the decision is made, if at all, even though they frequently support and care for the baby.

It is not at all clear how one would develop guidelines that would help practitioners or policymakers accord proper weight to the family's interest in the decision of what to do when an adolescent in the household becomes pregnant. However, a first step would be to learn more about the roles that families presently play in their decisions, since our present knowledge on this topic is minimal.

TEENAGE PARENTHOOD

Caring for the Child: Relations between the Baby's Father and the Family

A focal concern evident in many of the families we interviewed was whether or not to permit the father of the child access to his offspring. This decision, usually made by the mother's parents, involves a delicate balance of interests. Although we issued invitations to include the fathers in the "family interviews," in no instance did he come to the interview. Thus, it must be noted that our information about the fathers was filtered through the mothers and their families.

Unlike the conventional process of family formation, the families we studied had to decide whether or not to incorporate the child's father as a family member. Apparently, as the father became aware of his tenuous position, he often entered a bid to help support the child. If his offer was accepted by the adolescent and her family, he was accorded certain rights to call upon the mother in the home, to help in the selection of the name, and to visit the child after delivery. Accordingly, his family was extended the privileges of kinship, symbolized by an invitation to the baby shower or by the prerogative of caring for the child.

Frequently, adolescents who remained in their family's household found themselves in the difficult position of balancing the claims of the father, who often wanted to be included, against the demands of her parents, who frequently wanted to restrict the father's access to the child. In the case quoted below, a prospective grandmother is discussing the possibility of involving the father's family in the plans for the child. The father had expressed a strong desire to help support the child, but the pregnant adolescent's mother clearly had some misgivings about counting on his support or on the assistance of his family:

> *What are the plans for the father, financially, you know, as far as the baby's father helping out or anything?*
> Grandmother: All I know, I can say right now, is the

baby will be most likely our responsibility and nobody else's. I don't know if he will contribute to the child's welfare. Now, I have not spoken with them, the baby is due next month and they haven't come forward to state anything. So therefore, I don't imagine they will. We will do our best for the baby. I don't want to sound a little selfish, but unless somebody comes forward and claims the baby or what have you . . .

If they come, will you let them take over?

Grandmother: Since Robin is pregnant, no one has asked her if she needs coffee, or, "When are you going to the hospital?" They haven't asked anything about the baby's future. But if they feel like they want to come here and take over. . . . My daughter is the one who is pregnant, and they will not take over. I won't allow it.

Marriage provides a formula for establishing family boundaries. When it does not occur, the interested parties must arrive at an informal settlement, establishing rights and obligations to the child. The material from our interviews suggests that an agreement is not easily achieved in some families. Parents set limits, sometimes unrealistic ones, on how often the father may visit the child in "their" home. The adolescent mother is sometimes forced to choose between intermittent support from a father who would like to support his child but is in no position to do so, and the steady support of her family. If they opt for the latter, they must accept the parents' conditions, which may include disengaging themselves from the father.

I should point out that not all families discouraged continued contact with the father. Among the participants in our pilot study, there was a great deal of variation in the permeability of the family boundaries. Clearly, the relationship between patterns of kinship support and paternal involvement deserves further investigation. On the basis of this preliminary research, I would suggest that we are not likely to achieve an adequate un-

TEENAGE PARENTHOOD

derstanding of the seemingly unpredictable patterns of paternal participation without examining the extended family's role as a regulatory agency.

Family Participation in Childcare

If difficulties exist in setting external boundaries on claims to the child, the difficulties of working out a division of labor within the family may be even greater. Most families we interviewed seem to have successfully worked out a way of distributing responsibilities for childcare among the family members. In some instances, assignments were made as a result of explicit discussions: "I told her [the adolescent mother] that I was not going to get up in the middle of the night; it was her responsibility." In another household the negotiation process was implicit: "No, she didn't say anything. I knew she [the grandmother] would take care of Tania if I went back to school." A sign of successful collaboration was the existence of a hierarchy of responsibility, with an executor overseeing the arrangements. The executor was not invariably the individual who occupied the role of principal caretaker, nor did particular family members always assume either of these roles. We simply do not have a sufficient number of cases to examine how these determinations are made or to assess what these arrangements tell us about general family dynamics or how they affect the prospects for childhood socialization.

Although our data suggests a cautious approach to these questions, I cannot resist some preliminary observations. There was great variation in the divisions of labor devised even in the fifteen families we observed. Some took the form of a pyramid, with the mother or grandmother, or occasionally the grandfather, occupying the position at the top; others might resemble a series of concentric circles in which family members were ringed around the child.

There were also differences in the number and type of caretakers. Some families were highly specialized in the assignment of child-rearing tasks, giving almost complete responsibility to one member, usually the mother or grandmother. In other instances, responsibilities were widely distributed among a large number of relatives, both inside and outside the home. Within this latter group, a further distinction can be made. Some households had synchronized childcare duties to a remarkable degree, while others were unable to achieve any semblance of coordination. Harmonious arrangements did not necessarily imply a neat division of labor. Certain families devised arrangements in which there was a considerable amount of overlap and redundancy, possibly as a means of ensuring that the infant received more than minimal care.

Not only do collaborative childcare arrangements protect the infant; they also protect the young mother from having to assume the full brunt of parental responsibilities. Although most of the young mothers in our sample had clearly had some prior experience caring for young children—siblings, nieces, nephews, neighbors—in general it was clear that parents or other family members provided considerable direct supervision and tutelage to the new parent. Indeed, it seems the family frequently served as a system of apprenticeship for early childbearers. Apprenticeship can be either educative or exploitative, depending on whether there is opportunity for promotion. Even with meager evidence we were able to discern differences in the degree to which families promoted growth in maternal role performance. Most families just supervised, but a few took over, assuming most parental prerogatives, treating the adolescent parent as if she were the baby's sibling.

In one family, for example, when the interviewer asked who cared for the child, all five members of the family sitting in the room raised their hands. In unison each began to insist that she or he did the largest share. It was probably not coincidental that during the interview the baby was passed from one member to the next during the first hour and ended up on the floor during much of the second hour. From these observations it would seem likely that this family had been unable to work out a hierarchy of responsibility.

When the structure of authority is unclear, or at the other extreme, excessively rigid, the young mother's relationship to her child may become precarious. Consider the following example of a mother, joined by her parent and one of her sisters in the interview. The new mother is describing her childcare experiences in the month or so after delivery:

> *So do you feel you're getting the chance to be the mother that you want to be, right now?*
> Mother: They are—everybody. Her [pointing to her sister sitting in the room], my other sister [Janine], my mother, everybody . . .
> Sister: Yeah, Janine [the oldest sister not in the room], she spoils the kids.
> Mother: Janine don't have any kids.
> Sister: And she just love them all.
> *So how do you feel about all that, that you're not getting a chance?*
> Mother: Well, I'm going to let them do it while they's doing it 'cause [laughs] ain't nobody that's going to want to do it. And, I know I'm going to have to do it. So let them do it while they doing it. Later on they ain't going to want to, so.
> *How do you know?*
> Mother: 'Cause I know them [laughs]. Janine might still want to do it. [Looking at sister in room.] I don't know about you. She might.
> Sister: I like little babies. When they get big like mine, little monsters . . .
> Grandmother: And I get tired of them all.
> Mother: I ain't even counting on her [laughs].

On the basis of this small fragment, it is difficult to say whether the strategy adopted by this young mother is realistic or not.

Rather than entering a supervised apprenticeship that might ease the transition to parenthood, she appears to be in a less advantageous position. Her mother and sisters seem to be willing to care for the child as long as he is sweet and adorable, but when the child becomes more demanding, he will probably be turned back to the mother for care. How this developmental program will affect the relationship between mother and child, we can only speculate.

These conflicts over divisions of labor and authority may indeed reflect deeper structural properties of the family system. The ways in which responsibilities for childcare are allocated will often be an indication of the family's preexisting capacity to respond to a new and unexpected task. When a new member must be incorporated, rigidities become manifest, and untapped flexibilities are revealed. Our preliminary data, once again, point to the need for a more systematic study of how organizational features of the family and household promote or impede the adaptation to early parenthood.

The Consequences of Family Involvement: Some Short-term Benefits

In examining the ways that families were drawn into the child-rearing process, we began to look at what this meant for the particular members involved and the functioning of the family. I alluded to the finding that young mothers generally benefited from residing with their parents during the early years of parenthood. Whether this is because of the support rendered by the family, or because of the special difficulties encountered by the young woman who sets up an independent household is a question which requires further empirical attention.

We also need to learn more about how children fare in differing family circumstances. In general, the dangers of detachment—inadequate ties to the extended family—appear to me to be much greater than the dangers of enmeshment—envelopment by the extended family.[11] One suspects, however, that the costs of over- and under-involvement might vary for both mother and child, at different developmental stages.

But, putting aside the well-being of the parents and children for the moment, what do we know about how early childbearing affects other members of the family? With some confidence, I can report that virtually nothing is known. In the survey analysis reported earlier, we attempted to discover how early childbearing affects the socioeconomic position of the family. While our findings indicated little overall impact, I am not confident enough of the quality of the data to put much faith in this conclusion. A similar analysis was attempted to see if early childbearing had any effect on the fertility of the young mother's siblings. Our results showed little effect, but again, I do not feel secure about these findings.[12]

Turning to the clinical data, I was particularly impressed with the range of sequelae that family members report following a pregnancy, varying from improving the quality of parent-child relations to restoring a flagging marriage. In the discussion that follows, I will stress again that the pregnancy can produce dividends for the family as a whole, and, at the same time, impose certain costs for individual members.

In most families we observed, the pregnancy clearly elevated the status of the young mother. By her own account, and according to the reports of other family members, she was accorded more respect and "treated less like a girl and more like a woman." At the same time that the pregnancy brought more burdensome responsibilities to the adolescent, she was accorded greater recognition by parents and siblings for producing a precious object, a baby.

In our case studies, regardless of the hardships it imposed on the mother and family, the infant was universally esteemed. In part, attitudes toward the child reflected the view in the larger culture that children are lovable and vulnerable creatures who must be cherished and protected. In many instances the infant apparently also bestowed particular benefits on the family. For example, the baby could serve to solidify a family that was experiencing conflicts or was under the threat of dissolution. Sometimes, the baby seemed to serve as a replacement for a family member who had recently departed from the home. In several instances, the advent of a baby restored the grandmother's place in the family by filling a nest that had recently become empty. Thus, even though it was often disapproved of, because it was a premature event, the pregnancy was valued for helping to restore the integrity of the family system by shoring up its foundations.

Not all grandmothers were as unambivalent about resuming the maternal role as the woman in the family quoted below, but several others shared this middle-aged respondent's view that having a baby in the household had a rejuvenating effect on her:

> *How has it* [the baby] *changed your life?* [Directing a question to the family.]
>
> Mother: She [referring to her mother] feels younger.
>
> Grandmother: Not only that, but I just feel . . . happier inside . . . not as nervous. I used to be very tense all the time. . . .
>
> *Is that right? It has a calming effect?*
>
> Grandmother: Yeah, yeah.
>
> Mother: When I came out of the hospital, and I had him, she wanted to get up with him [at night]. Every time he cried, she would go right up.
>
> Grandmother: I still do.
>
> *Is that right?*
>
> Mother: She wanted to take care of him and all.
>
> *So you didn't have to get up?*
>
> Mother: No. [The adolescent goes on to explain how she and her mother take turns sleeping with the baby.]

Some interpreters may wish to argue that the daughter in this family became pregnant in order to redeem her mother's declining position in the family. I regard such ex post facto explanations as hazardous; but it is clear that many families can "put the pregnancy to use" even if they do not always anticipate the benefits before conception occurs.

The grandmother was not the only person affected by the pregnancy. Several older women remarked with some surprise that their husbands seemed more involved in the family than they had been for some years. One grandmother, whose husband had earlier abdicated his parental role, described how having a grandchild in the home had revived his sense of responsibility to the family:

> Well, my husband seems more . . . he pays attention to me which I didn't expect. He brought some things which I didn't expect him to do. [Later in the interview, she added a further comment on the effect the child had on her husband.] I think eventually, maybe Joseph [the baby] will have something to do with [my husband] growing up . . . maybe as a grandfather.

Not coincidentally, a few parents reported an improvement in their marital situation. "The baby has brought us all closer together" was a refrain in more than a few interviews.

The senior generation were not the only ones to notice heightened family solidarity. Siblings, too, reported that the climate of relations improved after the pregnancy occurred. In an earlier paper, I speculated that one explanation for this common occurrence might be that a pregnancy increases the level of exchange within the family, thereby improving the quality of relations. A number of respondents, for example, recounted that having a child strengthened their family because they had to pitch in together to support the child. Adolescents who were dependent on their siblings for babysitting or other kinds of help in childcare tasks were accordingly beholden to them.

There are still other reasons that might account for the improvement in family relations following a pregnancy. Sometimes it seemed that the infant was a diversion for families who had been locked in longstanding conflicts. The child may have rearranged established coalitions, at least temporarily, dampening strife within the family. Several adolescents who had occupied a marginal position or were in the process of exiting from the household were returned to the fold when their pregnancy occurred. Needless to say, their parents were pleased to report that a daughter who had rejected them a year ago suddenly expressed gratitude for their efforts on her behalf.

Long-term Costs

Lest we exaggerate the benefits of the pregnancy for the families in our pilot study, let me provide some qualifications to the rosy picture. In the first place, in these clinical interviews we were studying the families during what may have been a honeymoon period: the baby was still adorable; the young mother still grateful for the assistance she was receiving; and her parents were still prepared to extend material aid and services. This was a period of easy credit. We were not able to trace the long-term impact of the pregnancy on family relations, but it would not be surprising if relations deteriorated as the child matured, or when a second pregnancy occurred. Many of the parents stated in no uncertain terms that they would be unprepared to extend themselves if their daughter "made the same mistake again." In fact, the odds of a second pregnancy within a short period of time are quite high. Indeed, in the Baltimore study, more than half of the young mothers become pregnant a second time within three years. This may help to explain why many of the young mothers set up independent households around the time of the three-year follow-up. A study of the impact of repeat pregnancies on the family would help to clarify the sources of household division.

In addition to the attrition of resources, which might lead to a decline in family relations, it is also important to mention that many of the benefits observed in the clinical sample were two-edged. As the grandmother's role was restored, some of the adolescent parents indicated that they felt unable to leave their parents. While increased support had clear advantages for the young mother, it also put her in a difficult subordinate position at a point when a greater measure of independence may have been indicated.

A question that might be raised from our exploratory study is whether a prolonged period of dependency on the family of origin complicates the transition to a family of procreation or the establishment of an independent household. Do some young members become trapped in the family of origin because they lack the psychological or material wherewithal to move out?

Our culture is deeply ambivalent about dependency on the family. At the same time that we harshly label as pathogenic the (usually black) female-headed, non-nuclear household, which often relies upon support of extended kin or non-relatives, we romanticize a distant past when families were self-sufficient, and protected their own. Like most social institutions, families can be viewed as either benevolent or oppressive. For the adolescent mother, a supportive family clearly provides a series of invaluable services during the transition to parenthood. Nevertheless, it is possible that the same structure that nurtures and promotes the development of the young mother at one stage in her life may thwart and frustrate her growth at another. We must be prepared to conduct careful longitudinal research to document shifts in family functioning, as the young mother matures, before we can reach any firm conclusions about the long-term consequences of family involvement for her well-being.

Similarly, we must withhold judgment about the impact of the pregnancy on relations among siblings. While some siblings were admitted into a network of exchange, as we noted earlier, others found themselves excluded or displaced by the new object of family interest. In one interview, the youngest sibling, a ten-year-old boy, sat mute, and sullenly observed the attention showered on the infant, his nephew. When asked about changes he had noticed since the baby was born, he replied curtly and in an apparently disingenuous manner, "None."

We observed the families during the honeymoon period in the transition to parenthood, either late in the pregnancy or just after the birth of the child. The parents and siblings were still enjoying the novelty of the event. Relatively speaking, the newborn was still undemanding and easily controlled. As discipline becomes more challenging, the potential for conflict within the family may increase. Recall the case quoted earlier, in which an older sister pointedly reminded the young mother that her adorable baby would become a "monster" in several years, and that childcare would become less attractive. Collaborative childcare arrangements, I suspect, are less easy to maintain as the infant reaches the toddler stage.

The issue of who exercises authority over the child also may become more conspicuous as the child advances in years. Several adolescents anticipated a time when they would have to protect the child from being spoiled by other family members, in particular, the grandmother. At present, careful ethnographic studies on how children are raised in non-nuclear families are lacking. This is an area of research that deserves more attention, particularly if the trend towards diversification in family forms continues.

While the initial pregnancy often brings some unanticipated positive consequences for the family, it is not at all clear that a second pregnancy will do the same. In fact, it is easy to speculate that while the first pregnancy may serve to intensify family bonds, a second may loosen them, propelling the young mother from her parents' household.

Conclusion

Scattered throughout this essay are a series of questions for researchers, and issues for policymakers, involving the role of the family in mediating the impact of early parenthood. This paper is admittedly replete with loose ends. It may be useful, however, to reiterate some of the points and discuss some of the implications of these observations for policy and programs.

I began the essay by asserting that researchers suffer from the same limitations of vision as social practitioners when they approach the subject of teenage childbearing. That is, we locate the problem in individuals, the adolescent mother or her child, rather than in social systems, such as families. As a result, our prescriptions are highly individualistic. This approach is not so much wrong as it is restricted, for we are bound to miss the systemic causes and consequences of childbearing, and to overlook the necessity of altering social and family arrangements in order to change the behavior of individual actors.

Researchers, naturally enough, are predisposed to advocate further studies. This paper has been built on a shaky empirical base: the survey material provides only fragmentary evidence on the family's role; the case studies are rich enough but limited in number. I have mentioned a number of areas that have not yet received adequate attention by researchers: (1) the meaning of the pregnancy to various family members; (2) the family's role in resolving an unplanned conception; (3) how the family's response to the event influences the father's involvement in the child-rearing process; (4) styles of collaboration in caring for the newborn; and (5) the short- and long-term effects of early parenthood on relations between the adolescent, her siblings, and her parents. Each of these topics, given cursory treatment in this paper, has obvious importance to practitioners attempting to design ameliorative programs.

Since research can be extended indefinitely, and programs cannot be delayed, a few summary observations may be in order. In devising measures to prevent early childbearing and to alleviate its deleterious effects, policy planners and practitioners have neglected families.

A commitment to appreciate and recognize the role of families has many practical implications for policy programs. Most of our meager efforts at sexual education either ignore or deliberately bypass the family. Teenagers, not their families, are the designated target group. Family planning programs expect parents to make referrals, but frequently do not help them play a role in the sexual socialization of their offspring. Despite our knowledge that parents' attitudes toward sexuality and birth control have a powerful influence on the likelihood that a teenager will use contraception successfully, we continue to overlook the family in the services we provide.

No wonder, then, that parents object to, or at best, passively comply with, efforts to promote sex education in the schools or in birth control clinics. The public questions why sex education does not have more immediate effects in preventing unwanted pregnancies. Programs of sex education equip adolescents with information, but they return them to a context that often undermines use of that knowledge. Instead of utilizing the potential of parents and siblings to help the adolescent gain control over their sexual behavior, and to reinforce the teenager's decision to contracept, we are inclined to view the family as an adversary to be counteracted.

Similarly, most pregnancy counseling does not take into account the fact that parents, and perhaps other relatives, are interested parties in the decision. If they are not consulted, or at least considered, the decision reached may be disruptive, unrealistic, or perhaps even destructive to the interests of both the adolescent and her family. For example, is it realistic or fair to effectively deny the family a role in making decisions about the pregnancy when society benefits from the family's assumption of responsibility for the child who is born? From our evidence about the extent of families' assistance, is it sensible to provide welfare assistance only to teenage parents who live apart from their families? Is it effective to design childcare and education programs to help the teenage girl be a better parent without determining who else in the family may be providing care for the baby, and offering instruction and advice to the adolescents' siblings (female and male) to help prevent additional teenage pregnancies, their own as well as their sisters'?

If our neglect of the family as a context for both understanding and treating early childbearing is as persuasive and blatant as I have claimed in this paper, what can the explanation be? Is the importance of the family so much taken for granted that policymakers are merely uncomfortable about belaboring the obvious? A more likely explanation for why we have not designed our programs to include the family is that it is cumbersome to do so. Developing programs that are directed at the family rather than single individuals requires much greater coordination, and, probably, greater resources, as well. But an even more fundamental reason for our disregard of the family is the deep cultural ambivalence we have about the relative virtue of individual autonomy and collective responsibility. Planners, policymakers, and practitioners do not know how to weigh the varied and potentially competing interests of different family members. In part, the neglect of the family is, then, an unconscious abdication more than a deliberate oversight. Unless we are prepared to correct this individualistic bias in our programs, we must be willing to concede that our efforts at intervention will be slight. At the same time, we will be continuing to run the risk of undermining a potent source of assistance.

NOTES

1. This chapter reports on research originally commissioned by the Family Impact Seminar in 1978, and supported by a federal grant (no. 1-HD-72822). It builds on two earlier versions, the first entitled "Burdens and benefits: The impact of early childbearing on the family," *Journal of Social Issues* 36, no. 1 (1980): 64–87; and "Family adaptations to teenage parenthood," a paper presented at the Society for the Study of Social Problems, Boston, 1979. I would like to thank the editor, Theodora Ooms, for helpful advice in drafting this chapter.

2. M. A. Vinovskis, "Adolescent pregnancy: Some historical considerations," *Journal of Family History* (in press).

3. C. S. Chilman, "Social and psychological aspects of adolescent sexuality: An analytic overview of research and theory," report prepared for the National Institute of Child Health and Human Development (contract no. 1-HD-52821), Institute for Family Development, Center for Advanced Studies in Human Services, School of Social Welfare (Milwaukee: University of Wisconsin, 1977).

4. For the exceptions, see K. Cannon-Bonventre and J. R. Kahn, *The ecology of help-seeking behavior among adolescent parents* (Cambridge: American Institutes for

Research, 1979); and also H. Presser, "Sally's corner," *Journal of Social Issues* 36, no. 1 (1980): 107–129.

5. Frank F. Furstenberg, Jr., *Unplanned parenthood: The social consequences of teenage childbearing*, chapter 11 (New York: Free Press, 1976).

6. The idea for this pilot study came from Theodora Ooms, who sensed the desirability of an interdisciplinary effort to collect clinical data on the impact of early childbearing on the family of origin. I owe special thanks to Lynda Butler, who undertook the difficult task of organizing the research and coordinated the team of clinicians from the Philadelphia Child Guidance Clinic; and thanks to the team—Jay Jemail, Barbara Penn, and Iolie Wallbridge—who, with Butler, conducted the interviews. I am grateful to Salvador Minuchin, who enriched this project by sharing with our team some of his insights into family functioning.

7. Frank F. Furstenberg, Jr., and Albert G. Crawford, "Social implications of teenage pregnancy," in *Adolescent pregnancy: New perspectives for the health professional*, ed. P. B. Smith and D. M. Mumford (Boston: G. K. Hall, 1980); and Frank F. Furstenberg, Jr., Richard Lincoln, and Jane Menken, *Perspectives on teenage sexuality, pregnancy, and childbearing* (Philadelphia: University of Pennsylvania Press, 1981).

8. M. H. Cantor, K. Rosenthal, and L. Wilke, "Social and family relationships of black teenaged women in New York City," paper presented at the 28th Annual Scientific Meeting of the Gerontological Society, Louisville, 1975.

9. E. Bott, *Family and social network*, 2d ed. (New York: Free Press, 1971); and C. Stack, *All our kin* (New York: Harper and Row, 1974).

10. P. M. Rains, *Becoming an unwed mother: A sociological account* (Chicago: Aldine/Atherton, 1971); and Kristin Luker, *Taking chances* (Berkeley, Calif.: University of California Press, 1975).

11. S. Minuchin, *Families and family therapy* (Cambridge, Mass.: Harvard University Press, 1975).

12. Furstenberg and Crawford, "Social implications," pp. 70–71.

5

Government Policies Related to Teenage Family Formation and Functioning: An Inventory

Kristin A. Moore

Every year the federal government spends billions of dollars on programs that affect families. In some cases, programs are explicitly designed to have a particular impact on family formation or functioning; however, it is not usually clear whether or not that impact is achieved. Furthermore, many programs achieve other or additional goals that may not have been foreseen or even desired by those who initiated the program. There are also numerous instances in which the same outcome is sought through several similar and overlapping programs. This paper represents an initial attempt to catalogue those governmental programs that seem particularly likely to affect the formation and functioning of teenage families.

The types of programs that might affect teenage families range from welfare assistance, through Aid to Families with Dependent Children and health care programs like Medicaid, to social services, school lunches, public housing, and job training. The Stanford Research Institute recently estimated that the 600,000 births each year to teenagers may cost federal, state, and local governments as much as $8.3 billion each year in welfare and medical costs alone.[1] The low educational and occupational attainments of many teenage parents, coupled with the large size and instability of families formed by teenagers, make this a particularly vulnerable family form—one likely to require a variety of governmental services over a prolonged period.[2] Developing an understanding of how government programs affect the functioning of families formed by teenagers is an important task.

However, government programs also affect the formation of teenage families. Eleven million teenagers have been estimated to be sexually active and in need of various services to control their fertility and safeguard their health.[3] Therefore, this paper considers programs that affect either family formation or functioning.

It is difficult in many cases to distinguish between these two types of impact. For example, the provision of prenatal care affects family formation in that improved care reduces the probability of miscarriage and stillbirth. It can also affect family functioning, however, if proper prenatal care prevents the occurrence of retardation or handicapping conditions. Similarly, Aid to Families with Dependent Children has provisions that can theoretically affect a teenager's decision about abortion or marriage. However, the primary purpose of the program is to provide income to enhance family functioning. Because of these overlappings, this paper is organized according to the programs themselves; and the various potential impacts are discussed within these sections.

The inventory presented here identifies and describes a total of approximately thirty-five separate programs, located in five federal agencies as they existed in 1978. (A few additions have included developments in 1979 and 1980.) Since change is one of the most dependable characteristics of any government program, the reader is cautioned not to assume that the government programs still exist as they are described on the following pages. In general, this inventory has been organized as a listing of individual programs under broad topic areas designating which department or division of the agency is responsible for administering the program. However, at a couple of points it seemed best to identify all the programs administered by a specific governmental unit that might affect teenage pregnancy and parents, causing some duplication of entries.

Aid to Families with Dependent Children

In 1977, nearly $10.3 billion were expended nationwide through Aid to Families with Dependent Children (AFDC); a budget of $11.2 billion was forecast for 1979. Over eleven million recipients in 3.6 million families received cash assistance through AFDC.[4] AFDC is located in the Social Security Administration of the Department of Health, Education, and Welfare (HEW).

It has been estimated that approximately half of the money expended through this program in 1975 went to households in which the mother was a teenager at the time of her first birth. Sixty percent of the women, aged fourteen to thirty, living in AFDC households bore their first child as teenagers, compared to 35 percent among women living in households with no AFDC recipients.[5] The Department of Health, Education, and Welfare estimates that 10 percent of all families receiving AFDC will be headed by women in their teen years, if current trends continue.[6] Teenage parents clearly have an impact on AFDC. How does AFDC affect teenagers?

The belief that the availability of welfare benefits provides an economic incentive for childbearing is quite widespread. It seems somewhat unlikely that the meager benefits available to welfare mothers would actually induce a young woman to become pregnant, particularly in those states in which payments fall below the need standard; and researchers have not yet found strong or consistent evidence of such an association. Nevertheless, anecdotal evidence for such incentives can be found. For example, AFDC money is referred to as "crib money" in some Georgia high schools, when the mother splits her payment with the father while the grandmother rears the child.[7]

Even though welfare may not represent a sufficient incentive to conceive, the availability of welfare support may encourage a teenager once she is pregnant, to bear a child when she might otherwise have obtained an abortion (particularly if prenatal care is free, while an abortion can only be obtained with personal funds). Welfare may also make it possible for a woman to avoid marrying the father of her child if she has doubts about his stability or earning ability. A teenager may see any amount of money as a source of independence, since it enables her to set up her own household free of parental control and supervision. On the other hand, it has been suggested that an aging welfare mother might encourage her daughters to become pregnant in order to sustain welfare support to the extended family.[8] In addition, the availability of welfare may be a deciding factor in whether an unwed mother keeps her child or gives it up for adoption. The attractiveness of the welfare option is affected, of course, by the size of the welfare benefit, and the rules implemented by the state welfare authorities, as well as by the attractiveness of her alternatives, such as the wage that she could earn in the labor market.

The goal of Aid to Families with Dependent Children is to provide cash assistance to families requiring financial support due to a parent's death, disability, or prolonged absence from the home. Initially, this meant coverage of widows; however, most children receiving AFDC benefits at present are in need because of divorce, desertion of a parent, or out-of-wedlock birth.

Several additional contingencies also qualify a child for benefits in some states (see Table 5):

- Unemployed father coverage: A father is present in the home, but he is unemployed. Coverage was available under these circumstances in twenty-seven states in 1978.
- Emergency assistance: Emergency coverage is available for up to thirty days, once during a twelve-month period, at the discretion of AFDC officials. In 1978, twenty-one states had such a

program. No eligibility rules are applied, since the program is intended to cover in cases of emergency. Federal and state/local governments each provide half of the funds for this program.
- Unborn child coverage: Unborn children are automatically covered unless they are first children. Coverage of first-born children varies from state to state, though most states do pay at least some pregnancy and delivery costs, either before or after the child is born. First children are covered before their birth under some circumstances in thirty states. In addition to the cash benefits to which the unborn child and its mother are entitled under this state option, this is an important benefit because extension of AFDC benefits to pregnant mothers automatically entitles them to Medicaid. At the present time, an unborn child can receive cash payments under AFDC or Medicaid services. Thirty-three states provide one or both of these types of coverage (see the list below). In addition, ten states cover unborn children under legislation that permits coverage of individuals who meet state income tests, regardless of whether they meet other criteria; in these states, unborn children conceived by married, poor parents can be covered even when the couple has no other children. (These states also appear in the list):

- *States that provide coverage for an unborn child: Either AFDC cash payment or Medicaid coverage of individuals who could not meet AFDC requirements:*

Alabama	Minnesota	Pennsylvania
California	Mississippi	Rhode Island
Colorado	Montana	South Carolina
Delaware	Nebraska	South Dakota
Florida	Nevada	Tennessee
Hawaii	New Jersey	Utah
Kansas	New Mexico	Vermont
Kentucky	New York	Washington
Louisiana	North Dakota	West Virginia
Maryland	Ohio	Wisconsin
Massachusetts	Oregon	Wyoming

TABLE 5
SUMMARY OF CHARACTERISTICS OF STATE PLANS FOR AID TO FAMILIES WITH DEPENDENT CHILDREN (AFDC), AS OF APRIL 1978*

State	Coverage			Percentage of Payment	
	Unborn Child Coverage	Unemployed Father Coverage	Emergency Assistance	Payment for Caretaker and One Child (Oct. 1976)	Average Monthly Payments per Family
Alabama	Yes	No	No	61.5	$112
Alaska	No	No	No	100§	296
Arizona	No	No	No	70	141
Arkansas	No	No	No	69	143
California	Yes	Yes	No	†	318
Colorado	Yes	Yes	No	100	203
Connecticut	No	Yes	Yes	100	311
Delaware	No	Yes	Yes	100	214
District of Columbia	Yes	Yes	Yes	90	239
Florida	No	No	No	83	145
Georgia	No	No	No	65	109
Hawaii	Yes	Yes	No	100	375
Idaho	Yes	No	No	87	251
Illinois	No	Yes	No	100	262
Indiana	No	No	No	90†	191
Iowa	No	Yes	No	100	274
Kansas	Yes	Yes	Yes	100	235
Kentucky	No	No	Yes	100§	172
Louisiana	Yes	No	No	40	125
Maine	No	No	No	90	212
Maryland	Yes	Yes	Yes	80	191
Massachusetts	Yes	Yes	Yes	100	319
Michigan	No	Yes	Yes	100	334
	Yes	Yes	Yes	100	289

State				
...ippi	No	No	†	47
Missouri	No	Yes	65	179
Montana	Yes	Yes	†	189
Nebraska	Yes	Yes		266
Nevada	Yes	No	81	186
New Hampshire	No	No	100	234
New Jersey	No	Yes	100	284
New Mexico	Yes	No	†	154
New York	Yes	Yes	100	385
North Carolina	No	No	100	157
North Dakota	Yes	No	100	244
Ohio	Yes	Yes	62	211
Oklahoma	No	Yes	100§	225
Oregon	Yes	Yes	91	280
Pennsylvania	Yes	Yes	100	293
Rhode Island	Yes	No	100	267
South Carolina	No	No	†	85
South Dakota	Yes	No	100	200
Tennessee	Yes	No	64‡	107
Texas	No	No	75‡	109
Utah	Yes	Yes	77	260
Vermont	Yes	No	75.6	267
Virginia	No	Yes	90	193
Washington	Yes	Yes	100§	294
West Virginia	Yes	Yes	†	179
Wisconsin	Yes	No	85	312
Wyoming	No	Yes	100	204

Source: State Plan and Program Characteristics Branch, Office of Family Assistance, Office of Research and Statistics, Social Security Administration, "Public Assistance Statistics," ORS rep. A-2, HEW (April 1978), Table 4.

†Full standard not met. Income is applied to the full standard. Payment is limited by maximum on the money amount, by family size, or the deficit; rules vary by state.

‡Or $275 for family of four in Indiana; $220 in Tennessee; or $300 in Texas.

§Full standard not met for very large families.

- *States that cover unborn children under legislation permitting coverage for those meeting state income test, regardless of family status:*

California	New Jersey	Vermont
Hawaii	New York	Washington
Massachusetts	Pennsylvania	Wisconsin
Minnesota	Utah	

- *Pregnancy-related medical care provided in states without unborn child coverage to babies who are AFDC-eligible when born (telephone interviews conducted by Dr. Martha Burt in fall 1979):*

  Alaska: first of month rule

  Arizona: county health clinics provide care

  Arkansas: ninety days retroactive

  Connecticut: delivery only

  Delaware: ninth month only

  Florida: unborn child coverage since July 1, 1978

  Georgia: first of month rule

  Illinois: eligible at delivery—lump sum retroactive for delivery and prenatal care

  Indiana: first of month rule

  Iowa: since October 1979, last trimester covered

  Kentucky: all prenatal care and delivery covered

  Maine: first of month rule

  Michigan: since early 1979, covered from time of application

  Mississippi: since July 1, 1978, all prenatal care from fourth month of pregnancy

  Missouri: first of month rule; pay all delivery and prenatal charges presented

  New Hampshire: ninety day retroactive

  New Jersey: since July 1, 1979, coverage back to date of conception

  North Carolina: only care to baby covered (not delivery or care to mother), beginning at time of delivery

  Oklahoma: month of delivery, but retroactive if lump sum bill presented

Texas: hospital and medical expenses from moment of birth only covered

Virginia: month of delivery; cover all bills presented by delivery physician, including prenatal care

Most of the remaining states also pay the costs associated with delivery of a child, as well as some or all of the costs of prenatal care, but only after the child is born, if the baby is eligible for AFDC once it is born. A number of these states will pay expenses back to the first of the month of application, a period that will include delivery if the mother applies for AFDC promptly. In a number of other states, this retroactive coverage extends ninety days; and in several states the entire bill for prenatal care will be picked up by the state, particularly if the physician presents a lump sum bill. The net effect of these varied policies is that in all of the states, the state will cover all or most of the dollar costs of delivery for an unmarried teenage mother, as long as she applies as soon as she becomes eligible in her state. (It should be noted, however, that after 1980, the information in the list may be of historical interest only, if legislation is passed to mandate coverage of unborn children regardless of family status when the family meets the income test.)

Since retroactive coverage represents only a "back door" approach to coverage of prenatal care, it is not known whether pregnant teenagers or social workers are aware of this type of coverage or of the importance of filing for AFDC immediately after childbirth. In addition, teenagers from middle-class families may not know they can get AFDC for their baby if they remain unmarried. Although the teenage mother living with her parents may not be eligible for AFDC if the grandparents' income is too high, the grandparents are only responsible for their minor child, not their grandchild. Therefore, the baby is automatically eligible for AFDC if it is deprived of a father, regardless of whether the teenage mother herself is eligible. Since the baby is not deprived of a father if the marriage takes place, marriage typically means that the baby is not eligible for AFDC. But it is also not known whether teenagers consider eligibility for AFDC as they reach a decision regarding marriage.

If these AFDC and Medicaid policies serve as incentives to resolve a pregnancy one way rather than another, the incentive seems to lie more in the direction of discouraging marriage and making out-of-wedlock parenthood financially possible than in encouraging the teenager to move out of the grandparents' home. The teenager can receive a grant for herself and the baby, if she lives in a low-income family. Even if she lives with middle-income parents, she will be eligible for a grant on behalf of the baby. There is, of course, an increase in the amount she receives if she moves away from her parents' home; however, this gain is offset by the loss of many in-kind sources of support. Consequently, the economic gain of moving out is probably small, particularly in middle-income homes.

In the case of the young pregnant woman deciding about marriage, however, numerous economic incentives exist that might weigh against such a decision. If she lives in a state that does not provide coverage to families with unemployed fathers, or if the father does not qualify as unemployed, the teenage mother who marries has to forego government assistance; consequently, her decision to marry may be affected by the father's earnings or his earning potential. Also, coverage of prenatal care and childbirth from either the government or private parental insurance would have to be given up in the event of marriage (unless the father qualified as unemployed in a state with unemployed father coverage). If he has a job, it has to provide maternity coverage as part of his health insurance if it is to compare with AFDC and Medicaid coverage. Thus a number of the features of programs could affect the young woman's decision to marry, particularly among social subgroups in which men have low earnings and lack prepaid health coverage. Finally, the existence of numerous forms of support for pregnant teenagers deciding to carry to term, at a time when abortion is not subsidized in many states, may also lead some young women to view out-of-wedlock parenthood as a more financially feasible pregnancy resolution.

At the present time, evidence that the benefits provided under the AFDC program affect teenage family formation and composition is lacking. Since most teenage parents indicate that their pregnancies were unintended, any impact that benefit characteristics have is necessarily fairly limited.[9] However, the net impact of several interrelated regulations may play a role in some cases. For example, a state that pays recipients the *full standard* (the full cost of living needs that the state recognizes as essential), provides coverage for an unborn child, does not cover unemployed fathers, and does not pay for abortions may in effect be creating incentives for out-of-wedlock childbearing. Likewise, a state that pays for abortion but not coverage of unborn children may be encouraging abortion. Whether such effects occur is an empirical question; however, states might consider the potential unintended effects that could result from providing a particular array of benefits but not all benefits.

Family Planning

Family planning assistance is funded through four separate programs, all located within the Department of Health, Education and Welfare:

- Title V of the Social Security Act (Maternal and Child Health)
- Title X of the Public Health Service Act
- Title XIX of the Social Security Act (Medicaid)
- Title XX of the Social Security Act (Social Services)

Although these four programs provide money for family planning in different ways, are oriented toward somewhat different populations, and do not represent a coherent, unified program, on the service provider level the four programs function more or less as one program. Nevertheless, they will be described separately because of their different intentions and regulations.

Title V: Maternal and Child Health (Bureau of Community Health Services)

In Fiscal Year (FY) 1977, approximately $26 million were expended for family planning under Title V. Money is provided through a formula grant program administered by the Office of Maternal and Child Health of the Bureau of Community Health Services. Formula grants typically go to state health departments that establish or provide funds to clinics. Each state must have one or more Maternal and Infant Centers, one or more Children and Youth Centers, as well as one or more projects for family planning, high-risk infants, and dental care. Not less than 6 percent of the formula grant in each state is to be spent on family planning.

This is not a reimbursement program; however, providers may seek reimbursement for services to low-income patients from other sources (such as Medicaid). Low income patients themselves are to receive services without charge; and there are no restrictions concerning the age or marital status of recipients. No reliable data exist on the national level as to the number of patients served; therefore, it is not clear how many teenage patients receive Title V services. Low-income adolescents can receive services through this program if a facility is accessible; this may pose a problem to many teenagers, since states are only required to have one such facility. Many states do have numerous Title V providers, however. Higher income teenagers may also receive services, but often fees will be charged according to income. Because eligibility rules are made by individual projects, they vary widely. Since this program was initiated to serve children and pregnant women, prevention of initial pregnancies among teenagers was not an explicit purpose; however, it undoubtedly now serves this goal to some extent.

Title X: Public Health Service Act (Bureau of Community Health Services)

Under the Family Planning Services and Population Research Act of 1970, Title X of the Public Health Service Act, $135 million were expended during FY 1978. Congress authorized $205 million for FY 1979, a substantial increase. This program accounts for about half of the federal funds allocated for family planning. Like Title V, it is a grant program. Monies are expended for "voluntary family planning services personnel, grants and contracts for services delivery improvement research, and grants and contracts for family planning information and education."[10] Although low-income people are to be given priority, services are not restricted to the poor. In addition, services are explicitly to be made available regardless of age, marital status, or parity. Indeed, in 1978, $7.8 million was earmarked for services to teenagers. Because teenagers have to meet the eligibility requirements of Title XIX or XX in order to receive family planning services under those titles, Title X represents an important source of financial assistance to teenagers seeking contraception. Title X guidelines state that "charges should not be made in a manner that will constitute a barrier to services. No patient should be denied services because of inability to pay."[11]

Title X funds are allocated by the Bureau of Community Health Services (which also administers Title V) to the ten regional offices of HEW. Regional officials award grants to individual providers, such as hospital clinics, health departments, planned parenthood facilities, neighborhood health centers, private non-profit agencies, and private physicians under contract to organized provider agencies. In 1978, more than 2,500 agencies that provide services in 4,900 clinics received Title X funds. The expansion of service and improved accessibility are explicit goals, as is service to teenagers: "Emphasis will continue on reducing the incidence of unintended adolescent pregnancy through the expansion of services in areas with high teenage birth rates and the improvement of outreach and counseling services. It is recognized that adolescent clients require more extensive counseling and follow-up than most older patients in order to effectively utilize family planning services."[12] To improve services to teenagers, four regional conferences were held to alert providers to the importance of "a positive course of action to address the adolescent pregnancy problem"; programs to reach males are being developed; and four innovative projects were funded to test ways of serving and informing adolescents.[13]

Title XIX: Medicaid (Health Care Financing Administration)

The Social Security Amendments of 1965 established Title XIX (the Medicaid program). States participating in the program are required to provide medical assistance to all AFDC recipients of cash assistance. At state option, they can also finance medical care for the medically needy, that is, people who would be eligible for cash assistance, except that the level of their income is, though sufficient to sustain themselves, too low to provide necessary medical care. In addition, states can opt to provide coverage to all children under twenty-one from low-income families, regardless of welfare status or program eligibility.

Under the original legislation, the inclusion of family planning services was a state option. However, Public Law 92-603, passed in 1972, made coverage of family planning services for cash assistance recipients under Title XIX mandatory for the states. In addition, the rate of federal financial participation for both the categorically and medically needy was increased from the regular Medicaid match of 50 to 83 to 90 percent.

At present, Medicaid reimbursement is mandated, in all states with a Medicaid program, for family planning services obtained voluntarily by any woman in a family receiving Aid to Families with Dependent Children (AFDC), and in 35 states, by individuals receiving Supplementary Security Income (SSI; Arizona is the only state without a Medicaid program). In addition, in thirty-three states, as noted above, an eligibility category has been created for the medically needy. The criteria vary greatly from state to state. State variation is increased by the option of offering Medicaid coverage to several additional groups; such as children under twenty-one who meet the AFDC income and resources limits, but are not dependent children (e.g., they may be emancipated minors or live with two employed parents); children in families that are eligible for benefits, but have chosen not to receive them; or persons eligible in states with broader coverage (e.g., coverage of unborn children in families with an unemployed father).[14]

Title XIX legislation explicitly includes "minors who can be considered to be sexually active." Since all family members covered by AFDC or SSI (in those states that cover SSI) are also eligible for Medicaid, a teenager who has never been pregnant can receive family planning services paid for by Medicaid as long as she has access to a Medicaid card. In FY 1976, over $40 million was spent on family planning within Title XIX, approximately 18 percent of the federal total.

Medical assistance for family planning includes payments for appropriate medical examinations, diagnosis, medical counseling and treatment, laboratory services, surgical procedures, drugs, supplies, and devices. These services may be provided in doctors' offices, clinics, hospitals (on both an in-patient and out-patient basis), family planning centers, or any other suitable settings. Thus, persons with access to Medicaid coverage should be able, theoretically, to obtain medical family planning services.

Title XX: Social Services (Administration for Public Services, Office of Human Development Services)

Family planning is one of the social services provided under the Social Security Amendments. In 1978, all states provided family planning to the eligible population, except Nebraska. Although nine states did not provide medical services under Title XX, all but two indicated that such services are provided under Title XIX. States have the option of providing family planning services on a universal basis (that is, without regard to income), a feature that not only makes services available to teenagers from non-poor families but enhances confidentiality, since documentation of family income is not necessary. Seventeen states have chosen the option of universal coverage: Alabama, Alaska, Arizona, Connecticut, Delaware, District of Columbia, Florida, Indiana, Kansas, Maryland, Mississippi, New Mexico, Oregon, South Dakota, Virginia, West Virginia, and Wisconsin.[15]

Thus, in 1978, poor teenagers could receive family planning services under Title XX in all states except Nebraska, while all teenagers could receive services in the seventeen states above. An additional seventeen states provided coverage without regard to income in cases of neglect, abuse, or exploitation: Arkansas, California, Georgia, Illinois, Kentucky, Louisiana, Minnesota, Missouri, Nevada, New Jersey, North Carolina, North Dakota, Ohio, Oklahoma, South Carolina, Tennessee, and Wyoming.[16]

As administered by the Office of Human Development Services through the Administration for Public Services, a state designates a state agency to supervise the Title XX program. Services can either be provided directly or contracted out to public or nonprofit, private agencies. Approximately $35 million was expended on family planning through Title XX in FY 1976, with about 17 percent of the federal expenditures on family planning. (There is a ceiling on total Title XX expenditures nationally of $2.5 billion, with ceilings on state expenditures as well, based on state population.)

Despite the fact that there are several programs with different rules and eligibility standards operating under different authorities, it is generally conceded that this fact is not felt very much on the clinic level, at least not by the patient. If the patient has a Medicaid card, Medicaid can be billed for reimbursement. For other women seeking family planning services, the provider typically seeks information to determine which program she can receive services under. Title XX can be billed for services to

GOVERNMENT POLICIES 181

low-income women; however, the expenditure ceiling limits use of this program. Recent increases in Title X appropriations, if funded, will probably enhance reliance on that program. Women are not turned away by clinic providers because they do not meet the specific regulations of one of the titles. Their bill is paid by another title or absorbed by the clinic. Thus, the young woman who presents herself at a clinic is likely to receive services. The barriers are that she may not know that she will receive services; the clinic may not be accessible; she may be afraid of parental discovery; or she may feel that even a fee assessed on a sliding scale is too high for a teenager to pay. Only a fraction of the teenage population at risk of unintended pregnancy is currently receiving services.[17] Clearly, barriers to contraceptive accessibility still exist. However, one would have to conclude that the efforts of the government to provide family planning services on a voluntary basis have been laudable, and have undoubtedly served to reduce the number of teenage families formed during the seventies.

Federal family planning services are provided to minors without a requirement of parental consent or notification. However, some states still have such requirements. Moreover, legislation has been introduced into Congress on several occasions to require parental notification for all minors served under Title X. Considerable controversy exists about this issue, but it seems clear that such a law would deter many minors from seeking medical contraceptive services and result in other unwanted consequences.

Abortion

At present, as a result of the Hyde Amendment attached to the HEW appropriation bill in 1977, and passed yearly since, the federal government funds only a small number of abortions. The District of Columbia, and several states have opted to pay for abortions themselves, some under court order; but the trend toward less public funding of abortion has continued with attempts to place restrictions on the District of Columbia, Defense Department employees, and government workers. It appears that this controversy will continue for some years in the courts and legislatures at both federal and state levels.

The impact of this exception to the reimbursement of medical services under Medicaid is clear, in one sense. It seems highly probable that the incidence of teenage family formation will increase. It also seems possible that the incidence of poverty associated with teenage parenthood will increase, since personal access to funds probably has a greater impact on whether a young woman obtains an abortion. Although statistical evidence on this question is limited, an initial examination of this issue suggests that most Medicaid-eligible women seeking abortion do manage to obtain an abortion.[18] Perhaps a third overall carry the pregnancy to term; an unknown proportion of these are teenagers. Clearly, the ban on Medicaid payment has not deterred as many women as some had feared, nor been as effective as others had hoped.

Health Programs

Medicaid (Health Care Financing Administration)

Title XIX of the Social Security Act of 1965, as amended, provides funds to states on an open-ended entitlement basis. State and local governments administer the program. Each state designs its own programs; and there is substantial flexibility concerning eligibility, benefit levels, and scope of coverage.

The goal is to provide health care services to the low-income population, specifically all those receiving, or eligible to receive, Aid to Families with Dependent Children or, in most states, Supplemental Security Income. This categorically eligible population is entitled to receive all mandated services, such as hospitalization, family planning, X-rays, lab costs, Early and Periodic Screening, Diagnosis, and Treatment services. Inclusion of the medically indigent, those made poor by heavy medical expenditures, is a state option.

The federal government pays for more than half of the administrative expenditures. The federal share of medical services varies from 50 to 83 percent, depending on relative per capita income in the state. In FY 1977, total funding was $17.7 billion, with the federal government contributing $10.2 billion.

Three million adolescents are estimated to be eligible for Medicaid, making this a highly important source of medical assistance (as well as family planning) for low-income teenagers.

Early and Periodic Screening, Diagnosis, and Treatment (EPSDT)

States are currently mandated to provide screening services to Medicaid-eligible children in order to identify physical or mental problems and to provide follow-up treatment for problems discovered in the assessment within the scope of the state plan through EPSDT. This program is administered by the Office of Child Health, within the Health Care Financing Administration.

Currently, legislation is being considered that would increase the eligible population for these services. The Child Health Assessment Program (CHAP) would strengthen and subsume the existing EPSDT program. Under the proposed legislation, it would be mandated that all states make eligible for Medicaid all individuals under the age of twenty-one who meet state income tests, regardless of their family status. In addition, CHAP would make all children assessed eligible to receive all medically necessary services covered under Medicaid (with some limitations on mental health and dental services). Introduction of this program would increase the number of children from poor two-parent families eligible for services, including family planning services and prenatal care under Medicaid.

Maternal and Child Health (Bureau of Community Health Services)

Title V of the Social Security Act has the goal of improving services to reduce infant mortality, and enhance the health of both mothers and children. The reduction of mental retardation and other handicaps, and promotion of health among young children and school-age children, also represent critical goals.

The Office of Maternal and Child Health, as noted in the discussion of family planning, has been concerned with preventing the occurrence of teenage pregnancy. Assistance is also provided to the teenage mothers who wish to carry pregnancies to term. This office has recently expanded its role in the delivery of medical services to teenagers and their babies by funding comprehensive programs that deliver social, economic, educational, and medical services to teenagers.

Administered by the Bureau of Community Health Services (BCHS) within HEW's Public Health Service, the Office of Maternal and Child Health Services funds totaled $315 million in FY 1977. States are awarded formula grants to provide services regardless of the income of the recipient. States are required to establish at least one Maternal and Infant project and at least one Children and Youth project. Nearly a third (55,000) of those receiving services in Maternity and Infant projects are adolescents.

Community Health Center Program (Bureau of Community Health Services)

Administered by the Bureau of Community Health Services, the Community Health Center Program was designed to bring medical care to underserved areas. In the late 1960s, programs were established in urban areas under the Office of Economic Opportunity. During the early 1970s, numerous non-urban centers were established under a different program. In 1973, all the health centers were folded into one program, and about 400 more medical centers were established, primarily in rural areas.

Services are provided to people with third-party payers (such as Medicaid); however, a center can also provide services with its own funds. Fees are assessed according to a sliding scale. Family planning services, prenatal care and pediatric care are all provided. There are no family structure requirements, such as those found in the AFDC regulations, and no age requirements. Teenagers are able to receive family planning services regardless of their income, though they might have to pay a charge based on the fee schedule.

The existence or absence of such a center could greatly affect whether a teenager is able to obtain family planning services, particularly in rural areas. In addition, location of such centers in medically underserved areas increases the probability that a pregnant teenager will obtain an early diagnosis, appropriate prenatal care, and pediatric care.

In FY 1977, funding stood at $215 million. Program staff anticipate that 11 percent of those served will be adolescents by the end of FY 1978.

Uniformed Services Health Benefit Program (Assistant Secretary of Defense, Health Affairs)

Medical services to the military are primarily offered in the form of direct care in military facilities. Out-patient services are provided free, while small fees are charged for some in-patient services. For active military personnel and dependents who do not have military facilities available to them, and dependents of retired, deceased, and totally disabled veterans, the Civilian Health and Medical Program of the Uniformed Services (CHAMPUS) is available. This cost-sharing program allows military families to obtain civilian sources of medical care. Although data are not available on the number of teenagers receiving services, there are no age restrictions on the types of services that dependents can obtain. However, the offspring of military dependents (the grandchildren of military personnel) are not covered; if a teenage dependent bears and raises a child while remaining a military dependent, the grandparent would have to adopt the grandchild before it would be eligible for military health coverage. Funding for the total military health program totaled about $500 million in 1978.

Social Services

Enactment of the Social Security Act in 1935 represents the initiation of federal participation in income assistance, social security, and unemployment compensation. Amendments to the basic law have been numerous; and this act, as amended, now provides the basic legislative authority for social services and Medicaid as well as Aid to Families with Dependent Children and Supplemental Security Income. The major social services program was authorized under Title XX of the Social Security Act, although other titles also offer social services. Since Title XX became effective in 1975, the social services program has been administered by the Administration for Public Services, Office of Human Development Services, within the Department of Health, Education and Welfare.

Title XX

Under Title XX, persons eligible for social services are current recipients of AFDC or SSI, and, at state option, other persons who meet state and federal income limitations. States may set any income limit that does not exceed 115 percent of the state median income for a family of four (adjusted for family size). States must impose reasonable, income-related fees for services furnished to persons with income over the 80 percent level. States may impose such fees for recipients and persons with income below the 80 percent level.[19]

After 1962 and particularly in the early 1970s, a rapid growth in expenditures occurred under Titles IV-A and VI. Concern over rising costs led to the establishment of a $2.5 billion ceiling on expenditures. Within this total, the federal government contributes 75 percent of a state's funds (except, as noted, in the case of family planning, which is reimbursed by the federal government at 90 percent).

The $2.5 billion is divided among the fifty states and the District of Columbia, according to population. While all states and the District have Title XX programs, the types of services offered and their administration vary greatly from state to state. However, each state Title XX plan offers at least one service directed to each of the following five goals:[20]

- Economic self-support
- Personal self-sufficiency
- Protection of children and handicapped adults from abuse, neglect, and exploitation
- Prevention and reduction of inappropriate institutionalization by providing community care services
- Arrangement for appropriate institutionalization and services when in the best interest of the individual.

There are few restrictions on the uses of Title XX funds; and consequently, states have been free to develop whatever programs they have seen fit. With Title XX monies, states have helped fund adoption services, homemaker/home management services, counseling, programs for unmarried parents, and varied services for children and youth. Two other Title XX services (described elsewhere individually) are day care and family planning. Although some services are delivered directly, Title XX funds are used, in many cases, to purchase services from other providers.

Approximately 5.9 million people are receiving some form of service annually from social services funded under Title XX. However, since Title XX is not the only source of funds for social services, the same or similar sets of services may be provided under different titles. Examples of other relevant services to children and youth funded under other titles are noted below. At the federal level, all of these programs are administered by the Administration for Children, Youth, and Families, within HEW.

Title IV-A: Foster Care Segment, AFDC

Federal funding assists states in paying for foster care and day care services of eligible children placed in the state's custody by the courts. Approximately 100,000 children are served monthly by this program.

Title IV-B: Child Welfare Services

Under Title IV-B of the Social Security Act, formula grants are awarded to state welfare agencies to assist in establishing, extending, and strengthening child welfare services that prevent the neglect, abuse or delinquency of children. Grants are used to pay personnel who provide protective services to abused and neglected children and their families, to license and set standards in private child care agencies, and to help pay the costs of foster care, day care, homemaker services, return of runaway children, and placement of children in adoptive homes. Most of the $56 million in FY 1977 funds were expended on foster care services.

Title V, Part A, Public Law 93-644—Head Start

The program provides funds to the states for the establishment of pre-school compensatory education programs for children of low-income families. Services are also provided for necessary health, nutrition, and social services to the child and the family. Ten percent of the children served must be handicapped. Approximately 350,000 children are involved in Head Start programs.

Child Abuse Prevention and Treatment Act

Federal funds are authorized for grants and contracts for research purposes and demonstration projects for child abuse, ne-

GOVERNMENT POLICIES

glect, prevention, and treatment programs. Funds enable states to make provisions for the investigation of reported cases and for the protection of the health and welfare of the abused or neglected child.

Runaway Youth Act

Funds assist states to establish homes for runaway youths that provide shelter, guidance, and counseling services. Approximately 160,000 youngsters are served yearly. In 1977, funding was $7 million.

The range of social services provided to children, the handicapped, elderly, and other adults is extensive and includes: foster care and adoption, day care, home chore services, transportation, protective services, homemakers, congregate meals, employment and other kinds of counseling, and information and referral. Unfortunately, no estimate is available of the numbers of people served, because certain people receive several of these services.

Since there are no data on the age of recipients, it is not possible to know how many teenagers receive services. One would assume that, to the extent that teenage families have particularly strong needs for social services, counseling, and economic assistance, the presence of these programs represents an important set of programs for teenagers. The enormous variability among programs, however, makes assessment of the overall impact of the social services package impossible.

Day Care

Day care services are provided under Titles XX, IV-A, IV-B, and IV-C of the Social Security Act.

Title XX

Day care is one of the most important services provided with Title XX monies. In fact, in terms of dollars expended, day care ranks number one; approximately $600 million per year have been expended under this program recently. In terms of persons served, day care has ranked third, with approximately 420,000 children served at a time. Since this is not typically a cash program, the usual procedure is to reimburse a formal day care provider, such as a day care center. Programs that are at the Title XX ceiling for their state often move day care funding into other programs, programs that tend to provide cash grants to people who then purchase their own day care, most often informal day care.

All states provide day care services to income maintenance recipients, and all but three states also provide services to people having a specified level of median income. The exceptions are: South Dakota, which limits the service to AFDC and AFDC service recipients; Montana, which limits the service to AFDC recipients and those whose income is below 150 percent of the level for eligibility; and Alaska, which provides the service, without regard to income, as a component of Child Protective Services.

Although all other states provide day care services to those with an eligible income, many also use non-income criteria to determine eligibility. Such criteria include: single-parent families; two-parent families with one parent incapacitated; parent(s) involved in an employment training program; parent(s) employed and requiring day care to maintain employment; and parent or child with a mental or physical handicap.[21]

In 1978, forty states provided day care services, without regard to income, in documented cases of abuse, neglect, or exploitation of children. The exceptions are: Alabama, Connecticut, Delaware, the District of Columbia, Idaho, Minnesota, Mississippi, Oregon, Pennsylvania, Rhode Island, and South Dakota. Thirty-three states will charge fees for day care services. Of these, thirty states are imposing fees below 80 percent of median income.

Title IV-A: Administration for Children, Youth, and Families (ACYF)

People who are receiving AFDC, or who are eligible for AFDC but, for some reason, are not receiving benefits, constitute the eligible population. Two forms of day care assistance are provided. First, all states provide a cash disregard for work-related expenses. This allows working recipients to deduct all expenses incurred in earning their income from their earnings, including day care, up to the amount that they earn. Second, a cash grant is sometimes provided when a special need exists, such as the need to attend school. This feature is, however, at the option of the state. Since the parent purchases day care, this program theoretically permits parents to select their preferred form of child care. Typically, informal care is utilized. This tendency is deplored by those who feel formal care is more carefully regulated and of higher quality.

Title IV-B: ACYF

Because Title IV-B provides unrestricted monies to states, day care services can theoretically be funded under this aegis. However, in 1977, only $57 million were expended in all; and day care represents only about 1 percent of all day care expenditures; therefore, this is not currently an important source of day care funding.

Title IV-C: ACYF

Title IV-C provides social services for Work Incentive Program (WIN) job trainees. Day care is one of the major services provided to trainees; and all recipients are eligible. However, the number receiving day care is not known.

Title I of Public Law 93-644

The Head Start program provides pre-school programs directed toward the low-income population. These programs have an explicit child development orientation to help low-income children, which may particularly include the children of teenage mothers.

Despite the size of these programs, it is clear that they would not begin to serve the needs of all school-age parents. More than 225,000 babies were born to girls seventeen or younger in 1976, young mothers who will need day care services for several years if they are to complete a high school education.[22] Therefore, even if the 420,000 slots funded under social services were allotted to teenage mothers, they would not provide enough children with day care services. Since the utilization of day care social services by teenage mothers is unknown, the actual impact of these programs on the school attendance, job training, and employment of teenagers is not known. Moreover, since state regulations vary greatly, the overall impact cannot be stated. It is known, however, that in Delaware, at least, a couple is forbidden from receiving day care if there is a husband present in the home, a disincentive to marriage. The availability of day care—especially infant day care—can be crucial to teenage parents who wish to acquire the education and job skills needed to be self-supporting, or who wish to take paid employment. The lack of such services undoubtedly condemns many young parents to welfare dependence.

Nutrition

Special Supplemental Food for Women, Infants and Children (WIC)

WIC, a program of the Department of Agriculture, provides funds to state health departments, or their equivalent, to provide food supplements, first, to women who are pregnant, post-

GOVERNMENT POLICIES 193

partum up to six months, or breast feeding up to twelve months, and, second, to children up to age five who are determined to be at nutritional risk according to state-set medical criteria. Studies have shown that foodstuffs are shared among the whole family, so targeting does not work as it is supposed to.[23] Nevertheless, pregnant teenagers represent a significant proportion of the clients for this program, although exact numbers are not known.

Programs operate in every state; despite spotty coverage, over 1.1 million people are served monthly with products such as milk, iron-fortified infant formula, iron-fortified infant cereals, fruit juices, eggs, and cheese. Between October 1, 1977 and June 1978, nearly $277 million was expended to provide such food supplements. Given the recognized nutritional risks of pregnant teenagers, participation in this program can improve the chances for a successful pregnancy and a healthy child.

Commodities Supplemental Food Program

This Department of Agriculture program makes surplus agricultural products available, first, to women who are pregnant, post-partum, or breast feeding; and second, to infants or children who are both eligible for benefits in federal, state, or local food, or health or welfare programs for low-income persons, and who are determined by a physician or other designated person to be in need of the nutrients in the supplemental food. Forty-one projects in thirteen states allow mothers, and children up to seven years of age, to receive canned meats, canned vegetables or fruits, cereals, milk and juices. Service sites do not overlap with WIC sites. Approximately 100,000 participants receive supplements, at a cost of $17.6 million.

Child Nutrition Program

The Child Nutrition Program of the Department of Agriculture finances part of the cost of meals for children in schools, day care centers, and some recreation centers. It includes: National School Lunch Program ($1.7 billion in FY 1977), School Breakfast Program ($151 million in FY 1977), Special Milk Program ($153 million in FY 1977), and the Food Service Equipment Assistance Program ($27,169,000 in FY 1977).

Meals are provided free to low-income students, and at a price to higher-income students; since all children enrolled in school up to age twenty-one are eligible, the program provides an excellent way for pregnant teenagers to receive one or more meals a day.

Office of Child Support Enforcement

The Child Support Enforcement program, within HEW, was initiated in August 1975, to assist states in enforcing the support obligations of absent parents, locating absent parents, establishing paternity, and obtaining child support. Each recipient of, or applicant for, AFDC is required to make an assignment of support rights to the state, and to cooperate with the state in establishing paternity and obtaining support. Child support payments made on behalf of AFDC children must be paid to the state. "If the child support payment collected is insufficient to make the family ineligible for public assistance, the family receives its full welfare grant and the child support is distributed as required . . . to reimburse the State and Federal governments to the extent of their participation in the financing of current and past assistance payments to the family."[24] The program does not, therefore, increase the income of AFDC families, but it does reduce the cost of AFDC to the public. States are also required to make their child support services available to individuals who are not AFDC recipients. An application fee and a charge for costs incurred may be charged of applicants.

The Office of Child Support Enforcement is required to review and approve state plans; establish standards and staffing requirements; provide technical assistance to states; and maintain records of program operation, expenditures, and collections. Linkages within states, between states, between state and

GOVERNMENT POLICIES

federal governments, and between federal agencies have been established to assist in locating absent parents. The salaries or retirement benefits of federal employees may be garnished to obtain child support monies.

During 1977, $410 million were collected. States collected an average of $1.58 for AFDC families for each $1.00 spent nationwide to implement the program. The success of the program in obtaining child support payments has encouraged the development of new legislation to assign rights to medical support as a condition of Medicaid eligibility. Information is not collected nationally on the age of fathers who are compelled to pay child support, nor are there any policies specifically regarding efforts to collect from teenage fathers. However, in 1979, a renewed emphasis was placed on establishing paternity for out-of-wedlock children; and thus, it seems reasonable to expect that more vigorous efforts are being made to collect from teenage fathers. Although some concern has been expressed that the government's pursuit of money from absent fathers may actually discourage fathers from acknowledging paternity and providing social or emotional support to children, overall, the program is extremely popular, due to its success in obtaining financial assistance from absent parents.

Administration for Children, Youth, and Families

The Administration for Children, Youth, and Families is housed within the Office of Human Development Services, HEW; it is not a program but an office administering various programs. Its mission involves the expansion and improvement of the range of human services to encourage the development of children and youth, as well as families.[25] Ten regional offices are coordinated through the federal Office of Regional, State, and Community Affairs.

A variety of research activities are funded and monitored through the Research, Demonstration, and Evaluation Division of the Office of Planning, Research, and Evaluation. Numerous research projects dealing specifically with teenage parents have been funded by this office. (See the list below for recent studies.)

The Day Care Division and the Head Start Bureau are housed within the Office of Developmental Services. Day care policies, standards, manuals, and guidance materials are produced by the Day Care Division. This Office also serves as an advocate for quality day care, coordinates interagency activities relating to day care policy, designs legislation and programs, and identifies training and technical assistance needs for states and local communities. The Head Start Bureau maintains statistics on Head Start programs, develops the annual budget, provides guidance and technical assistance to regional offices and local programs, and develops policy relating to Head Start.

The Children's Bureau, located within the Office of Services for Children and Youth, focuses on conditions that affect the general well-being of children. Policies, procedures, training, and statistical data relating to child welfare services (funded under Title IV-B of the Social Security Act) are developed by this bureau. The Children's Bureau has maintained a continuing interest in the implementation of parenting education within the high schools. Prevention, identification, and treatment activities related to child abuse and neglect are centered in the National Center on Child Abuse and Neglect and the National Clearinghouse on Child Abuse and Neglect.

The Youth Development Bureau, also within the Office of Services for Children and Youth, is responsible for programs relating to runaway and homeless youths, and serves as an advocate for youth both within ACYF and within other federal agencies. Programs for delivering services to youths are developed and evaluated within this bureau. In 1979, its grants program provided funds to 166 community-based public and private agencies that offer temporary shelter, counseling, and after-care services to approximately forty thousand young persons. Five hundred seventy-five of the clients were females whose average age was sixteen. It is estimated that for at least 10 percent of these young women, pregnancy is an actual or feared issue.

The Runaway Youth Act of 1974, which established this program, requires that within seventy-two hours of coming to ask for help, the youth's parents have to be notified, with his or her knowledge. Eleven million dollars have been authorized for this program annually.

The breadth of activities relating to both adolescents and the children of teenagers makes ACYF a potential focal point for services and research oriented toward teenage families. As yet, no formal overall statement focusing ACYF's attention on teenage parents has been issued. However, many of the individual programs address the concerns and needs of teenage parents. Moreover, within specific programs—for example, the runaway program—agency concern has been explicitly directed toward teenage parents.

National Institute on Drug Abuse

Although only about 10 percent of the population served by the treatment program of the National Institute on Drug Abuse is eighteen or younger, the adolescent is a high-priority target for the program's prevention effort. In FY 1977, $200 million were expended on programs that identify, treat, and rehabilitate narcotic addicts, drug abusers, and people with drug dependencies. Project grants are awarded for payment of the costs of treatment, rehabilitation, subsequent care, innovative prevention projects, and the evaluation of new approaches to prevention and treatment. The National Institute on Drug Abuse is part of the Alcohol, Drug Abuse, and Mental Health Administration in HEW.

The incidence of drug abuse among teenage parents is unknown; however, the consequences of any such abuse for pregnancy outcome and the quality of parenting seem especially serious. Particular stress on educating pregnant teenagers regarding the potential consequences of drug abuse seems warranted, as does special attention for the drug abuse problems of teenage parents.

Office of Education

Although HEW's Office of Education has not funded a large organized program dealing with teenage parenthood, the Bureau of Special Projects Program subsidizes small projects, surveys, and studies in areas designated by Congress to be of special concern. (This description of education programs is as they existed prior to the government reorganization, which established the new Department of Education on May 6, 1980.) Projects can be federally or state funded; the role of the Office of Education is to pay salaries of people who provide technical assistance. This program is designed to improve the quality of education in selected areas by experimenting with new educational and administrative methods, techniques, and practices. Several programs of the Office of Education seem potentially important sources of training for teenage parents who wish to improve their educational backgrounds and job skills. Among those are programs for vocational and adult education.

Vocational Education

Funded under the Vocational Education Act of 1963, as amended, the program provides training for youths and adults to improve their occupational skills and competitive position in the labor market. State programs include basic grants, program improvement and supportive services, special programs for the disadvantaged, and consumer and homemaker education. In FY 1977, the funding level for this program was $422 million.

Adult Education

Under Title III of the Adult Education Act, the program has been funded to encourage establishment of public educational programs that provide adults the opportunity to achieve basic and secondary-level educational competency, including training that will lead to meaningful employment. In FY 1977, $81 million were expended for this program.

Some education-related services are provided to the many community-based programs for pregnant teenagers under Title III of the Elementary and Secondary Education Act. Title IX of the Education Amendments of 1972 also deserves mention as the legislative authority requiring schools to provide an education to pregnant students who wish to attend school. Although schools are now prohibited from discriminating against pregnant students, the absence of needed services, such as infant day care, nevertheless interferes with school attendance for many young mothers.

Exploring Childhood and Education for Parenthood

The Administration for Children, Youth, and Families (formerly the Office of Child Development) funded two curricula dealing with parenting education. The Exploring Childhood curriculum was designed for schools to use with teenagers and young children; parents and nonparents, males and females are involved. This curriculum is now available commercially, through the Education Development Center. A similar Education for Parenthood curriculum was developed for use with national, private youth-serving organizations, such as the Boy Scouts and the Salvation Army. Private groups are now conducting this program on their own.

Department of Housing and Urban Development

Two of HUD's major housing programs may affect the housing of teenage families—public housing and Section VIII housing.

Public housing includes units that are provided to low-income households for a rent that is not to exceed 25 percent of a family's income. In the year ending on September 30, 1977, over

750,000 households participated in the low-rent public housing program. Section VIII operates in the private housing market. Participants select housing on the open market, and HUD underwrites part of the rent. Section VIII is a more recent and, as yet, a smaller program. In the six-month period ending on December 31, 1977, over 200,000 households received Section VIII assistance.

Eligibility for housing assistance in either program is based on income. Families with an income less than, or equal to, 80 percent of the median income for a family of four in the local area, adjusted for family size, are eligible for Section VIII housing. Although this implies that teenage heads of families are theoretically eligible for publicly subsidized housing, relatively few appear to actually receive assistance. The elderly receive a very large share of housing assistance. Only 10 percent of the household heads in public housing are estimated to be under the age of twenty-five, suggesting that few teenagers are heads. Although HUD regulations do not preclude assistance to teenage families, local constraints, such as the legal authority of a minor to enter a contract, might affect the ability of teenagers to form households of their own.

Department of Labor

Youth Employment and Demonstration Projects Act (YEDPA)

Since 1977, the Department of Labor has developed a series of initiatives designed to address the problems of youth unemployment: the Youth Employment and Demonstration Projects Act, amending the Comprehensive Employment and Training Act (CETA); and expanded funding for existing programs. This act incorporated many of the features of more than 100 bills that had been introduced in the Congress, into four separate subprograms. Together they provide job training, supervised work experiences, remedial education, and other supportive services for in-school and out-of-school youths. Eligibility requirements have been made deliberately stringent, often using family income of 85 percent of the poverty level for the previous six months.

Although the programs clearly had the potential to serve teenage parents, it was difficult to estimate how many were doing so, since the data were not being collected by prime sponsors. A few recent studies, however, do indicate that although a substantial number of teenage parents are being served, considerably more are eligible that are not being enrolled.

Since 1979, attention has been drawn to the need to use these programs as a vehicle for serving the special needs of teenage parents. In a field memo dated February 13, 1980, the department's Office of Youth Programs listed young single parents as its highest priority target group.[26] This new emphasis is reflected in the Administration's proposed youth legislation, the "Youth Act of 1980," which was introduced in Congress in March 1980, to replace the existing Youth Employment Demonstration Projects Act scheduled to expire on September 30, 1980. In the proposed legislation, pregnant teenagers and teenage mothers are exempted from CETA income eligibility requirements. The Hawkins amendments to the Administration's bill, which is receiving serious congressional consideration, does not specifically mention teenage parents, but it does allow prime sponsors to use 20 percent of their funds to serve youth with special needs.

The National Association of Counties' report on CETA's services to teenage parents discusses the many supportive services—especially day care—that the teenage parents need to be able to benefit from these programs.[27] And although the legislation authorizes using funds for these services, most prime sponsors are in fact ill-equipped to provide them. (The report describes several model programs that have developed innovative special efforts to enroll teenage parents.)

The largest of the YEDPA programs is the Youth Employment and Training Program (YETP); its goal is to provide the training and support needed to help participants complete school and/or gain unsubsidized employment. (In FY 1978 it was funded at

$537 million.) Other programs include: the Youth Community Conservation and Improvement Program (YCCIP), which provides subsidized work experiences ($115 million in 1978); the Youth Incentive Entitlement Projects (YIEPP), which is to provide part-time and summer jobs and training for school students ($115 million in 1978); and the Youth Adult Conservation Corps (YACC), which, in collaboration with the Departments of Agriculture and Interior, provides conservation-related jobs to out-of-school youth ($233 million in 1978).

Job Corps

The intent of the Job Corps—an older program—is to provide job skills together with a set of motivational and attitudinal characteristics that are conducive to satisfactory job performance—for example, punctuality. Training may take the form of basic education, including some college courses, or vocational training toward acquisition of a specific job skill. Job placement and counseling may also occur. Enrollees are frequently referred to other services, as necessary; in some cases, Job Corps pays for these services. In 1978, 31 percent of the enrollees were female. The goal of half male/half female is closer to being reached in urban than in rural areas. (In FY 1978, funding was $417 million.)

Office of Youth Programs (OYP)

The Department of Labor's Office of Youth Programs currently has three major discretionary efforts underway to develop information for the CETA system on how to best serve pregnant adolescents and young parents. Below are brief descriptions of the initiatives.

The Women's Bureau

OYP has funded the DOL Women's Bureau in FY 1980 to administer five to eight eighteen-month demonstration programs

GOVERNMENT POLICIES

that address the employment needs of adolescent mothers. The goal is to develop several possible models of intervention to be replicated eventually by prime sponsors. Contracts to operate the program models will be awarded to community-based organizations and public school systems.

Manpower Development Research Corporation (MDRC)

MDRC, a nonprofit corporation that designs, manages, and evaluates social programs, has been awarded a contract by OYP in FY 1980 to fund eighteen-month demonstration programs at six sites, for pregnant teenagers and teenage mothers who are on welfare or are members of welfare families. Community-based organizations will operate the programs, and special emphasis will be placed on developing and examining new links between the Work Incentive Program (WIN) and other existing service delivery mechanisms. The programs will identify local community women to work individually with teenagers and their families and coordinate the delivery of needed services.

Youthwork, Inc.

In FY 1980, Youthwork, Inc., a nonprofit intermediary set up by the Department of Labor, conducted a national competition to identify and fund exemplary programs for high-risk youth. Three of the fourteen proposals funded are programs directed toward pregnant adolescents and young parents.

Work Incentive Program (WIN)

This program is jointly funded and administered by the Employment and Training Administration of the Department of Labor and the Office of Human Development Services of HEW. In FY 1978, $365 million were expended; $385 million were budgeted for FY 1979. The program provides employment, training, job referral, and supportive services for members of households receiving Aid to Families with Dependent Children. All household members who are not exempt under law (such as mothers of children under age six, and disabled persons) must register if they are over the age of twenty-one, or between sixteen and twenty-one, but not enrolled in school full-time. Approximately 16 percent of the registrants were under twenty-two. Although the legislation specifically designates unemployed male household heads as the number one priority, this program has the highest proportion of females among its participants of all the programs—73 percent in 1976.[28] Many WIN registrants receive training through other programs, such as CETA. WIN registrants are referred to a WIN sponsor, typically a state employment service. Registrants are appraised, and, if accepted, they are provided with a job placement. If training or supportive services are necessary for job placement, they are provided. These support services are provided by the state welfare department on a 90:10 federal/state matching basis. The state administrative unit services are provided under the auspices of DHEW under the Social Security Act. In FY 1977, nearly 300,000 WIN registrants entered unsubsidized jobs, and half of these earned enough to leave welfare.

Miscellaneous

It needs to be mentioned that the child labor standards and minimum wage law administered by the Department of Labor also affect teenagers' employment—their relative attractiveness to employers—and their ability to earn income.

Research

Research on the topic of teenage childbearing and teenage family functioning is taking place in numerous departments of the government. A summary of project titles for 1977 and the department funding the research is presented in the list below. Several organizations have emphasized teenage childbearing:

- Bureau of Community Health Services:
Maternal Intervention to Aid Development in Prematures

Follow-up of Young Mothers Served by Special Programs
Jackson Comprehensive Health Education
- National Institute of Mental Health:
Psychological Studies of Minority Mental Health
Prenatal Parent Education and Family Relations
Behavioral Development: A Prospective Adoption Study
Human Predicaments and Human Services
- National Institute of Child Health and Human Development:
Family Formations and Fertility: Key Trends and Patterns
The Value of Children in the United States
Developing Measures of Parenthood Motivation
The Consequences of Early Childbearing: An Analysis of Selected Parental Outcomes
Consequences of Adolescent Pregnancy and Childbearing
Sequelae to Teenage Pregnancy
Long-term Study of the Success of Contraceptive Planning
Social and Demographic Consequences of Teenage Childbearing
Long-term Consequences of Adolescent Childbearing
Effects of Induced Abortion on Subsequent Reproductive Functions
Resolution of Adolescent Pregnancy: The Danish Experience
A Comparative Study of Family Planning Clinic Users
Consequences of Adolescent Childbearing
Endocrine Status of Young v. Mature Primagravida
Consequences of Late Adolescent Childbearing in the United States
Consequences of Teenage Motherhood for Mothers, Children, and Infants
Early Childbearing and Kinship Relations
Relations Between Teenage Pregnancy and Neonatal Behavior
Adolescent Pregnancy and Mother-Infant Relationships
- Administration for Children, Youth, and Families:
A Study of Child-rearing by Young White Mothers
Demonstrations in Education for Parenting
Ecology of Help-seeking Behavior among Adolescent Parents

Study of the Use of Support Services by Young Families
Assessing the Child Development Information Needed by Adolescent Parents with Very Young Children
Legal and Social Benefits of Paternity Establishment
Project TAPP: Teenage Pregnancy and Parenthood Program
Teen Parents Project
Intervention for Teenage Offspring Born Prematurely
- Bureau of Education for the Handicapped:
Developmental Education: Birth through Two
Infant Special Education Project
A Community-based Model for Intervention with Infants, Toddlers, and Pre-schoolers
Williamsburg Pre-school for Special Children: Model Program
- Title III: Division of Supplementary Centers and Services:
A Competency-based Program for Personnel for the Education of Exceptional Children
- Department of Agriculture:
Nutritional Status Studies of Adolescent Girls in Selected Areas of South Carolina
A Study of Factors that Influence Human Food Habit Formation and Change, Phase II
Factors Affecting Dietary Habits of Teenage Families
Teenage Pregnancy: Related Factors in School, Contraceptives, Family, Personal, Attitudes, and Values
Nutritional Status of Pregnant Adolescent/Adult Pregnant Women
Changes in Food Practices for Better Nutrition
A Study of Factors that Influence Human Food Habit Formation and Change, Phase VI
- Youth Development Bureau:
State of the Art Paper on Youth Development, and Assessment of Exemplary Youth Development Programs
- Office of Indian Education:
Support for Early Childhood Education Programs, Project SECEP

Reservation Education, Rosebud Sioux Tribe
Tribal Home Base
- State and Local Educational Program:
School-age Mothers Reentry Project

The Center for Population Research within the National Institute of Child Health and Human Development has issued several requests for proposals on the antecedents and consequences of teenage childbearing:

> Research on problems associated with adolescent pregnancy and childbearing involves efforts to understand the determinants of this phenomenon and its consequences. The continuing rise in the birth rates of adolescent girls is a matter of much public concern. . . . These developments have serious implications for the well-being of young mothers, who are socially, psychologically, and economically less well equipped to assume the responsibilities of parenthood. . . . Research is emphasized which is designed both to provide baseline data concerning adolescent sexuality and childbearing, and to isolate those factors that influence adolescent decisions concerning their sexuality and possible subsequent fertility. Emphasis is also on studies that analyze the contraceptive patterns of teenagers and examine how and why they resolve any subsequent pregnancies.[29]

In addition to research on social aspects of population issues, the Center for Population Research also supports fundamental biomedical research on reproductive processes relating to fertility and the regulation of fertility.

During the past several years, the Administration for Children, Youth, and Families also has placed special emphasis on research concerned with teenage families. In FY 1977, high priority was given to studies on the informational needs of parents of young children that emphasized the needs of teenage parents. In 1978, special mention of teenage parents was made when grant proposals on the family and child development were invited. More than ninety proposals were received; several new studies are likely to be found relevant to this topic.

Recently the National Institute of Education issued a request for proposals on the educational implications of pregnancy and parenthood among youth. Studies examining the relationship between education, pregnancy, and subsequent life-changes and the school policies that affect pregnant teenagers will be funded.

The Department of Agriculture has also funded a number of studies that concern the nutritional status and needs of teenage mothers. Overall, it is clear that numerous governmental departments have concerned themselves with aspects of teenage families. As yet, however, it does not appear that the data and results are being integrated and made readily available.

Discussion and Conclusions

From this bewildering array of programs, policies, and services, it is possible to extract at least a few organizing principles and conclusions. One clear trend is the overwhelming number and variety of programs in existence that could potentially affect teenage family formation and functioning. Many of these programs are not available to all teenagers, either because of eligibility requirements or inadequate funding; nevertheless, it seems likely that teenage parents represent a significant portion of the population receiving government services. Unfortunately, this statement cannot be documented with statistics because the data do not presently exist.

This fact suggests a second conclusion. It is clear that, for the most part, teenage parents are not a visible target group for government programs, compared, for example, to the unemployed or veterans. The Department of Housing and Urban Development, for instance, does not separate out teenagers anywhere in its program statistics. The Department of Labor is taking some first steps in considering the needs of teenage parents—for example, in experimental day care projects. However, conversations with government officials repeatedly confirmed the impression that teenage parents are viewed as a small and special group. Since data from the National Longitudinal Survey of Young Women[30] suggest that, among young women who are eighteen and of low socioeconomic status, over one-third of the blacks and about 20 percent of the whites are already mothers, it appears that low-income teenage mothers actually constitute a sizeable group. Given their low levels of schooling and their consequent difficulties on the job market, teenage mothers are also particularly likely to require the kinds of special training offered by the Department of Labor, but their needs are not widely recognized.

Therefore, although teenage parents appear to represent a sizeable, if unknown, proportion of the group receiving government services or in need of government services, their visibility tends to be low, and they tend not to be targeted specifically. Such tendencies undoubtedly lead to the neglect of their special needs.

This situation leads to a third general conclusion. Based on data-gathering interviews conducted for this inventory, it appears that few government officials possess an overview extending beyond their particular area of expertise. Management of programs seems to be conducted in a highly segmented way. Almost inevitably, conversations with a variety of people were necessary in order to gain information on any single program. This suggests that the young person in need of services is not considered as a "whole person" at the federal program planning level. They are seen as persons without job skills, or as persons without adequate housing, or as persons who need an IUD (intrauterine device), rather than as whole persons with interrelated problems and needs. Beyond this, the problems or needs of the person's family are, essentially, unknown. Perhaps at the level of service providers, the multiple needs of a person are met in an integrated manner. Presumably there is great variation in this from program to program, and from community to community. But few federal programs take an integrated approach.

Moreover, the present review did not uncover a single instance in which the parental family—the family of origin—is explicitly involved. Participation of the family is neither encouraged nor prohibited. As Furstenberg notes, "Policies and programs are designed to serve individuals, not families."[31] Since the family has been ignored, we do not know whether family involvement would be good or bad, efficient or inefficient, helpful or harmful. Presumably the effects of family involvement depend highly on circumstances such as the type of program, the form of involvement, the health of family members, and the age of the teenager; however, we have very little information on these kinds of issues.

Several recommendations inevitably flow from the above conclusions. More data specifically focusing on teenagers is needed. There is a need for data that addresses teenagers from a perspective that is broad enough to answer more than one question at a time. For example, data on education, labor market experience, fertility, attitudes, and family background should be gathered together, so that the interrelationships between different aspects of people's lives can be studied.

Similarly, there is a need for more coordination between government programs, a view that clearly underlies the recently enacted Adolescent Health, Services, and Pregnancy Prevention and Care Act. Although it is not clear that the services presently available are adequate to meet the needs either of teenagers as a group or teenage parents, only half of the monies expended will go toward provision of new services where needed. The other half is specifically directed toward the linkage of existing services. Helping the teenager sort through the maze of programs, policies, and regulations should improve program outcomes. It is extremely difficult and inefficient to expect each individual to figure out the system independently. One of the effects of encouraging such linkages, of course, is likely to be an increase in the utilization of existing services, which may create pressure toward additional funding for programs such as day care, job training, and family planning. While this may increase the costs of these programs in the short run, the costs of teenage childbearing to the public may fall in the long run, if teenagers are helped to complete their schooling, obtain employment, and avoid unwanted initial and repeat pregnancies.

NOTES

1. Stanford Research Institute International, *An analysis of government expenditures consequent on teenage childbirth* (Menlo Park: Author, 1979).

2. Kristin A. Moore, Sandra L. Hofferth, Steven B. Caldwell, and Linda J. Waite, *Teenage motherhood: Social and economic consequences* (URI no. 24300; Washington, D.C.: The Urban Institute, 1979).

3. Alan Guttmacher Institute, *11 million teenagers: What can be done about the epidemic of adolescent pregnancies in the United States* (New York: Alan Guttmacher Institute, 1976).

4. *The budget of the United States government: Fiscal year 1979*, App. (Washington, D.C.: GPO, 1978).

5. Kristin A. Moore, "Teenage childbirth and welfare dependency," *Family Planning Perspectives* 10, no. 4 (July/Aug. 1978): 233–235; and Kristin A. Moore, "The economic consequences of teenage childbearing," testimony presented on Feb. 28, 1978, to the Select Committee on Population, House of Representatives, 95th Congress, vol. 2, no. 3 (Washington, D.C.: GPO, 1978), p. 34.

6. Julius B. Richmond, testimony presented on March 2, 1978, to the Select Committee on Population, House of Representatives, 95th Congress, vol. 2, no. 3 (Washington, D.C.: GPO, 1978), p. 496.

7. Linda Walters, Personal communication, Sept. 1978.

8. James Storey, Personal communication, Sept. 1978.

9. Melvin Zelnik, and John F. Kantner, "Contraceptive patterns and premarital pregnancy among women age 15 to 19 in 1976," *Family Planning Perspectives* 10, no. 3 (1978): 135–142 and table 14.

10. Office of Population Affairs, *Report on population and family planning activities*, Report to the House Committee on Appropriations (Washington, D.C.: HEW, 1978).

11. Bureau of Community Health Services, *Program guidelines for project grants for family planning services under Section 1001, Public Health Service Act* (Washington, D.C.: HEW, 1977), p. 4.

12. Office of Population Affairs, *Report*, p. 49.

13. Office of Population Affairs, *Report*, p. 49.

14. Bruce Spitz and John Holahan, *Modifying medicaid eligibility and benefits*, paper 986-13 (Washington, D.C.: The Urban Institute, 1977).

15. Eileen C. Wolff, *Technical notes: Summaries and characteristics of states' Title XX social service plans for fiscal year 1978* (Washington, D.C.: HEW, 1978).

16. Wolff, *Technical notes*, p. 72.

17. Joy G. Dryfoos and Toni Heisler, "Contraceptive services for adolescents: An overview," *Family Planning Perspectives* 10, no. 4 (July/Aug. 1978): 225.

18. James Trussel, Jane Menken, Barbara L. Lindheim and Barbara Vaughan, "The impact of restricting Medicaid financing for abortion," *Family Planning Perspectives* 12, no. 3 (May/June 1980): 120.

19. Administration for Public Services, *Social services U.S.A.: Statistical tables, summaries and analyses of services under Social Security Act Titles XX, IV-B, IV-C for fifty states and D.C., April–June 1976* (Washington, D.C.: HEW, 1976).

20. Administration for Public Services, *Social Services U.S.A.* (OHDS no. 77-03300; Washington, D.C.: HEW Office of Human Development Services, April/June 1976), p. 94.

21. Wolff, *Technical notes*, p. 56.

22. National Center for Health Statistics, "Final natality statistics 1976," *Monthly Vital Statistics Report* 26, no. 12 (1978): 9, Table 2.

23. Marc Bendick, Jr., "WIC and the paradox of in-kind transfers," *Public Finance Quarterly* 6 (July 1978): 359–380.

24. Office of Child Support Enforcement, *Child support enforcement*, Second annual report to the Congress for the period ending Sept. 30, 1977 (Washington, D.C.: HEW, 1977).

25. *Federal Register* 43, no. 147 (1978): 33336–33337.

26. Stephen Boochever, *Improving services to young parents through C.E.T.A.* (Washington, D.C.: National Association of Counties, 1980), p. 15.

27. Boochever, *Improving services*, p. 15.

28. Lorraine A. Underwood, *Women in federal manpower programs* (URI no. 24400; Washington, D.C.: The Urban Institute, 1979).

29. Office of Population Affairs, *Report*, pp. 18, 32.

30. Kristin A. Moore, Linda J. Waite, Steven B. Caldwell, and Sandra L. Hofferth, *The consequences of age at first childbirth: Educational attainment*, working paper 1146-01 (Washington, D.C.: The Urban Institute, 1978).

31. Frank F. Furstenberg, Jr., "Burdens and benefits: The impact of early childbearing on the family," paper originally prepared for Conference on Teenage Pregnancy and Family Impact, Washington, D.C., Oct. 1978, published in *Journal of Social Issues* 36, no. 1 (1980).

6

Sex Education and the Prevention of Teenage Pregnancy: An Overview of Policies and Programs in the United States

Peter Scales

Introduction

Sex education as a concern of federal, state, or local policy is a topic surrounded by considerable ignorance, confusion, and mythology.[1] A wide variety of material relating to sex education has indeed been published since 1970. A recent project has produced over twenty bibliographies of material on sex education published since 1970—the references included in these lists number in the thousands.[2] In all these years, however, there have been few attempts to describe or analyze the variety of sex education programs being offered throughout the country in terms of the following questions:

- What kinds of sex and family life education are being offered today? In what contexts and under whose sponsorship?
- What is the role of federal, state, and local policy regarding sex education in schools?
- What are the goals of sex education, and do we know how effective such programs are in achieving these goals? Specifically, is it effective in reducing teenage pregnancy?

This chapter attempts to begin to answer these questions. Sex education provided under public sponsorship continues to evoke considerable controversy. Although the debates are often focused on the content of sex education, the central question of values concerns whose responsibility it should be to teach sex education to children and adolescents. Thus, this chapter puts the debates concerning public support of sex education in the context of the role of schools, churches, nonprofit community service organizations, and particularly, parents themselves. It asks what parents' views on sex education are, and how they participate in sex education programs.

Although many conclusions of this review are couched in necessarily qualifying language, one thing is sure: there is a great deal more formal sex and family life education occurring today in schools, churches, and communities than is usually recognized; and it has the support of the great majority of parents. In the absence of state mandates, in the face of small but vocal groups of opponents, and in the middle of a debate over what values will be taught and whether the family will thereby be preserved or destroyed, a solid array of models exists that suggest reasonable approaches for the future.

These efforts have proceeded largely without widespread coordination. Coordination among health and education providers, parents, and teachers tends to be localized and fueled by a few determined and dedicated individuals rather than the result of strong institutional backing involving states, regions, or the nation. There are exceptions, of course, and some of these will be described.

But the overall policy direction—the guidance backed up by legislation, sufficient funds, and a general consensus on goals—is missing, in part because a perspective beyond the evaluator's, the teacher's, or the individual participant's has been missing. Educators and policymakers can no longer ignore the clear social trends. The pattern today is for young people to have their first sexual intercourse earlier than in previous generations.

Twenty percent of teens under fifteen have had intercourse; and each year, one in ten teenage women becomes pregnant.

It is ironic that approval of sex education, including the teaching of contraception, has jumped dramatically since 1970—70 percent of Americans believe contraception should be taught in the schools, according to a 1977 Gallup Poll—yet there has not been a corresponding rise in the extent to which states require even the most basic education in human reproduction. In Massachusetts, for example, the State Department of Education reports that only fifteen of the state's 428 school districts offer some formal sex education. A department spokesperson was recently quoted as saying that "there are just too many other important things for educators to worry about today." Perhaps one of those worries should be that, in Massachusetts, the only significant increase in teenage births over the last two years has been an 18 percent jump in births to girls under fifteen.[3]

We can trace the lack of initiative in the schools back to the controversy in the late sixties, when the battle cry of some was that sex education caused promiscuity and unwanted pregnancies. Research shows this to be untrue, but for years, we have allowed this charge to define what is meant by "sex education."[4]

The following review will attempt to fill in some of the gaps in our knowledge of sex and family life education. First, some of the problems surrounding the definition and goals of sex education, issues of values, and program evaluation will be discussed. Then some basic information on the extent, sponsorship, and content of these programs will be presented, including a description of some approaches that might be considered exemplary models. The next section will consider parent involvement in sex education, leading into a brief analysis of the nature of the opposition to school-based programs and how such opposition has been successfully met in many communities. Finally, the role of the federal government is discussed; and a concluding section makes some recommendations for federal leadership in this arena.

What Is Sex Education?

For purposes of this chapter, *sex education* will be used as a shorthand term to cover a comprehensive view of the topic. Sex education has been defined by a leading professional association as "any information and opportunities for discussion about the process of reproduction, human sexual development, sexual functioning, sexual behavior, sex and gender roles, interpersonal relationships, sex and health, and the sociological study of sex."[5] Most professionals in the field, including this author, and many educators, church leaders, parents, and most adolescents themselves would concur with the view of the World Health Organization that sex education programs "should be far more broadly and imaginatively conceived to deal, not only with reproductive physiology, but with questions of ethics in interpersonal relationships."[6] The intent of sexuality education ideally should be to contribute to the development of mature people capable of making wise and responsible decisions. Some prefer to use the term family life education, but many courses entitled "family life education" or "education for parenthood" do not deal with anything but the biological facts.

The goals for sex education programs implicit in the above definitions are clearly broad, and encompass many aspects of human relationships. However, many have clearly expected and hoped that sex education programs would help to accomplish the specific goal of a reduction in the present levels of adolescent pregnancy. (See Figure 5.)

While prevention of teenage pregnancy may be an implicit goal, the explicit content of many programs has not been designed to reach this goal. It is clear, for example, that by excluding discussion of birth control and failing to provide decision-making practice in sex education programs, teenagers have been prevented from preventing pregnancies. Our review of many programs indicates that the majority of teenagers do not get the tools that allow them to consider their sexual and reproductive options and act on the decisions they have made. Sex education can have an ultimate effect on teenage pregnancy only in two ways: by reducing the amount of intercourse, and/or by increasing the use of contraception. We have enough studies now to indicate that "knowledge" about sex (often measured by a single item on the "fertile" period, hardly a respectable knowledge domain) can be high without the use of contraception. Education cannot hope to provide the tools for everyone to avoid premature pregnancy. There seem to be as many "reasons" for pregnancy as there are people and instances of sexual intercourse. Eugene Sandberg, Stanford University obstetrician/gynecologist, describes sixteen different classes of reasons, and he readily admits that the list is incomplete.[7] No facile categorization can do justice to the variety of human motives governing sexual behavior, but programs must cover those issues that are motivationally useful rather than politically safe before it is fair to rigorously evaluate programs against a complex criterion such as teenage pregnancy.

Evaluation of Sex Education Programs

If the goals of sex education are as broad and diffuse as indicated above, it is clearly not surprising that evaluations of sex education have suffered most from this lack of clarity and consensus on goals; that is, what effects do we want sex education to have? How can we expect to measure and document effects if we have no agreement on what effects are desirable? Many programs clearly are based on unrealistic expectations, and few are studied for a sufficiently long time to accurately assess their impact.

Dale and Chamis provide some caveats with regard to expectations of sex education programs, and list as "common misconceptions of a sex education program" the following:

- that it will relieve the parents and the church of responsibility for guiding young people and building values;

FIGURE 5
FEATURES, OUTCOMES, AND GOALS OF SEX EDUCATION PROGRAMS*

Important Features ⟶ **Important Outcomes**

Topics for discussion

Physiology
Skills
Values
Sex and personality
Sex-related activities
Pressure, exploitation, and assertiveness
Contraception
Myths

Teacher characteristics

Knowledge
Enthusiasm
Supportive discussion skills
Trust of administration and community

Classroom characteristics

Supportive atmosphere
Freedom to explore student issues
Resources
Activities
Co-ed classes

Program characteristics

Course credit
Time and place
Vertical integration
Involvement in development of program
Evaluation
Counseling
Provisions for disadvantaged

Knowledge about social and sexual topics

Physical development and reproduction
Social and sexual aspects of adolescence
Sexual activity
Birth control
Probability of becoming pregnant
Adolescent marriage and parenthood
Venereal disease

Understanding of self

Clarity of long-term goals
Clarity of sexual values
Understanding of emotional needs
Understanding of personal social behavior
Understanding of sexual response

Values and attitudes

Attitude toward sex roles
Attitude toward sexuality in life
Attitude toward the importance of birth control
Attitude toward premarital sex
Attitude toward different sexual life styles for others
Opposition to force in sexual activity
Recognition of role of family

Satisfaction with self and relationships

Self-esteem
Satisfaction with personal sexuality
Satisfaction with social relationships

Interaction skills

Taking responsibility for personal behavior
Taking responsibility for personal sexual behavior
Decision-making: social
Decision-making: sexual
Communication

Source: Adapted from Douglas Kirby, Judith Alter, and Peter Scales, *An analysis of United States sex education programs and evaluation methods* (final report), vol. 1 (Atlanta: Center for Disease Control, 1979).

Important Outcomes (cont.) ⟶ **Important Goals**

Social and sexual behavior

Communication: parents
  Frequency
  Comfort
Communication: friends
  Frequency
  Comfort
Communication: date or boyfriend/girlfriend
  Frequency
  Comfort
Communication: sexual topics
  Frequency
  Comfort
Communication: birth control
  Frequency
  Comfort
Communication: assertiveness in saying no
  Frequency
  Comfort
Communication: assertiveness in demanding birth control
  Frequency
  Comfort
Social interaction with members of the same sex
  Satisfaction
  Frequency
Social interaction with members of the opposite sex
  Comfort
  Frequency of group activities, parties, and dates
  Satisfaction with frequency
Social interaction: feeling concern and caring about others
  Frequency
  Comfort
Sexual interaction
  Comfort with level of sexual activity
Sexual intercourse
  Frequency
Use of birth control
  Comfort
  Frequency

Reduction of unwanted teenage pregnancy

Improvement in social, sexual, and psychological health

- that it will either lessen sexual "promiscuity" or stimulate sexual play through the stimulation of natural curiosity;
- that it will automatically reduce the incidence of venereal diseases or unwanted pregnancies;
- that it will prevent hasty, ill-advised marriages.[8]

Any program adopting these expectations, say Dale and Chamis, is "idealistic and unrealistic." Rather than seeking moral indoctrination, sex education should "seek to equip young people with the skills, knowledge and attitudes that will enable them to make intelligent choices and decisions."

The review of literature in the present paper indicates that decision making is not emphasized in most sex education programming, yet it is apparently this area that is one of the crucial antecedents to a variety of choices that can lead either to abstinence or to sexual experiences, with or without protection. What, then, is the point in demanding sophisticated and detailed evaluation from programs that, by excluding key concepts and experiences, are almost guaranteed to be ineffective?[9]

Early in 1978, Mathtech, Inc., of Bethesda, was awarded a contract by the Center for Disease Control (CDC) to compare successful and unsuccessful sex education programs and evaluations. They extensively searched the relevant literature since 1965, in cooperation with the Institute for Sex Research; conducted site visits to programs around the country; developed a criteria set for evaluating the success of programs; and assessed the evaluations typically used in sex education. Programs were evaluated on a variety of dimensions: goals and objectives, format, content, materials, personnel, accessibility, confidentiality, community support, and support for minorities. An extensive, though not exhaustive review of this literature by Gordon, Scales, and Everly supports the hypothesis that evaluations in sex education are still in their methodological infancy, and the Mathtech report concurs.[10] Frequently, reliabilities are not reported; no controls, either by subjects or by statistical analysis, are included; samples are drawn nonrandomly, or are too small for generalizability; and the basic question of appropriateness of evaluation to intended outcome is rarely addressed. Research has shown several intermediate variables to be important in understanding contraceptive use, and perhaps this is where our effort should now be directed. University of Washington researchers were recently awarded a National Institute of Mental Health grant to give young people practice in decision making and verbalizing about birth control. The group will be followed for several years to determine if this experience, as the literature would imply, has some effect on subsequent avoidance of ill-timed or unplanned pregnancy. As absurdly obvious as it seems, two University of Pennsylvania researchers have demonstrated that talking about contraception before intercourse has a significant association with whether or not contraception is used.[11]

Finally, evaluation in sex education needs to take into account the local context in which it's conducted. As important in any predictive equation as are the program topics are the pushes and pulls of the community—who is in favor of the program, and how do they back up that sentiment? Who is opposed, and what mechanisms, with what degree of success, do they use to prevent, circumscribe, or eliminate programs?

Mathtech's overview of sex education programs and evaluation methods addresses many of these issues. They first conducted a survey of sex education leaders in order to clarify the important features and outcomes of programs. Approximately one hundred professionals rated the importance of several hundred characteristics and consequences of programs in both reducing unplanned pregnancies and facilitating a positive and fulfilling sexuality. These ratings were then used in other contract work, including the identification of exemplary programs. (Nearly fifty exemplary programs were identified and described, including schools, Planned Parenthoods, church groups, youth agencies, state and local governments, and others.)

A comprehensive review of the empirical evidence for the success of sex education programs was conducted, and concluded that: sex education classes improve the knowledge of the students; some programs make the students more tolerant of other people's behavior, and possibly more responsible for their own behavior. Few studies have adequately examined behavior, however, and thus, these conclusions are tentative.

A review and critique of previous evaluation techniques was also completed, and new evaluation strategies were suggested, including a basic set of questions with which to distinguish adequate and inadequate evaluation.[12] The Mathtech project has also developed and tested several new questionnaires for students, teachers, and school principals to be used in several new models of good program evaluation. In addition, new tables were developed for estimating the proportion of young women in a program who are likely to become pregnant in a given period, without necessitating the collection of vital statistics that have assorted weaknesses.

Mathtech is applying all of these improvements in evaluation and program identification in a long-term evaluation of fifteen programs around the country under another Center for Disease Control contract.

How Much Sex Education Is Being Provided and by Whom?

First, before reviewing the extent and sponsorship of the sex education young people are currently receiving in formal programs given in schools, churches, and community-based organizations, it is important to note that the majority of them get their sex education from informal sources—primarily their friends—but also films, television, and magazines.[13] These patterns, of course, have been the basis of peer sex education programs. Few adolescents report that their parents have been a source of sex information; and even fewer say that clergy or physicians have been much help. As data reported below indicate, far more young people say that they have learned something about sex from school and from books than from their adult sources. This does not mean that students have anything resembling a comprehensive sex education program, but merely that, at some point in some course, they received some facts about human sexuality or sex-related issues.

Second, the research undertaken for this chapter revealed that there is very little systematic national data collected on sex education in schools, and what there is sometimes is contradictory. Though case studies and journalistic accounts are common, systematically collected and nationally descriptive data are also scarce on the following: sex education offered through religious organizations, family planning clinics, or youth agencies; and sex education for parents. There is a substantial amount of information available on curriculum packages or guidelines developed by a professional and/or interest group. There is little more than anecdotal or superficial information available on community and family involvement with sex education. Finally there are only rough guesses as to the numbers of children and adolescents reached by any of these programs.

School-based Sex Education Programs

The first issue to confront in estimating the amount and kinds of sex education taking place in public schools is how many states mandate such education. Several recent studies present a confused and contradictory picture, suggesting that this is a rapidly changing area and studies may quickly become outdated. For example, a Mathtech survey in 1979 found only two states that required sex education (Maryland and Kentucky). A 1976 survey conducted by the American School Health Association (ASHA) found that six states and the District of Columbia require some form of sex education (Hawaii, Kentucky, Maryland, Michigan, Missouri, and North Dakota). Another survey in 1978, receiving replies from only forty-three states, found that only five states require sex education at the high school level, but except for Maryland, their list of states was different from ASHA's.[14] Many other states have legislation permitting sex education or administrative guidelines recommending it, but it is fair to say that the decision to include sex education in schools is most often made at the district level. It should be noted that although fifteen states require "comprehensive" health education, ASHA reports that there is no requirement that "comprehensive" automatically includes sex and family life education.

Thus, mandates are only part of the picture. Many programs occur in areas with no mandates; and there are even individuals covering "forbidden" topics quietly and entirely on their own in highly restrictive areas. There is some indication that districts have been providing more sex education in the last few years. In 1974, for example, the National Education Association reported that, in a random sample of over eight hundred public school systems, about 70 percent said there was some "limited" provision of sex education, and only 10 percent said it was "fully" provided. The preferred mode was integrating sex education into "regular" courses, reported by over 80 percent of those who offered sex education at all as their approach.[15] In a 1978 study sponsored by the National Institute of Education, however, about 35 percent of 454 private, and 1,448 public schools in a random sample said that they offered sex education as a separate course.[16]

Regarding sex education in parochial schools, data are not yet available on the extent to which the Catholic part of this sample offers sex education. In March 1978 testimony to the House Select Committee on Population, however, Msgr. James McHugh, former director of the Family Life Division of the United States Catholic Conference, estimated that perhaps 50 percent of parochial schools have adopted some sort of program, many using a model developed by the Catholic Conference. (The model consists of a grade-one-to-eight program of texts for the teachers and children and accompanying guidelines for parents.)

Another indication of how much sex education is being taught in school is provided by a survey conducted in 1975–1976 of a random sample of 1,700 teachers in secondary schools about the extent to which they taught any topics relating to "population education." The findings indicated that, even most broadly interpreted, such topics consumed only a very brief unit—from five to ten hours within the curriculum—and only about 25 percent of all secondary school teachers were covering, within the population education area, topics that could be considered related to sex education itself.

In another study examining national curriculum variety, Hottois and Milner mailed questionnaires to superintendents of all school districts with more than five thousand students in 1968.[17]

About 55 percent of the 540 responding school districts said they had sex education programs. Again, the content varies dramatically. Over two-thirds of those districts with programs reported covering "human reproduction"; but only 57 percent covered "ethical standards"; a mere 39 percent considered "planned parenthood."

These figures are similar to the findings of Kirby, Alter, and Scales in their survey of state departments of education and the guidelines states produced on sex education. They concluded that contraception, masturbation, abortion, and homosexuality are clearly the least likely topics to be included; while venereal disease, the anatomy of reproduction, and family roles and responsibilities appear quite likely to be covered.

Another source of information about the extent of sex education taught in schools is to turn to the students themselves to see what they think they learn from school. Again the data provide a rather incomplete picture, and do not provide much detail about how much sex education is taught, or what was learned.

Looking at reports from students that Abelson and his coauthors conducted in a 1969 national probability study of several thousand adults (over twenty years of age) and young people (fifteen to twenty) for the United States Commission on Obscenity and Pornography,[18] less than 10 percent of the adults said schools were a source of sex information. The schools' contribution was increasing, however, since 38 percent of the younger respondents said the school was a source. In an attempted national probability study in 1972, Sorensen studied over 400 teenagers, but sampling problems raised some doubts as to the generalizability of his data.[19] Nonetheless, he reported that nearly 40 percent had "never read a serious magazine article about sex" and that just over half had never read a serious "educational book" about sex. In 1978, Gallup reported that about 40 percent of teenagers, thirteen to eighteen, say they have had a school sex education course; about 30 percent say they have had a course that covers contraception. Encyclopedia Britannica Corporation conducted a nonprobability survey of "more than a thousand" junior high school students in forty schools in cities where the company has local contacts. Among this limited group, 52 percent said that sex education was taught in their schools (and over 70 percent said it should be taught). Most often mentioned as preferable grades for sex education were the sixth and seventh.[20]

This finding agrees with the sentiments of 5,000 students, kindergarten through the twelfth grade, surveyed over ten years ago in Connecticut by Byler and her co-authors.[21] Their work, *Teach us what we want to know*, is a poignant cry for sex education to start no later than the fifth grade, because "that's when some kids begin, and after that it's too late." Adults are more likely to agree that later grades, typically early high school, are the most appropriate starting points.

In a 1976 national probability sample, Kantner and Zelnik studied over 1,800 never-married women, fifteen to nineteen years old.[22] Percentages of those having a sex education course can be computed from their published data. Asking respondents if they had ever had a course in which the menstrual cycle was covered, they found that 65.5 percent of the whites and 73 percent of the blacks had had "sex education." These figures seem quite high, if taken to mean a comprehensive course. It seems more likely that these respondents remembered covering menstruation in some unit or segment of a course; it appears unlikely that such a high percentage had a separate course or a full presentation.

Given these findings, is it really so surprising that a recent study of thirty-one books on sex education for adolescents found, by looking at "key words" and index listings, that most were inadequate because they didn't cover content that was interesting to their intended adolescent audience?[23] Gallup's 1978 survey also found that students whose sex education course included contraception were twice as likely as other students to rate those courses "helpful." Clawar also sheds some light on this area of sex education content.[24] He found that parents and children tend to prefer different topics. Parents become more uncomfortable with topics that relate to actual behavior; while this is what most interests young people.

Clawar also made an observation that will be important to consider when reviewing "Education for Parenthood" programs —many students find the emphasis on "family living" in sex education boring: "The theme of family living is mentioned over and over again. However, many of these courses fail to mention the alternative forms of the family that are operating in America today. The students are aware of this and feel it is just an attempt by the school to reinforce traditional values." In addition, Clawar noted that students are frequently more concerned with their short-term problems than with rather long-term considerations, such as marriage.

In spite of these many limitations, and the narrowness of much of what passes for sex education in schools, encouraging examples of innovative models exist. All exemplary programs share: an involvement of parents and community groups; careful, long-range planning focusing on the training of teachers and detailing of curricula; and a conviction that sexuality education, to be adequate, must go beyond the mere provision of facts, and enable students to clarify their values in life and about sexuality. These programs, like many others, find that inviting parents to review materials and make suggestions about content gives parents a chance to consider what their sex education needs are, and frequently results in requests for parent sex education sessions.

All of these programs approach sex education, not in terms of separate courses divorcing sexuality from other aspects of growth and development, but "in terms of the larger ideas of human personality and sexual identity."[25] Each carefully gears the curriculum to the levels of the students. Earlier grades (roughly, those below the fourth) concentrate on feelings—how students feel about themselves and parents, siblings, and so forth, and how different feelings are expressed; simple facts of reproduction—such as that all living things can reproduce other living things of their own kind, and that there are differences between animal and human reproduction; and basic questions about bodily differences between boys and girls.[26] At about the fourth- or fifth-grade level, changes that accompany puberty are discussed, and it is common for more depth to be given to relationships, choices and responsibilities, and the nature of values development. In about grade five or six, the human reproductive system is covered, and the specifics of fertilization are introduced. In later grades, more advanced information is offered; and issues such as male-female relationships, what love is, sexual attraction and interest, concerns about body size or proportion, and questions of "normal" behavior are covered.[27]

The successful programs tend to have periodic reviews and continued contact with parents and the community, not simply a one-shot working relationship. And they have benefited both from surveying what other communities have done and from using the kinds of decision-making forums discussed later in this chapter.

Thoms and Tatum, drawing on their experience of a very successful program that is now in its eighth year at George Mason Junior-Senior High in Falls Church, Virginia, outline a model of steps for developing a sex and family life education program: it begins with assessing the community's needs and interests, moves to examination of what others have done, and only after this preparation, considers the formation of a mixed committee.[28] It is suggested that the fifteen- to twenty-member committee include several teachers whose disciplines would be involved, representatives of the local clergy, a pediatrician or other doctor, the school nurse and school psychologist, the PTA president, and several parents.

At this point, the main tasks become selecting the teachers and detailing the curriculum; and this step can take a year of biweekly meetings to accomplish.

To summarize the extent of sex education in schools, it appears that between one-third and one-half of schools are offering some sex information, although sex and family life education are rarely offered as separate courses. Yet, it is probable that no more than 10 percent of students receive comprehensive sex education.[29] What is provided seems to occur within other courses, and to take up a small amount of classroom time. In addition, there are wide variations in the extent to which particular topics are covered. Elementary schools are less likely than secondary schools to have sex education, and schools in the South are less likely than schools in other regions to offer it. In general, students find schools to be a more frequent source of sex information than parents or other adults, but less frequent a source than friends.

Voluntary Organization Involvement in Sex Education

Many national voluntary organizations that serve youth are involved in sex and family life education for teenagers, parents, community leaders, and professionals, such as teachers, doctors, and clergy. Among these groups are the National Congress of Parents and Teachers (PTA), with two major projects; seven leading youth organizations involved in a project sponsored by the Administration for Children, Youth, and Families (ACYF); roughly twenty national groups offering sex education programs through their affiliates in three cities, in a pilot project of the Center for Population Options, formerly the Population Institute; and Planned Parenthood Federation of America, which offers sex education through many of its approximately 190 affiliates. In addition, other groups are involved at the level of producing pamphlets or booklets, holding health fairs, and providing speakers in their communities.

For example, several years ago the Red Cross developed a detailed guide on sex education for parents that was complete with discussion plans, curriculum suggestions, and bibliography.[30] The YWCA of New York City attracted over 4,000 people for a three-day health fair in 1978; among those exhibiting was Planned Parenthood. Future Homemakers of America trained youth and adult teams from forty-five states in the areas of birth defects and their prevention, attitudes about teenage pregnancy and parenting, and communication skills. Their mission was to reach their peers with projects about the consequences and responsibilities of teenage pregnancy and parenthood. The January/February 1977 issue of their publication, *Teen Times*, was devoted entirely to teen parenting; and provided a wealth of examples of young people reaching other young people through puppet shows, slides, radio spots, and many more activities. A selection of these programs will be described in a little more detail to provide a flavor of the range of activities such organizations are conducting.

- *Parent Teacher Association*. For many years, both nationally and in individual states, the PTA has had a strong interest in, and commitment to, promoting improved education for parenting, and has been concerned with teenage parenthood. For example, in recent years, collaboration with the March of Dimes through a series of national conferences resulted in a resource kit entitled *How to Help Children Become Better Parents*; a range of PTA activities in Utah resulted in a secondary-level parenthood education program, although even the word "parenting" raised a "red flag" for some people; the April 1978 issue of *PTA Today* called for sex and family life education in all grades; and the PTA is currently implementing a Bureau of Health Education pilot project to establish comprehensive health education—including curriculum guidelines—in six states.[31]
- *Education for Parenthood*. A consortium of seven voluntary orga-

nizations (including the Boy Scouts, Girl Scouts, Boys Clubs, National 4H Clubs, Salvation Army and the National Federation of Settlements), through grants from three federal agencies, conducted a variety of parenthood education projects for teenagers over a three-year period, but only ten percent of these included some sex education.

- *The Population Institute* (now the Center for Population Options) initiated projects with twenty-three groups in three cities, providing the groups with assistance to expand their efforts in sex education, which they had all rated as a top priority concern in an initial survey. The groups included the Red Cross, Boys Clubs, YWCAs, and many church affiliated groups. In the local projects, parents, teenagers, and other community representatives were invited into the planning process. Projects have included peer counseling, parent-youth discussions, sex education courses, and hot lines.[32]
- *Planned Parenthood.* In 1977, Planned Parenthood conducted a survey of its affiliates and found that about half of the 104 responding were offering sex education as part of their programs for teenagers, single adults, young married couples and parents, and also for the mentally retarded and physically disabled. Half of the respondents viewed their programs as "comprehensive," but one-third said programs were limited to biological information or facts on birth control. Unlike some of the school-based or other community programs, these projects were far more likely to cover topics of birth control and responsible decision making.[33]

A 1978 Department of Health, Education and Welfare survey of 100 clinics in nineteen states found that family planning providers, including Planned Parenthood, often provided the only school sex education in many communities.[34] However, this outreach would often be limited to only one or several sessions.

- *Teenage Health Consultants* (TAHC). A consortium of Minneapolis clinics banded together in 1972, and created a very successful peer education and peer counseling program that has become a model for others. The program has carefully trained over one hundred teenagers who, in turn, have reached over five thousand of their peers through rap groups, role playing sessions, and various community education activities. The program also lays out a series of steps for obtaining crucial parental support.[35]

- *Medical Students as Sex Educators.* In general, although doctors have been considered by parents to be among the most appropriate leaders of sex education programs, medical schools have only recently included human sexuality as a standard, albeit brief, element in their curricula; and neither general practitioners nor family practitioners have played much of a role in these programs (psychiatrists have tended to be more motivated).[36] However, one innovative program described by Quinn and Sklarew has involved Howard University third- and fourth-year medical students in conducting question-and-answer sessions for six weeks in twenty to twenty-five District of Columbia schools, with considerable success.[37] A national survey of medical schools in 1976, however, found that only 10 percent provided these kinds of "field experiences" in their sex education programs.[38]

It is difficult to estimate the extent to which young people are being reached by the programs of these voluntary agencies. Collectively, their influence potentially reaches to millions of teenagers; but what percentage of this total audience is receiving some sort of sex education program or material is uncertain. A very approximate guess is that about half are getting some kind of sex education from these agencies, although it is unlikely to be comprehensive, and a somewhat greater number are being reached through parenthood education programs that may or may not contain coverage of sex education topics.

Church-based Sex Education Program

Activities of organized religious groups are not easily summarized. For example, the National Council of Churches' Office of Family Ministries and Human Sexuality has not yet developed an overall statement of the efforts of its member churches. There are currently twenty different representatives from the Methodist, Anglican, Baptist, Presbyterian, and United Church of Christ groups on the official commission of family ministries and human sexuality, most of whom are engaged in some type of sex and family life education.

The efforts of most groups are directed by the Interfaith Statement on Sex Education, a 1968 document cooperatively prepared by the United States Catholic Conference, Synagogue Council of America, and National Council of Churches. This statement holds that the home is the most important locus of sex education; calls for religious organizations to provide resources, leadership and opportunities for young people; and maintains that schools and other community agencies also have roles in sex education. Rather than attempting to avoid discussions of values, the statement affirms that the most constructive tactic is to promote the understanding and acceptance of a wide variety of values. It goes on, however, to suggest that sexual intercourse within marriage is preferable to premarital experience. It does not mention specific topics such as birth control, abortion, or homosexuality.

A few selected examples of church based activities are described briefly below:

- *The United Methodist Church.* According to testimony presented before the Senate Human Resources Committee, the United Methodist Church is involved in training ministers and lay leaders in running sex education discussions.[39] Sensitivity to the primary role of the family is a main concern of this training. The April 1978 edition of *Engage/Social Action Forum,* a monthly journal, was devoted to adolescent sexuality; and featured six articles on values, abortion, legal issues, organizational policy statements, and sex education.
- The *Synagogue Council of America*. The Council is, like the National Council of Churches, an umbrella organization that coordinates, but does not represent, several groups of Jewish con-

gregations. Included in the Council are the Union of American Hebrew Congregations (Reform), the United Synagogues (Conservative), and the Union of Orthodox Jewish Congregations. Their efforts, aside from the teachings that all young people experience on the way to their bar or bat mitzvah, are mainly in the area of publications to be used in youth discussion groups. For instance, the reformed group uses *Love, Sex, and Marriage: A Jewish View*, by Rabbi Roland B. Gittlesohn.[40]

- *The United Church of Christ* (UCC). The church publishes the *Journal of Current Social Issues*, which frequently contains articles on adolescence and sexuality. Its Spring 1978 issue was devoted to sexuality, and its Fall 1980 issue to teenage pregnancy. UCC is also conducting the "Neighbors in Need" project, in which funds are granted to local organizations attempting to combat unplanned teenage pregnancy.

- The *Unitarian Universalist Association*. The Unitarians have produced (with Deryck Calderwood of New York University) a highly touted multi-media presentation entitled *About your sexuality*. Using filmstrips, discussion guides, and pamphlets, this program is designed for use with junior- and senior-high-age youths, as well as their parents. An evaluation study of this package, though marred by the methodological weaknesses of most sex education evaluation, found that a several month experience with the kit was associated with "increased family discussions" on sexuality topics.[41]

- The *United States Catholic Conference*. The Roman Catholic church has developed a curriculum that is used for grades one to eight, and features an accompanying parents' guide. At the heart of the Benziger Family Life Program is the "fundamental importance and sacredness of the family." Despite the heavy emphasis on the family, and the encouragement in general for the reader to form his or her own family, seventh-graders do learn that "they have a choice about someday establishing a family of their own."[42] They also learn, although inaccurately, of the "crime" of abortion. A 1979 survey of the dioceses found, however, that only 5 percent of church-based programs are considered "sex education"; but as stated earlier, an estimated 50 percent of parochial schools offer the Benziger Family Program.[43]

Characteristics of Successful Programs

Throughout this chapter a variety of sex education programs that serve as exemplary models have been mentioned and briefly described. Although we do not yet have evaluations that are able to relate successful outcomes to program characteristics, certain criteria of success can be pinpointed; namely, that programs are well accepted in the community over several years, are appreciated by the various participants, and are well rated by professional educators and community leaders. In addition to those already mentioned, there are other fascinating and valuable projects that cannot be described here for lack of space. Among these are the programs of Chicago Planned Parenthood's Teen Scene, the Teen Machine of New York Medical College's Family Life Theater, the Rock Project of the Center for Population Options (and its companion Sports Project), the High School Press project of the National Alliance for Optional Parenthood, the variety of projects in the Emory University Family Planning Program, the peer education projects of the Future Homemakers of America and the March of Dimes, Zero Population Growth's "Love Carefully Day," and numerous others. Whether school-based or community-based these programs share certain elements:

- The involvement of teenagers, parents, and community leaders in planning and ongoing support for these programs appears to be a critical ingredient for any successful program.
- Often as an outgrowth of parent participation, parents request activities that are designed to meet parents' own needs for information and to improve their skills in communicating with their children.
- The curriculum content of these exemplary programs ap-

proaches the topic of sex education broadly in the context of human growth, development, and relationships. They usually include discussions and activities that emphasize the examination of values and responsible decision making in the area of sexual behavior and developing communication skills. Most also include information about contraception.
- Training teachers is probably the single most crucial aspect of achieving success in any sex education program. It is the quality of the teacher that often creates the greatest parental concern about school-based programs, and, among the teachers themselves, there is doubt about their ability to teach sex and family life education.

In addition to numerous local or regional training opportunities offered through churches, universities, or family study/counseling centers, training is offered to individuals from around the country by the American Association of Sex Educators, Counselors, and Therapists (AASECT), by the University of Indiana's Institute for Sex Research, by Syracuse University's Institute for Family Research and Education, and by Planned Parenthood Federation of America. Each year, the March issue of *SIECUS Report*, an influential journal that goes to thousands of the top professionals in sex and family life education, contains a listing of upcoming summer workshops in sexuality; and the newsletter of the National Council on Family Relations (NCFR) also contains news of workshops and seminars around the country.

Parent Involvement in Sex Education

The issues regarding parent involvement concern the extent to which parents approve of or support sex education programs in schools, the extent to which they participate either as planners or as consumers themselves, and the occasions on which parents have expressed resistance or opposition to school-based programs. Again, there are no nationally generalizable data with which to provide an easy answer to these questions. Many school-based formal courses or programs appear to require parental permission; all permit children to be excused upon a parent's written request; and many build in review sessions in which parents can see the materials to be used, talk with the probable teachers, and raise concerns. (See, for example, the guidelines of the Board of Education, Prince George's County, Maryland.)[44] However, the majority of classroom sex education is occurring as part of other courses. In most of these cases, it is unlikely that parents are even consulted, much less required to give permission.

When permission is required, and where attempts are made to allow parents a review of materials, there are very few demands for a child's removal from a program. Jacobson described a Staten Island program begun in 1968 that continued its parental permission requirements each year.[45] A five-year pilot project, begun with a series of community meetings meant to share the program's development with parents, religious leaders, and other interested community members, was sufficiently successful to have resulted in the recommendation to adopt this curriculum in all the district schools (eventually reaching 10,000 of the 40,000 students). It was estimated that only 3 percent of parents refused consent; and "a great majority" requested instruction in the "Family Living Including Sex Education" course for their children.

This estimate coincides with figures from California. California does not require sex or family life education, but does require parental consent in writing for a child to attend any optional sex or family life education class. Fewer than 2 percent of parents refuse their consent.[46] Saxon also reports on a Connecticut school's human sexuality program in which parents were not involved in the planning; nor was their permission to attend required, although students themselves could choose not to attend.[47] In five years, only seven out of 2,500 students have asked to be excused, and only two cases of negative feedback have been received from parents.

One side effect of inviting parents into the process of planning and materials review has been requests by parents for their own sex education classes. A national study of more than a thousand parents of children between the ages of eight and thirteen indicated that 31 percent felt the need for classes and instruction in "teaching children about sex."[48] This is just what the NEA pamphlet "What Parents Should Know about Sex Education" advises: "Take a course in sex education." Kirkendall voices a similar note in the SIECUS study guide *Sex Education*: "It cannot be repeated too often that adults are the ones most in need of help."[49]

Several projects have been described in which parents have been the targets for sex education programs either preliminary to, or as a by-product of, programs aimed at the audience of children and adolescents. The NIMH sponsored a three-year program directed by the Institute for Family Research and Education (IFRE), in Syracuse, which reached over 1,200 parents in four- to six-week parent sex education programs led by trained community leaders.[50] This project, when evaluated, indicated that parents (mostly mothers) who took the courses reported improved ability to communicate with their children about sex, compared to a control group of parents who did not participate. In addition, impact was apparent in the community: about 40 percent of seventy trained community leaders also subsequently offered sex education to professionals, teenagers, and other community adults through church or club meetings.

In another example, the New York City Family Living and Sex Education Student Peer Information Project (1973–1975) was initiated by students who gathered some 9,000 signatures of support from other students, teachers, parents, and interested community members for a peer information and referral center in every high school. The total effort took three years before the City Board of Education gave its approval, and before private funding was secured for a pilot project in fourteen schools. The response of parents was tremendous, including parents in predominantly black communities, who have been considered (usually by white educators) "hard to reach": "So many of the black parents in our black communities requested adult sex education classes that our Family Living/Sex Education Citywide Advisory Council elicited the assistance of staff educators from local health agencies."[51]

Another successful effort to reach the wider community of parents—rather than specific parents who sign up for programs—is the National Family Sex Education Week (NFSEW), which has been conducted by IFRE yearly since 1975. The underlying assumption of this project is that parents are the main sex educators of their children; and that the schools, churches, and other community groups share in this task with the parents. The week is celebrated in October, and in 1978 was observed in approximately three hundred cities and communities. The projects in these communities have been varied, including articles in local papers and journals; spots on radio, TV, and talk shows; special seminars and discussion groups; book store displays; and community debates and surveys. The NFSEW has developed a newsletter, *Impact*, distributed to over 50,000 organizations and individuals; and an *NFSEW Notebook* has been developed as a guide for communities' future efforts.[52] A new effort in parent sex education is being conducted by Mathtech, with CDC support. Critical features of these programs are being identified; several model programs will be offered; and their impact on family communication about sex will be carefully measured.

If the large majority of parents are supportive of sex education programs in school, and many of these eager for information themselves, why, then, are so many school administrators reluctant to institute such programs?

Clawar studied literature on this issue and made the important distinction between resistance and opposition.[53] Resistance is frequently overcome when parents are appraised of a program's intentions, and have some knowledge about what will be covered. Parental resistance typically centers around three general concerns: (1) the qualifications, methods, and manners of the proposed teacher; (2) the content and focus of the course, including worries about stimulating children into sexual experiences they wouldn't otherwise have had; and (3) the fears related to dealing with children's anticipated increase in knowledge about sexuality. Administrators who oppose sex education tend to be concerned about a possible negative community reaction (which rarely occurs), while teachers worry about their own ability to teach sex education and about the timing of such a course.[54]

Kirkendall has offered some more possible sources of objection from parents, based on his fifty years of experience as a sex educator and counselor:

1. Parents alone know when sex education should be given; children are innocent and uninterested in sex until instruction is given; and parents will know when better than anyone else.
2. Children will take instruction for license and become sexually involved quite early.
3. Material will be offered value free, and taught without reference to religion or deity.
4. Parents are and should be held responsible for any misbehavior on the part of their children.
5. "We got no sex education when we were growing up and we got along all right."
6. The teacher is trying to work through his or her own problems in instructing the children.
7. If anyone other than parents do it, it should be doctors and clergymen who teach children about sex.[55]

These are the kinds of concerns that can direct sex education for parents, and which, if confronted openly and honestly, encourage parents to more readily support sex education for their children.

Sources and Management of Opposition to Sex Education

If parents are not primarily in opposition to sex education, who is? Opposition seems to come, not primarily from parents, or even from administrators or teachers, but rather from "citizen groups" that have traditionally not been involved in a community's educational decision making. Hottois and Milner's 1975 book *The sex education controversy* is one of the best analyses of this issue, and the only one known to this writer that is based on systematic survey research. About half of the 540 responding districts had sex education programs. In about half of the districts with programs, school officials were responsible for initiating sex education programs, while 32 percent were prompted by a broad-based PTA–like group. In this survey, "citizen groups" comprised nearly 60 percent of the opponents of sex education, but only 17 percent of the proponents.

A similar account of the nature of the opposition to sex education programs was provided by the proponents who responded to the author's survey.[56] The single most frequently cited obstacle to offering sex education was school administrators' reaction to vocal minorities. The group Parents Who Care was mentioned several times as successful in swaying administrator opinion out of proportion to its small number. Other more practical obstacles mentioned by surveyed respondents include: too many "dos and don'ts" regarding what teachers can include; lack of funds for running an expanded or new program; teens' embarrassment about signing up for a course; the failure of program planners to involve a wide range of community members, including young people; the inability to find a resource person to coordinate a full program (i.e., staff training, materials acquisition, parent workshops, and so forth; and the "inability to get qualified teachers who are at ease with both sex and students."

Hottois and Milner demonstrated that sex education opponents, more often than not, are ineffectual in influencing major policy decisions regarding sex education, and that media coverage tends to give the opposite impression by accentuating the actual level of "sensational" cases of successful or victorious opposition. The IFRE project came to the same conclusion. Upon analyzing letters to the local newspaper editor over the three-year project period, it was found that opponents of sex education had been given 50 percent more coverage (and half of their letters had been written by members of one right-wing group—Catholics United for the Faith). Yet, a random telephone survey conducted well into the project's first year showed that most community adults (over eighteen) approved of sex education. In fact, less than one-fifth agreed that providing information would stimulate "irresponsible" sexual behavior; and two-thirds said sexually active teenagers should have access to birth control services.[57]

In Hottois and Milner's survey, opponents were not highly successful in getting districts to refuse to consider a sex education program: three-fourths of the districts had at least considered a program by 1970. And three-fourths of these adopted a planned sex education program on the first consideration. Once a program got underway, opponents were even less successful. Similar to the NEA findings, only 5 percent of existing programs were eliminated on a second consideration; and less than 10 percent made their programs less comprehensive—almost half expanded the comprehensiveness!

In their book, Hottois and Milner discuss at some length the difficult philosophic and political issues found by those proponents of sex education who recognize the importance of respecting diverse values within the community, and want to encourage community input into a discussion of plans for new sex education programs, yet realize that it is not possible to satisfy every conceivable point of view in the development of these programs. Thus, the authors found that when opponents of sex education are unsuccessful, it is more likely that the dynamics of community conflict have been mismanaged than that the opponents have successfully convinced the majority of the rightness of their views.

They also found that, in general, the initiative for new sex education programs tends to come from innovative superintendents who may have been influenced by the spate of favorable professional articles appearing in journals in the early sixties. Articles in lay magazines appeared in the late sixties, after most of the programs were initiated. These innovators are successful in dealing with the community conflicts and disagreements by setting up working committees of laypersons and professionals, and avoiding forums of mass participation, such as public meetings, to consider such programs. This allows minority viewpoints to be expressed without exerting disproportionate influence on policy.

Most parents are eager to help provide sex education for their children, and, when included in the planning process, tend to request their own sex education classes. The media have tended to overplay the sensational successes of sex education opponents, creating the impressions that there is typically negative reaction to sex education, when the reverse is more accurate. Opponents tend to be comprised of political "out-groups" not ordinarily consulted in the usual bureaucracy of educational decisionmaking. Communities with something approaching "comprehensive" sex education have tended to utilize mixed committees of lay and professional persons in the development of such programs, and to eschew mass meetings.

The Role of the Federal Government

Numerous examples of federal financial support for sex education programs and research have been alluded to in this review. It is difficult to estimate the federal dollars spent on sex education-related activities, partly because such activities are carried out in many different programs and are mixed in with other activities. However, the total amounts are, in general, low. For example, a 1972 study of programs for school-age parents and their infants found that only 12 percent of programs reporting multiple-level funding included federal monies; and only 14 percent of single-level funded programs received federal funds.[58]

Potentially many of the programs listed in Kristin Moore's inventory of federal programs (see Chapter 5) and in a similar inventory compiled by the Special Programs Staff of the Bureau of Elementary and Secondary Education (BESE) could be used for supporting various kinds of sex education-related activities or research.[59] However, the major sources of support to date include: family planning funds (Title X), in which an increased effort in recent years has been made to target the adolescent population and provide information and education to them; health education monies, which have included a special emphasis since 1977 on teenage pregnancy; and some vocational education monies supporting consumer and homemaking education programs that sometimes focus on different aspects of parenting education. Federally supported school health programs (through formula grants to the states) sometimes support adolescent health projects; and there are several references in the 1979 reauthorization of the Title I of the Elementary and Secondary Education Act (ESEA) that suggest more emphasis being placed on family life and sex education, parenting programs, and population education.

In terms of research, the federal government has supported, and continues to support, several important studies concerned with improving our knowledge of prevention of adolescent pregnancy (notably projects funded by the National Institute for Child Health and Human Development, and the Administration for Children, Youth, and Families). Most recently, the Center for Disease Control has supported several new contracts to look specifically at various aspects of sex education (evaluation, barriers, parent-child communication, and model approaches).

Often, federal government support of demonstration programs and research has been joined by private sector support, and together they have funded the efforts of voluntary nonprofit organizations.

In sum, the federal support of sex education programs has been disbursed in many different departments; has had no coordinated leadership; and although the legislative potential for an expanded level of support in many programs is present, there has been no priority given to committing authorized funds to support such efforts. Furthermore, even with regard to information gathering, it can be said that there has been a distinct lack of awareness of, or priority given to, sex and family life education. For example, the National Longitudinal Study of the high school class of 1972, a study of 22,000 young people, did not contain a single question on their experience with sex education and their impressions of its value in their lives. The 1976 National Panel on High School and Adolescent Education talked only vaguely of the school's responsibility to prepare youth for "future family roles." And it is only in the last two years that the National Assessment of Educational Progress has begun to consider some venereal disease knowledge questions in its tests of basic skills. These examples represent missed opportunities that can be easily corrected.

In like manner, the legislation creating the Public Health Services' Office of Adolescent Pregnancy Programs failed either to stress the importance of primary prevention of teenage pregnancy or to demonstrate an awareness of the role which education plays in it. For instance, "prevention of adolescent pregnancies" was number fourteen in a list of fifteen components outlining a comprehensive approach to teen pregnancy that was presented in Congressional testimony, surpassing in its obscurity only the traditionally hard-pressed category of "evaluation." While education was mentioned as important, especially in terms of linking educational services with health care providers, the effectiveness of varying kinds of education or content was not acknowledged.

Conclusions and Recommendations

This review of the field of sex education has suggested several conclusions and recommendations for policymakers at federal, state, and local levels of government.

The federal role should be one of providing leadership, information, and coordination to those at the state and community levels who are committed to improving and expanding sex education efforts within schools and in the community.

Perhaps what is needed is a legislative initiative similar to the Educational Amendments of 1976, which revised vocational education laws with regard to sex bias and discrimination. Those amendments charged the Commissioner of Education both with developing a vocational education data reporting system, and with investigating the extent of sex bias. It included, as an explicit purpose, the overcoming of sex discrimination; mandated five-year state plans for accountability; and provided for revising curricula to eliminate sex bias. All these provisions can be readily applied to similar activities in the area of sex and family life education; that is, state boards of education could be held accountable for five-year plans of progress in sex education, could be charged with developing or revising curricula, and the Secretary of Education could be held responsible for developing and maintaining a data reporting system on sex education activities.

Sex and family life education is a classic case today of everyone reinventing the wheel. There is an urgent need for some kind of central clearinghouse that would provide easy access to research results and program descriptions, and a vehicle for communication between those working in the field. The government should build on and expand the preliminary efforts of the BESE Special Programs staff to catalogue and describe innovative programs and curriculum guidelines.

Vehicles already exist in the federal education field that could incorporate such an information network—for instance, the National Diffusion Network, budgeted at $10 million annually, whose purpose is to identify and evaluate exemplary programs in education; and the Child Welfare Resources and Information Exchange, which publishes bimonthly abstracts of programs that affect child welfare and are judged easily replicable. But to date, neither vehicle has given any emphasis to sex and family life education.

In the area of research support, in addition to current emphases, policymakers should urge that more priority be given to research and evaluation that will strengthen the ability of supporters of sex education to answer the myths touted by opponents (that parents are not in favor of sex education, and therefore, it undermines the family; or that sex education promotes promiscuity); and to determine what the effects are on children and family relationships when parents either do or do not permit their child to participate in a sex education program. The results of such research and evaluation projects need to be disseminated widely.

In addition, this author recommends that increased federal funds be used to support the following: teacher training for sex education programs directed at parents; employment programs for youth working in areas of sex and family life education (using CETA or YEDPA funds, for example, for peer counseling programs); more assistance in developing comprehensive curriculum guides and special curricula geared to the needs of special groups (such as Hispanics and the disabled); and public awareness campaigns with regard to the need for sex education, the levels of parental and community support for such programs, and the apparent effects of such programs. In addition, a broader interpretation may need to be made explicit in some existing enabling legislation. For example, although Title IV-C of the ESEA can be used for dropout prevention projects, only 2 percent of the funds are so utilized, in part because no such priority has been set.[60] Yet this seems a natural mechanism, for pregnancy is still the number one cause of school dropout among females.

At the state level, most states have policies permitting sex education in schools, but few have provided the kinds of information and leadership needed to enable district administrators to overcome some of their reluctance to initiate new or strengthen existing sex education programs. Some states are already active in developing comprehensive curriculum guidelines that provide helpful directions, or even mandates, to local school districts; but even these states fail to provide funds for sound training of teachers. In addition, even the "progressive" states fail to build into their curriculum expansions, workshops, or materials that would help local administrators deal with controversy. Such steps are vital to successful use of any guidelines.

The critical leverage in giving more priority to sex education exists at the district and community levels. Several of these points have been made earlier in this chapter. When public schools do not provide sex education—or when what they provide is minimal and perfunctory—it is largely because administrators are concerned about possible negative community reaction. Thus, much policy in this area seems to derive from concern for the "community," including the anticipated responses from parents. Yet, data and experience show that parents rarely oppose sex education, although they may temporarily resist it because of quite legitimate concerns about staffing and content. When these concerns are addressed, when the parents and other community leaders are brought into the planning from its initial stages, sex education programs are heartily supported, and even sought by the parents themselves. The barriers to sex education, and strategies for overcoming them, are the focus of a CDC contract being conducted by Mathtech, the heart of which is the case study of twenty-five communities across the country.

Many of the professional educators surveyed for this chapter felt that the churches in the community played a critical role in the development of school-based sex education programs. When churches in the community become aggressive supporters of such school programs, and when responsible church members are on task forces, school administrators, it is felt, are less fearful of incurring the community's wrath. Church leadership can lend credibility to the school efforts, and can reassure people that it is ignorance, as one survey respondent wrote, that promotes promiscuity; and that informed knowledge can strengthen the family and the very values the churches espouse.

As a nation we must decide whether "parenting" in the broadest sense is a basic skill akin to mathematics or reading comprehension, worthy of our monitoring and fostering from the earliest ages. This parenting includes all the knowledge and support needed to decide when, and if, to become a parent.

But we also need to remember that there is one issue on which both opponents and proponents of sex education agree, namely, that parents should play a major role both in the sex education of their children, and in preparing them for a possible parenting role. Without representation on committees, without an opportunity to meet teachers and review materials, and perhaps without an opportunity to explore their own sexual concerns, parents jealously guard the information flow towards their children. When involved, however, parents seem to accept the fact that they cannot be the sole source of their child's experience, in sexuality or any other area, and welcome a partnership with public school educators, church, and other community leaders in helping their children prepare to assume adult roles and responsibilities.

NOTES

1. This chapter is a considerably shortened and reorganized version of the complete paper originally prepared by the author. This complete document is available from the Institute for Educational Leadership, Suite 310, 1001 Connecticut Avenue, N.W., Washington, D.C. 20036.

2. D. Kirby, J. Alter, and P. Scales, *An analysis of United States sex education programs and evaluation methods* (Center for Disease Control contract no. 200-78-0804; Bethesda, Md.: Mathtech, 1979); available from the Bureau of Health Education, CDC, Atlanta, Ga.

3. C. Hartman, "Sex," *Boston Magazine* 70, no. 5 (1978): 104–113.

4. S. Gordon, P. Scales, and K. Everly, *The sexual adolescent—communicating with adolescents about sex* (North Scituate, Mass.: Duxbury Press, 1979).

5. From the definition developed by the American Association of Sex Educa-

tors, Counselors, and Therapists in *Sex education for adolescents and youth* (Washington, D.C.: AASECT, 1976).

6. World Health Organization (WHO), *Education and treatment in human sexuality: The training of health professionals* (Technical report ser. no. 572; Geneva, Switzerland: WHO, 1975).

7. Ortho Pharmaceutical (Canada), Ltd., *An exploration of the limits of contraception* (Don Mills, Ontario: Ortho, 1975).

8. G. Dale and G. C. Chamis, "Family life education program," mimeo, Flint Community School System, Flint, Michigan, 1971.

9. P. Scales, "How we guarantee the ineffectiveness of sex education," *SIECUS Report* 6, no. 4 (1978): 1–3.

10. Gordon et al., *The sexual adolescent*, pp. 162–193; Kirby et al., *An analysis*, pp. 10–24.

11. J. Delamater and P. MacCorquodale, "Premarital contraceptive usage: A test of two models," *Journal of Marriage and the Family* 40, no. 2 (1978): 235–249.

12. Kirby et al., *An analysis*.

13. Anna M. Rosenberg Associates, "Today's teenagers have no heroes," press release, Nov. 21, 1975; available at 444 Madison Avenue, New York, N.Y., 10022.

14. J. Sullivan, B. Gryzlo, and W. Schwartz, "Certification of family life educators: A status report of state departments of education," *The Family Coordinator* 27, no. 3 (1978): 269–272.

15. A random sample of 839 school systems around the country was drawn, with 575 (68.5 percent) returning usable questionnaires. The NEA study considered both elementary and secondary schools, and also the relationship between the size of the school system and whether sex education was available. In terms of overall offering, the only difference appears to be whether sex education is "fully provided" or not, with systems having fewer than 3,000 students (as compared with systems having more than 25,000, or between 3,000 and 25,000 students) somewhat less likely to be full providers (no definitional guidelines were supplied for these categories, thus adding a further source of uncertainty to the figures). Among those offering sex education to some degree, less than 2 percent said there was a trend curtailing the sex education; in fact, nearly 5 percent of those not providing sex education indicated there was movement to add it.

16. Questionnaires were returned by 454 (75 percent) of the private schools, nearly 80 percent of which were Catholic schools. The suburban and east/midwest sample statifiers were substantially over-represented. In the public school part of the study, 1,448 of the 3,000 returned usable questionnaires (72.4 percent), with the majority (60 percent) being returned by suburban schools—only 7.5 percent of this sample represents urban schools. Two possible explanations for the disparity between the NIE and NEA studies are, first, that there is a four-year difference in the time the studies were conducted, and second, that the NIE study surveyed principals, whereas NEA questionnaires were completed by "someone" in the school district office. And principals seem to be more in touch

with what is actually occurring in their schools—district offices often get reports that contain what principals think they want to hear, not necessarily what is really going on (Abramowitz, 1978). Susan Abramowitz, "High school bureaucracy: A myth exposed," paper prepared for annual meeting of American Educational Research Association, Toronto, Canada, March 1978.

17. J. Hottois and N. A. Milner, *The sex education controversy* (Lexington, Mass.: D. C. Heath, 1975).

18. H. Abelson, R. Cohen, E. Heaton, and C. Sliger, "Public attitudes toward experience with erotic materials," in *Technical Reports of the Commission*, vol. 6, ed. United States Commission on Obscenity and Pornography (Washington, D.C.: GPO, 1970).

19. R. C. Sorensen, *Adolescent sexuality in contemporary America* (New York: World, 1973).

20. P. Scales, "A quasi-experimental evaluation of sex education programs for parents," Ph.D. diss., Syracuse University, 1976; also see G. L. Fox, Chapter 3 of this volume.

21. R. Byler, G. Lewis, and R. Totman, *Teach us what we want to know* (New York: Mental Health Materials Center, 1969).

22. M. Zelnik and J. F. Kantner, "Sexual and contraceptive experience of young, unmarried women in the United States, 1976 and 1971," *Family Planning Perspectives* 9, no. 2 (1977): 55–74.

23. J. S. Rubenstein, F. G. Watson, and H. S. Rubenstein, "An analysis of sex education books for adolescents by means of adolescents' sexual interests," *Adolescence* 12, no. 4 (1977): 293–311.

24. S. S. Clawar, "Resistance to sex education," *Journal of Sex Education and Therapy* 3, no. 1 (1977): 28–33.

25. G. H. Thoms and M. L. Tatum, testimony before the Senate Human Resources Committee, July 12, 1978, Ninety-fifth Congress (available from the Senate Committee).

26. A. Moore, "Programs, services, and approaches toward the reduction of adolescent pregnancy" (report prepared for the HEW Secretary's Advisory Committee on the Rights and Responsibilities of Women, by Health Education Resources, Inc., Bethesda, Md., 1977); J. M. Quinn, "Do animals have belly buttons? Sex education at the elementary school level," *Children Today* 36 (Sept.–Oct. 1976): 206.

27. See Prince George's County Board of Education's *Family life and human development (K–12)* PGIN 7690-0505, Upper Marlboro, Md.: Prince George's County Public Schools, 1977.

28. Thoms and Tatum, *Testimony*.

29. Kirby et al., *An analysis*, p. 7.

30. K. F. Brooks, *Sex education for parents* (Washington, D.C.: American Red Cross, D.C. Chapter, Nursing and Health Programs, n.d.).

31. Now in its fourth year, the project includes Arkansas, California, Colo-

rado, Georgia, Indiana, and Pennsylvania. Pilot projects in these states are now being replicated in Arkansas, California, Idaho, New Hampshire, New York, North Carolina, and Ohio.

32. J. Senderowitz, "Youth agencies are enthusiastic sex educators," in *Searching for alternatives to teenage pregnancy*, ed. P. Scales (Washington, D.C.: National Alliance for Optional Parenthood, 1978), p. 31.

33. Planned Parenthood Federation of America, unpublished survey of affiliates, 1978; available at Planned Parenthood, 810 Seventh Avenue, New York, NY 10019.

34. In studying over one hundred communities, the DHHS report found family planning providers were the sole offerers of sex education in more than 40 percent of the cases; "Family planning and the teenager: A service delivery assessment" (obtainable from the office of the Inspector General, the Department of Health and Human Services).

35. Peer Education Health Resources, *Teenage health consultants program guide* (St. Paul, Minn.: PEHR, 1976).

36. R. W. Libby, A. Acock, and D. Payne, "Configurations of parental preference concerning sources of sex education for adolescents," *Adolescence* 9 (1974): 73–80; H. I. Lief and K. Ebert, "A survey of sex education in United States medical schools," in *Sex Education in Medicine*, ed. H. I. Lief and A. Karben (Holliswood, N.Y.: Spectrum, 1976), pp. 25–34.

37. J. M. Quinn and B. H. Sklarew, "Practice meets theory: A new approach to medical sex education," *Journal of Medical Education*, 53, no. 11 (1978): 916–920.

33. Lief and Ebert, "A survey," pp. 25–34.

39. J. Blockwick, testimony before the Senate Human Resources Committee, July 12, 1978, Ninety-fifth Congress (available from the Senate Committee).

40. R. B. Gittlesohn, *Love, sex, and marriage: A Jewish view* (New York: Union of American Hebrew Congregations, 1976).

41. J. Carton and J. Carton, "Evaluation of a sex education program for children and their parents: Attitude and interactional changes," *The Family Coordinator* 21 (1971): 377–386.

42. United States Catholic Conference, "The Benziger Family Life Program, mimeo, U.S. Catholic Conference, Washington, D.C., n.d.

43. United Catholic Conference, unpublished results of diocesan survey on family life education, U.S. Catholic Conference, Family Life Division, (Washington, D.C., 1979); available at 1312 Massachusetts Avenue, N.W., Washington, D.C. 20005.

44. Prince George's, *Family life*.

45. S. Jacobson, "Sex education: a community project," *Journal of Research and Development in Education* 10, no. 1 (1976): 23–30.

46. S. Brill-Lehn, *Sex education: A resource and strategy guide for California communities* (Washington, D.C.: Population Institute, 1976).

47. B. Saxon, "Our first five years: Sex education at Lee High School," *Journal of Research and Development in Education* 10, no. 1 (1976): 30–36.

48. General Mills, Inc., *Raising children in a changing society* (Minneapolis: General Mills, 1977).

49. L. A. Kirkendall, *Sex education* (SIECUS Study Guide no. 1; New York: Sex Information and Education Council, 1965).

50. Institute for Family Research and Education, *Community family life*.

51. Parker, as cited in Moore, *Programs*, p. 53.

52. For additional details see Joseph P. Fanelli, "Family sex education is theme of national week," in *Searching for alternatives to teenage pregnancy*, ed. P. Scales (Washington, D.C.: National Alliance for Optional Parenthood, 1978), pp. 7–8; also, Gordon et al., *Sexual adolescent*, pp. 194–225.

53. Clawar, "Resistance," pp. 28–33.

54. The Mathtech, Inc., research has found that, at least on paper, states tend to recognize the need for special preparation for teachers of sex education. Nearly half of all those states with any guidelines on sex education note that sex education teachers need special training (Kirby, Alter, and Scales, 1979).

55. L. A. Kirkendall, Personal communication, July 26, 1978.

56. One hundred sixty-two questionnaires were sent to the following: attendees of a Region I, II, and III conference on teenage sexuality in Jan. 1978; 1977 endorsers of National Family Sex Education Week; and members of the Sex Education Coalition of Metropolitan Washington. Fifty usable questionnaires were returned; and another ten failed to reach the respondents (thus, of those reached, only one-third responded). Quantitative analysis was not conducted. Given the low response, a qualitative summary of apparent trends was undertaken, and is referred to at times in this chapter.

57. Institute for Family Research and Education, *A community family life education program for parents: Final report* (NIMH Grant 13710; Syracuse, N.Y.: IFRE, 1977).

58. Beryl Parke, "Federal programs of possible help to school-age parents, their children, families, or communities," unpub. report, Special Programs Staff, Bureau of Secondary Education, Office of Education, Washington, D.C.: Dec. 1977.

59. W. Stanley Kruger, "Federal agencies with an interest in sex education programs," memo, BESE, Washington, D.C., July 1978. (Separate document available on Foundations with an Interest in Sex Education, and Approaches to Sex Education, abstracts of federally-sponsored projects.)

60. Office of Human Development Services, *Current Programs*, Tap H, unpublished report, n.d. (c. 1978).

7

Adolescent Parent Programs and Family Involvement

Janet Bell Forbush,
with the assistance of Teresa Maciocha

Introduction

The 600,000 adolescent women who give birth each year constitute a large group of clients with multiple service needs. As the problems of pregnant teenagers and teenage parents have received increased attention, the numbers of service programs addressed to their needs have multiplied. Approximately 1,500 agencies located in communities throughout the United States are currently providing some kind of service—ranging from comprehensive multidisciplinary programs that provide a myriad of health, educational, and social services, to a single service provided by one small agency.

Very little quantitative information has been gathered on a national basis regarding these programs, or regarding the numbers and backgrounds of the clients they serve. Also, little is known about their quality or effectiveness. The first part of this paper consists of a brief description of what is known about the kinds of service programs available and the history of their development. The second part examines their relationship to the other primary source of support to adolescent parents, namely, their own families. Since the question of family involvement has not been addressed in any published information known to the authors, the views and experiences of a small but representative sample of service providers was drawn upon. In order to explore this relationship, these agencies were asked questions regarding how much help they felt their clients received from their own families, to what extent agency staff attempted to work with these families, and whether they felt it was important to do so.[1]

Service Programs

History of Services

The issue of adolescent pregnancy began to achieve national prominence in the 1960s as data relating to teenage fertility became more available.[2] Several developments contributed to the growth of the service network aimed specifically at adolescents, as it is known today. For example, as obstetricians and pediatricians documented high infant mortality rates and other health risks facing teenagers and their infants, hospital-based demonstration and research programs were established. Many of these were supported with funds from the Maternal and Child Health Services program of the Department of Health, Education, and Welfare (HEW). Likewise, with assistance from other federal funding sources, such as Title I of the Elementary and Secondary Education Act, education programs in a few communities were developed to ensure continued school attendance of pregnant teens and also to specifically address the high rate of school dropout experienced by pregnant teens.

Other concerns associated with adolescent pregnancy included the growing number of illegitimate births and resulting public welfare burden indicating that the problem was not to be addressed by health or educational programs alone. An important demonstration grant, which funded the provision of comprehensive health, education, and social services, was initiated in 1963 at Webster School in Washington, D.C. The project, which was in part a response to community concerns in Washington, acted to some extent as a catalyst to the development of similar programs in other parts of the country.

At the same time, two national organizations, both based in the District of Columbia, were established to address the nondirect service needs of adolescent parents. The Consortium on Early Childbearing and Childrearing focused primarily on research utilization and information sharing among researchers and policy officials concerned with adolescent childbearing. The National Alliance Concerned with School-Age Parents (NACSAP), as perceived in 1969 by its founders, was an organization that would provide technical assistance to those working with pregnant adolescents and school-age parents. Part of NACSAP's mission was also the development of advocacy strategies for preventing high-risk adolescent pregnancy.

By 1973, there were an estimated 250 comprehensive programs serving pregnant adolescents, yet, the quality of these programs was not uniform. In its *National Directory of Services for School-Age Parents*, published in 1976, NACSAP listed information on 1,134 agencies providing some type of specialized assistance to young people who were pregnant, already parents, or sexually active.[3] The introduction to the *Directory* cites the constant state of change among the staff and services listed, noting that support services for young people who become pregnant or parents are often considered "frills" rather than essential components of programs. A random sample survey of forty-two such programs that was conducted by NACSAP early in 1977 showed that few offered infant day care of interconceptional services, including birth control, and still fewer offered services for males. Counseling about options like adoption or abortion was also limited. Programs generally developed services around the chosen pregnancy solution. The majority of young women at this time were opting to keep their infants.

Kinds of Services Available

The needs of pregnant adolescents and school-age parents represent a formidable "shopping list" in terms of the services required, which result in extensive involvement of a variety of public and private agencies. The following list of forty-two services, illustrates the variety and extent of their needs:[4]

Abortion	Emergency
Counseling	Shelter
Services	Twenty-four-hour service
Adoption	Financial assistance
Counseling	Emergency
Services	Ongoing
Advocacy	Food
Birth control	Foster care
Counseling	Housing aid
Services	Information and referral
Child care	Language training
Clothing	Legal
Counseling	Counseling
Continued casework	Services
Divorce	Leisure-time activities
Family	Medical care
Group	Pediatric care
Marriage	Residence
Psychiatric treatment	Post-delivery
Education	Pre-delivery
Accredited	Self-help (mutual help) groups
Child development	Transportation
Consumer	Vocational
Health	Placement
Parenting	Training
Educational counseling	Young parents,
	special programs for

Whereas a few public and private agencies have developed a comprehensive approach to this population, offering several of the sources mentioned above, most of them are set up to serve only the health *or* education *or* social service needs of young parents. Even more important is the fact that few human service agencies have set the needs of school-age parents and pregnant adolescents as a priority.

Comprehensive services generally include: prenatal and postnatal health care; general academic and special parenthood education; counseling services; referrals; day care; and occasionally, post-partum follow-up. These services are offered by community and state agencies, as well as nonprofit, private organizations. In addition, universities, particularly those with medical centers, frequently offer a variety of services to pregnant teens.

Residential homes, promoted during the late sixties and early seventies, were the forerunners to comprehensive service programs. These include Florence Crittenton agencies, Booth Memorial Salvation Army homes, and various Catholic Charities agencies. The programs were customarily established for young women in their teens who were forced to leave their homes to have a baby. Today, given a somewhat more tolerant view of adolescent pregnancy and the availability of additional sources of funding, residential facilities are diversifying their programs. There are some that have retained their traditional approach; that is, they function as temporary, private homes for single mothers.

Some agencies offer more limited services, such as referrals, counseling, or education. This type of agency might be sponsored by a YMCA or a local church, or conducted under the auspices of state health, education, or social service agencies. Some of the agencies are day schools operating under the aegis of the public school system. They provide required high school courses, in addition to parenting education and counseling, prior to delivery.

In general, the array of services that may be available in any community varies tremendously, and forms an irregular patchwork of programs that may not be well coordinated. For example, pregnancy counseling services may have little to do with foster care in adoption services. Prenatal health services to the teenage girl may be quite distinct from postnatal care to her and her infant. Also very few programs are able to offer long-term follow-up services.[5] In one recent study in Boston, a comprehensive review of available services was conducted and matched against 100 adolescent parents' own assessment of the services they needed. This study found that whereas counseling was the most common service offered to teenage parents, the parents themselves said they most often needed concrete help that was usually not available—such as financial aid, child-care, job training, and job placement.[6]

Funding

There is no single or typical pattern of funding for school-age parent services. The different agency histories, services, and locations have generated a mosaic of funding patterns using federal, state, city, or county government, or private, United Way, or other sources. In many agencies the multiple funding reflects the multidisciplinary nature of the agency's effort to impact on the needs of pregnant adolescents and young parents. In others, it is a desperate attempt to find even makeshift funding to keep a program together. By contrast, an agency with only one major funding source may simply reflect a lack of awareness of what other support might be available. Whatever the circumstances, the very characteristic of multiple funding sources imposes difficulties in planning, administering, and evaluating the services provided to pregnant adolescents and school-age parents. Furthermore, funding is frequently committed for short periods of time; and the levels of funding tend to vary considerably from year to year.

The following example of one agency's funding profile and the ensuing difficulties was cited by the principal author in Congressional testimony in March 1979, as it was quite typical of the situation of agencies nationwide.

The School-Age Parent Continuation Program in Seattle,

Washington, opened in 1965, and serves approximately 300 students a year under the auspices of the Seattle public schools. During the 1978–1979 school year, the Seattle program was funded by eight different sources. The two principal sources were the State Department of Public Instruction, which provided special education monies, and the Seattle School District, whose support is predicated on frequent school levy votes. Three of the funding sources operated on an annual budget cycle commencing July 1. Three others began budget cycles on January 1. The coordinator of the program estimates that one-third to one-half of her time is spent on fund raising, record keeping, and the filing of statistical reports. No additional staff is presently available to assist in on-site administration, evaluation, follow-through or outreach to former students.[7]

Agency Characteristics

The following discussion of the characteristics of program staff and clientele draws on the senior author's experience at NACSAP and upon specific information obtained in the survey and telephone interviews of twenty-one agencies described later in this paper. However, these characteristics should be considered broadly representative of agencies across the nation.

- *Staff.* Agencies vary considerably in the size of their staff and the number of clients served. Generally, most agencies are prevented from employing as many staff as they feel they need due to a lack of sufficient funds.

Social workers or counselors are to be found on the staff of almost all agencies. The comprehensive centers and day schools usually have accredited teachers. The larger comprehensive centers have physicians and psychologists, along with substantial administrative and secretarial staff, an asset lacking in many programs that suffer from financial constraints. Several agencies have professionals unique to their programs. Examples of these are art therapists, community outreach workers, adaptive physical education instructors, infant stimulation providers, and nutritionists.

Some medical facilities employ midwives. Public health nurses, family planning technicians, sometimes on "loan" from public agencies, or even students from nearby universities provide supplemental, if only part-time, help. Otherwise, part-time employment seems to result from economic constraints rather than lack of need for services.

- *Volunteers.* Agencies were asked in the telephone survey about the use of volunteers. Their responses ranged from enthusiastic to rather strong opposition regarding volunteer involvement. A few agencies who use volunteers extensively even employ persons solely to supervise them. One comprehensive center tries to incorporate senior citizens, churches, and neighborhood merchants into their volunteerism. Such a wholistic use of volunteer human resources seems to be rare; most agencies have neither the time nor the funds for the supervision of volunteers.
- *Clientele.* While the agencies refer to serving teenage parents, that is, fathers and mothers, in reality, the clientele is almost exclusively female. Although the young women served by the sample agencies are predominantly high-school age, the median age being sixteen, there are several agencies who work with pregnant women beyond their teenage years. All the agencies point out that girls fourteen and under are seen, but much less frequently.

The agencies included in the survey are located in many parts of the country, in both rural and urban areas, and thus represent the distribution of agencies nationwide. The number of clients served in the sample agencies vary from six girls living in a private residential facility in the Midwest to the 1,500 who pass through a comprehensive care center in Chicago in the course of a year. Although, when taken together the programs serve girls of different races and economic classes, the administrators of several programs located in metropolitan areas characterize their clients as being predominantly black and from low socioeconomic backgrounds.

Evaluation

Since the last ten years have seen a substantial growth in the number and scope of service programs for pregnant girls and teenage parents—from 250 before 1970 to more than 1,000 in 1977—it is appropriate to consider what is known about their effectiveness. Policymakers who are being asked to support new or continued funding for these programs and those administering existing funds are expressing strong interest in their being evaluated.

Unfortunately, the number of evaluation studies of such programs is relatively small. According to a recent article by Klerman, which reviews twenty-eight evaluation studies conducted since 1970, most "were either very limited in terms of methodology . . . or when the methodology was reasonably strong, studied a very limited problem such as medical outcomes or return to school."[8] Klerman discusses problems of design and research methodology, and notes a lack of clarity about what is, or can be measured in a comprehensive services setting. She also comments that most of the programs that write up their results are providing services largely to minority populations.

Klerman concludes that, "If one accepts observations based on rather meager evidence, programs are reporting achievement in some areas." The strongest positive findings are related to medical outcomes: pregnant adolescents are receiving more prenatal care earlier in their pregnancy, and thus, are reducing pregnancy complications, prematurity, and infant mortality. In terms of education, results are less clear, but it seems that comprehensive programs are helping more pregnant adolescents stay in school during their pregnancy, and some to return to school afterwards. In terms of subsequent fertility, the results reported in the studies vary; short-term gains were not in general maintained. (A very high proportion of pregnant teenagers have a subsequent pregnancy within two years.)

It seems clear, as Klerman urges, that we need additional evaluation studies—especially those predicated on careful designs—of teenage pregnancy programs. Some steps have been taken to encourage the development of effective program evaluation; for example, a detailed training manual for service providers has been produced by the University of Pittsburgh Graduate School of Public Health.[9]

Family Involvement

Family involvement is defined in this study as the extent to which program staff interview, consult with, and/or offer specific services to an adolescent girl's parents, siblings, or boyfriend and his family, and/or other family members. The contacts with family members may be at the agency or in the homes of clients.

To the authors' knowledge, there have been no published reports on the nature and extent of family involvement, so defined. There have been, however, a few reports of attempts to involve the teenage father,[10] and on the need to recognize the role of the adolescent girl's mother.[11] To explore this question, the authors drew principally on two sources: first, an analysis of information that was collected from a direct mail questionnaire completed by a nationally representative cross-section of fifteen of the forty agencies originally surveyed by NACSAP in 1977; second, follow-up telephone interviews that were conducted by the authors in 1979 with agency administrators, and also, an additional six agencies. The total of twenty-one agencies thus included eight agencies providing comprehensive services, eleven agencies offering at least two services, and two offering only referral services. Together they represent a wide range of health, education, and social services. Two residential maternity homes are included in the study.[12]

NACSAP Survey Findings

The original 1977 survey was designed to learn about the program's overall scope, funding, variety of services, and the clients served. One section of the questionnaire sought information about family support and involvement. Questions asked whom the agency considered its primary client, and whether families served as a source of referral. To what extent did agency staff work with family members? To what extent were agency services paid for by the parents of the adolescents? Also, respondents were asked to indicate who provided primary care of the infant born to the teenager. And to what extent did the teenagers' parents, siblings, male partner, or other family members participate in any of the agency's programs?

Responses from the sample of fifteen agencies were tabulated and analyzed. Several agencies had found the questions quite difficult to answer: they often gave vague, general answers or left them unanswered. Clearly these agencies did not usually collect specific information on the topics of family involvement, and, therefore, the answers reflect general impressions or "best guesses." Some general findings did emerge, and they are summarized below.

- All agencies in the sample identified the adolescent female as their primary client. None of them view themselves as offering services to the family unit, including the pregnant teenager or teenage parent, her parents, siblings, or other family members.
- Three-quarters of the sample cited other agencies as the source of most of their referrals. Referrals from family members were uncommon, although there were a couple of notable exceptions that did cite family members as a common referral source.
- Most of the agencies reported very little staff time spent with the teenage client's family members, although all except a few agencies reported occasionally seeing another family member, usually the teenage girl's mother. The comprehensive programs

appeared to be the most likely to be involved with family members.

- Most of the agencies reported that Medicaid reimbursement and other public funds were the source of most of their payments for any medical or other services offered. In addition, about half the programs reported that the parents contributed a small portion of the fees.
- It was notably difficult for the agencies to identify who cared for the teenager's baby. Several reported that the majority of babies—90 percent, in some cases—were cared for by the adolescent mothers. But since these agencies also reported that the adolescents were usually living with their own parents, it seems likely both that in many cases, the care of the baby would have been shared with other family members, and that in some cases, the maternal grandmother could well have been the primary caregiver. The responses undoubtedly reflect the fact that very few of the agencies provided long-term services or extensive follow-up to their clients after the birth of the baby. It is important to note that the maternity homes and residential facilities included in the study reported a much larger proportion of the teenagers' babies being cared for in foster or adoptive homes.
- With regard to the issue of family involvement, agencies were asked to indicate which family members participated in various aspects of the agency's program. Almost half of the agencies reported that there was little or no involvement of anyone other than the teenage girl and her infant. Five reported no contact whatsoever with the father of the baby; and overall, it seems that only about 10 percent of the fathers participated. A couple of the agencies involved the fathers to a much greater extent, one reporting 50 percent of the fathers being involved in at least one aspect of the program.

When family members were invited, the maternal grandmother was the family member most likely to participate, especially in counseling sessions, at the time of labor and delivery, and in visits to the newborn nursery. The maternal grandfather was reported as occasionally participating. Other members of the family, such as siblings or aunts, rarely were seen, except in the newborn nursery. Similarly although two programs mentioned that the teenage girls' friends were frequently present at clinic visits, the usual response was to report very little involvement of friends.

It is important to note that three of the agencies in the sample deal with girls who have pathological home lives, some of them severe. These agencies responded that family involvement was usually out of the question. The teens who have no home life, or whose home life is beset with insurmountable problems, receive services from these agencies that are much more vital. Such young women appear to be atypical, but there are not sufficient data to be able to assess their proportion in the population of pregnant teenagers as a whole.

Thus, this small but representative sample confirms the general impression that families of adolescent clients are not involved by the service providers in the agency program. And yet, the exceptions to this practice—the few agencies that do encourage involvement of the male partner or teenager's mother more actively—suggest that a wide range of practice on this issue exists, and thus, that more family involvement may well be possible or desirable for a broader group of agencies.

Follow-up Telephone Interviews

The program administrators who were interviewed on the phone had been sent a copy of the follow-up questions that were to be asked them, in advance. As was explained to the administrators, the authors were interested in following up the written survey findings with a discussion of what the administrators perceived as the role that teenagers' families play in coping with pregnancy and parenthood. Of particular interest, therefore, was the extent to which programs are aware of this role and actually seek to involve families. A further objective was to learn how much importance agency administrators assign to family involvement and at what point—and for what reason—in the services they would involve parents, siblings, or other family members.

The informality of the telephone contact precluded the collection of any quantitative data. Since the intent was to gain more qualitative and descriptive information than was possible in the written questionnaire, the findings of these interviews, although they give a diverse and informative picture, may not be generalizable to other agencies across the nation.

Adolescent Clients' Family Situations

With the exception of the three previously mentioned agencies who work with teens from severely disrupted homes, the general impression of the administrators was that teenagers remained at home with their families during and after pregnancies. Even those adolescents living in residential facilities usually returned to their own homes after delivery. (A few girls returned to the foster care system.)

In almost all cases, family members were aware of the pregnancy by the time the girl came to the agency. In general, it was reported that the common reaction of parents to news of their daughter's pregnancy was shock. Very little was known about subsequent reactions or how the situation was worked out. Some administrators seemed to have a greater awareness of how parents felt; but certainly, this was not a concern (as long as the situation was not dangerous). And in general, when reference was made to the teenager's parents, the parent most likely to be known to the agency was the teenager's mother.

The comment was offered on several occasions that most families are supportive. Yet, several mentioned instances of foster care and references to family problems that would seem to preclude any such broad generalization. However, the admitted current trend of the increased numbers of adolescents keeping the baby would seem to indicate that most families are, indeed, supportive of their daughter's pregnancy in practical ways. The interviewers also frequently mentioned their awareness that, after delivery, the grandmother very often becomes the primary caregiver for the new baby, thus confirming impressions of the few researchers who have looked at this question.

Family Involvement in Services

The agencies' relationship to the families varied with the nature of the services. The closer they worked with the young women—that is, the more time they spent in providing the girls with counseling and educational activities—the more likely they were to be interested in involving family members. There appear to be no real indicators to predict why some agencies follow through with family involvement while others do not. At its current level, any kind of family involvement is unique and irregular. Since the teenager is the primary client, and any time spent with her is limited by pressures of staffing, inadequate funds, and numbers of teens who need services, the notion of involving family members is either alien or presents problems that most agencies cannot, or will not, confront.

Looking to another, less personal option of family involvement, we asked specifically if parents of teenagers in the community served as board members, volunteers, or on an advisory committee. Clearly, the cases in which such community members were included were inadvertent rather than intentional.

Almost all agencies conducted an "intake interview," usually involving an agency social worker and the pregnant teen. None of the agencies mandated interviews with other family members as part of the intake process or later. Most administrators said it was at this time that a family history was gathered from the adolescent. The exceptions in this sample were the two residential facilities. Although one facility does not take a history per se, the mother and daughter generally visit prior to enrollment. The other agency mentioned that it spent little time on this initial activity, so as to avoid stress. In several cases in which girls were referred to one agency by another, a family history was sent along with the girls' records.

A few of the agencies encouraged family involvement by offering counseling sessions, group and individual, to parents, siblings and boyfriends. Their enthusiasm for family involvement seemed to be a reaction to the success of the outreach. It is difficult to judge how much effort went into this outreach. From their replies to the questions, it seems that this kind of endeavor requires a long period of trial and error, and a strong sense of determination. Clearly, most of the agencies in the sample did not give family involvement a high priority. (It should be noted that there are some agencies that serve girls from distant localities, a condition that precludes family involvement.) Outreach efforts were much more common to comprehensive centers with large staffs and a great number of services. Of special interest were two agencies that have programs involving counseling and discussion for siblings, focusing especially on sisters, since they appear to be a particularly high-risk group. One program could only see selected families because of time limitations. Another agency admitted that lack of time and training prevented them from seeing families at all. They were cautious about family involvement in general, noting that unless a counselor could devote a great deal of time to a family and follow through properly, the impact of intervention could be negative.

The day school programs had the least family interaction. Interaction amounted to very limited and traditional programming like parent-teacher meetings or an annual open house. Most of the programs described family counseling either as taking place occasionally or when appropriate, or as an activity that they tried to engage in as often as they could.

Two programs were exceptions to this general rule. One administrator described an extremely active grandmothers' group that was supplemented with frequent home visits. This agency realized that the grandmothers were primary caregivers for the teenager's baby, and wanted to impress upon these women that the agency was trying to help the teenager and not usurp the grandmother's role. The administrator noted that many grandmothers seemed to feel threatened by the professionals. Visiting the family at home was a way of allaying such fears.

Another agency reported making attempts to see the families at least once a week, and minimally, three times during the course of the pregnancy. They were extremely supportive on the issue of family involvement and readily acknowledged the usefulness of working with the entire family rather than a single member taken out of the context of her home life. This agency was an exception in the study sample.

The residential facilities allowed or encouraged weekend visits from families. Apparently, this is the full extent of their family interaction. And this would seem to be primarily a social time for the girl and her family, not a time for the staff to meet with them all.

Home visits are even less common than instances of programming for family members at the agency. The restriction here seems to be staff time. One agency conducts weekly visits to those homes providing foster care for a teenager. In addition, they stress the large amount of time spent on telephone contact with other families. For those few agencies that mentioned incorporating home visits into their services, the value of viewing the girl with her family and baby in a natural setting was critical to their assessment of child care. From these visits, they learned who was really taking care of the baby, and thus gained a perspective that allowed them to more fully understand the extent of the needs of a particular family.

In one conversation with an administrator from a large urban agency, a theory about services was presented that bears credibility, in as much as it was mentioned or alluded to by others also. The administrator stated that from a teenager's perspective, a pregnancy is a very short-term crisis, the greatest hurdle probably being her family's reaction. Once the family is informed and accepts her condition—with or without the agency's help—the crisis is over. Even though the agency offers multiple counseling services to a community aware of their availability, teens and parents rarely take advantage of them. It seems that what the agency has to offer, and what the community of pregnant teens and their families have, or perceive need of, is simply not well matched.

The interviewees reported resistance to some services, counseling in particular. The inference of mental disorder requiring help from a counselor or psychologist was strongly resented.

One administrator's hypothesis, which was reported by several respondents, was that young people, especially poor young people, lack a sense of the future, which means that even a pregnancy is dealt with in a very short-term manner. Technically, a pregnancy is short-term, lasting only nine months. However, since most teens keep their babies now, it appears that the new generation of infants may be receiving insufficient consideration, both from the teenager who becomes pregnant and from service providers. The interviewers confirmed that follow-up services appear to be almost as infrequent as family involvement. And after delivery, when the teen mother is ready to complete her interrupted education or to find employment, it is dubious whether either of these options will truly be available to her. She and her baby will need good, reliable, and inexpensive day care—a rare commodity even for more mature mothers with greater financial resources. In those cases where the grandmother assumes responsibility for child care, the teenager may often see her own mothering role as being undermined. Several agencies noted that the resentment these teenagers feel may cause them to leave school or their jobs so that they can reinstate their motherhood.

Teenage Pregnancy as a Family Pattern

Through discussion or interviews with, or about, families, many of the agencies have uncovered a repetitive pattern of teenage pregnancy passed on to the next generation. That is, the mothers of the teenagers had themselves been pregnant as teenagers. Some of the agencies noted also that sisters often experience teenage pregnancy. Second and third pregnancies for the same girl are found to be common at the comprehensive centers. (The smaller agencies theorized that the girls were too embarrassed to return to them in the event of a subsequent pregnancy.) Again, these are important trends that are virtually untracked. That they exist tells something about the motivational level of the young mothers and the unsuccessful attempts at secondary prevention by service providers.

Teenage Fathers

One program director referred to teenage fathers as the "invisible commodity." By contrast, however, a few communities are making efforts to involve them to a much greater extent. Outreach to the boys, as to the families, requires a high level of motivation and an even higher degree of persistence. In this case, an easy generalization can be made: a teenage girl is much more likely to turn to her family than to her boyfriend. When he is an "invisible commodity," she has no choice. Several agency staff remarked about the anger they heard when the girls were trying to come to grips with their situation, and perceived virtually no consequences for their partner. A popular line of thinking is that many boys are afraid of being pinned with a paternity "rap" that they simply cannot afford.

Some agencies have tried to bring in the fathers and failed. The only day school that sounded at all progressive in its policy towards pregnant adolescents has recently had two fathers actually request to attend the alternative school program. One comprehensive program which successfully involves males probably does so because of its individualistic approach. Initially it deals with the boy and his own problems. Then, after he is assimilated into the agency and feels more comfortable, it involves him as a parent.

One program, mentioned previously for its more than usual family involvement, had counseling sessions for both of the teenage parents and their families together. Of course, not every family participated, but that such an option even existed was clearly unusual for these programs.

Summary and Conclusion

Information gained from this varied sample of programs across the country indicates that, in general, agencies have very little specific information about the kind and extent of practical help that families provide their pregnant teenagers, although it was the impression that most pregnant teens, and many teenage parents, continue to live with their families. If pressed further, most agency administrators would readily admit that it was their impression that the grandmothers tended to provide a great deal of the child care for the new baby.

Although many of these experienced programmers did recognize that the adolescent girl's family is much affected by, and involved in, her pregnancy and subsequent parenting, for the most part, services have yet to incorporate this realization into the design of their programs. There may be several reasons for this lack of involvement, particularly the lack of sufficient funding and staff to broaden services to include family members. However, several of the agencies interviewed on the telephone seemed unclear about the need to give family involvement any priority.

A clear distinction needs to be made, however, between the majority of agencies described in the sample and those few agencies who serve teenagers who do *not* have family supports available. A few of the programs interviewed serve adolescents who had come from severely disrupted family backgrounds and had come from, or would be moving into, foster or institutional care. These were the programs that reported virtually no involvement at all with the adolescents' families.

The interviewers, however, discovered several agencies that were exceptions to the more general lack of family involvement.

A few agencies have purposefully built into their programs individual and group counseling sessions for family members, including, in at least one case, groups for the sisters of the pregnant girls; these commonly reach out to involve the teenager's mother, and may also make home visits. Such programs clearly felt their involvement led to more effective and efficient services.

The teenager's male partner is also not usually involved in the program's services nor did such outreach have a high priority for most programs. Again a few programs were exceptions, and had been successfully working with the adolescent males and teenage fathers.

The first conclusion from this small survey is that more information is clearly needed. Given that pregnant teenagers appear to be so largely dependent on the support and help of their families, more information and research is certainly needed about the extent to which agencies work in partnership with the families, and plan their services to complement the families' own resources; or alternatively, whether their current practice of ignoring the family context may undercut family support relationships.

Second, those few programs that have already moved in innovative ways to become more involved both with teenage fathers and a teenage mother's parents and other family members need to share their experience with other programs that might want to move in this direction. It needs to be added that careful plans should be made to evaluate the effectiveness of any new program approaches to working with families of teenage parents.

NOTES

1. A secondary aspect of family involvement that is not discussed at any length in this chapter is the extent to which community family representatives, or adolescents themselves, are involved in the planning and direction of the overall program—on boards, committees, or as volunteers.

2. Wendy H. Baldwin, "Adolescent pregnancy and childbearing: Growing

concerns for Americans," *The population bulletin* 31, no. 2 (1976): 4 (Population Reference Bureau, Inc., 1337 Connecticut Ave. NW, Washington, D.C. 20036).

3. JBF Associates, *National Directory of the National Alliance Concerned with School-age Parents, 1976* (Washington, D.C., 1976); JBF Associates, available from 3746 Cumberland Street NW, Washington, D.C. 20016.

4. Marion Howard, "Young parent families," in *Child welfare strategy in coming years* (HEW publication no. [OHDS] 78-30158; Washington, D.C.: GPO, 1978). This list is adapted from those on pp. 213 and 216.

5. Lucy Eddinger and Janet Forbush, "School-age pregnancy and parenthood in USA," report prepared by NACSAP, 1977; available from JBF Associates, 3746 Cumberland Street NW, Washington, D.C. 20016.

6. K. Cannon-Bonventre, and J. R. Kahn, *The ecology of help-seeking behavior among adolescent parents* (Cambridge, Mass.: American Institutes for Research, 1979).

7. Janet Forbush, testimony on Titles VI, VII, and VIII of the Health Services and Centers Amendments of 1978, before the Senate Labor-HEW Subcommittee on Appropriations, March 28, 1979 (P.L. 95-626), Ninety-fifth Congress.

8. Lorraine Klerman, "Design problems in evaluating service programs for school-age parents," *Evaluation and the health professionals* 2, no. 1 (1979): 55–70.

9. E. L. Husting, E. C. Khoury, P. B. Cohen, J. R. Markel, and E. R. Schlesinger, *Guidelines for self-evaluation of programs serving adolescent parents* (Pittsburgh, Pa.: School of Public Health, University of Pittsburgh, June 1973).

10. Reuben Pannor, "The teenage unwed father," *Obstetrics and Gynecology* 14, no. 2 (1971).

11. Eleanor Wright Smith, "The role of the grandmother in adolescent pregnancy and parenting," *Journal of School Health* 45, no. 5 (1975): 278–283.

12. The following is a list of agencies who provided information for this survey: Numbers 1–15 are the sample of agencies selected from National Alliance Concerned with School Age Parents'(NACSAP) original 1977 questionnaire survey; numbers 16–21 are the additional agencies added for the follow-up telephone interviews. (*Note*: The NACSAP survey classified the agencies according to three broad categories thus: Class A agencies provided comprehensive services; Class B provided two different types of services; Class C provided only one service, usually referrals.) The agencies include:

1. Area Learning Center–Teenage Parent Program, St. Cloud, Minn. (Class B)
2. Catholic Charities, Sioux City, Iowa (Class B)
3. Catholic Social Service, Fort Worth, Tex. (Class B)
4. Chicago Child Care Society, Chicago, Ill. (Class C)
5. Delaware Adolescent Program, Inc.—Kent County Center, Dover, Del. (Class A)
6. Florence Crittenton Agency, Knoxville, Tenn. (Class B)
7. Inwood House, New York, N.Y. (Class A)
8. Martha Meilson School, Bronx, N.Y. (Class B)

9. Maternity and Infant Care Project, Los Angeles, Calif. (Class B)
10. Parent and Child Development Services, Inc. Savannah, Ga. (Class A)
11. Saint Francis Maternity Residence, LaCrosse, Wis. (Class B)
12. Sophia Little Home, Cranston, R.I. (Class A)
13. The Salvation Army—Booth Memorial residence and Hospital, Omaha, Neb. (Class A)
14. Villa Gerard—Catholic Charities of Lane County, Eugene, Oreg. (Class B)
15. Young Mothers Program, Fremont, Calif. (Class B)
16. Friends to Parents, Inc., San Francisco, Calif. (Class C)
17. Johns Hopkins Center for Teenage Mothers and Their Infants, Baltimore, Md. (Class A)
18. Park School, Grand Rapids, Mich. (Class B)
19. Teen Mother Program—Tracy Education Center, Cerritos, Calif. (Class B)
20. Chicago Comprehensive Care Center, Chicago, Ill. (Class A)
21. The Door: Center of Alternatives, New York, N.Y. (Class A)

8

Ethical and Legal Issues in Teenage Pregnancies

Margaret O'Brien Steinfels

Introduction

Of all the ages and stages through which human beings pass, adolescence, in recent times, has been the subject of more scrutiny, probing, puzzlement, and frustration than any other. Adolescents are often baffling to themselves, exasperating to their parents, puzzling to their own peers, and in matters of public policy and social customs, subject to a welter of confusing and contradictory traditions, practices, and regulations. Or, as the premier adolescent, Romeo Montague had it:

> Why then, O brawling love! O loving hate!
> O anything, of nothing first create!
> O heavy lightness! Serious vanity!
> Misshapen chaos of well-seeming forms!
> Feather of lead, bright smoke, cold fire, sick health!
> Still-waking sleep, that is not what it is!
> This love felt I, that feel no love in this.
> (Act I, Scene 1)

Even the exclamation points are characteristic of adolescence. Clearly the paradoxical and mercurial nature of adolescent emotions is not new. Nor is the concern parents feel for the dilemmas of their children. Witness the problem of Juliet's father:

> Capulet: My child is yet a stranger in the world—
> She hath not seen the change of fourteen years
> Let two more summers wither in their pride
> Ere we think her ripe to be a bride.
> Paris: Younger than she are happy mothers made.
> Capulet: And too soon marred are those so early made.
> The earth hath swallowed all my hopes but she,
> She is the hopeful lady of my heart.
> (Act I, Scene 2)

The source of our great dilemma, although hard to remedy, is not difficult to identify. It is the boundary-like quality of adolescence: first, it is a time of passage from childhood to maturity that, in the United States and most developed countries, is made rough and uneven by prolonged economic dependence and a high rate of youth unemployment; second, it is a time of extended schooling characterized by the inability of many to participate in schools; and third, it is a time of ambivalent roles for families attempting to mediate their offspring's choice of career, life style, and sexual or marriage partner. We have long abandoned the form or pretense of arranged (or approved) marriages; and legally, we appear to be on our way to severely restricting parental controls over the sexual and reproductive behavior of their minor children.

In a series of recent judicial and regulatory decisions, the courts and federal regulatory agencies appear to favor a policy that would require public agencies, and many private ones as well, to treat adolescents from puberty (at the age of eleven or twelve) through the age of majority (eighteen or nineteen) as if they were adults for the purpose of providing contraceptive services and performing abortions.[1] The Supreme Court decisions in *Planned Parenthood* v. *Danforth* and *Carey* v. *Population Services International* have made privacy rights applicable to adolescents, extending to them the constitutional protections, previously enjoyed by adults, to secure access to nonprescription contraceptives and abortions.[2] The Court, in effect, restricted parental knowledge and control, except when an adolescent voluntarily seeks parental help and advice. In addition, it cast into doubt the distinction between mature and immature minors, at least with respect to sex and pregnancy-related medical care.

The Court's extension of privacy rights is virtually without parallel in other areas of law or policy affecting minors. A ludicrous but telling example of the unbalanced state of the law in this area is suggested by the situation of the adolescent girl who can obtain an abortion without her parents' consent, but requires their permission to be absent from school in order to attend an abortion clinic.

The present state of the law raises serious legal and ethical questions, because it starts to unravel the tightly knit union of law, tradition, and custom that has governed the relationship between the family and the state, one in which the state has acknowledged the primacy of the family in raising and socializing children.

What has been remarked by one philosopher about teenage sex can be extended to the legal, ethical, and policy issues it raises: "One of the main difficulties of being a teenager is sex, at once a great discovery, a great mess, a great pleasure, a great frustration, and an all-around great muddle."[3] Whatever public policies we may devise to manage that muddle, such a muddle is a condition that the legal and ethical analyses in this paper tend to confirm rather than resolve. In fact, many issues raised here point to deep-seated ambiguities and conflicts in American law and social policy that the dilemma of teenage pregnancies simply serve to sharpen—for example, the conflict between individual rights and group rights. In a society in which the law recognizes individual relationships on the basis of contract and in the absence of a normative definition of the family, it is difficult to establish a ground in the law for talking about anything like family autonomy or parental rights.

Although the present state of the law seems to favor adolescent autonomy in sexual behavior and reproductive decisions, it is the argument of this chapter that it is possible that the impasse can be negotiated within the present legal framework, so that not only will individual rights be protected, but parental responsibilities can be exercised. It is important, however, to try to understand the sources and nature of the disagreements and conflicts; these are described in the sections on legal issues and ethical issues. And given the boundaries set by the law on the ethical issues open to governmental discussion, the few resolutions that appear to be legally permissible and politically feasible, are briefly outlined in the final section.

Legal Issues

Some commentators on families, children, and the state describe the relationship between parent and child as resting upon property rights, children being chattel property subject to the "ownership" of their parents.[4] The common law tradition, from which these property rights are said to derive, treats infringement of parental control and authority as a violation of property rights. Thus, for example, barring statutory exception, medical treatment of a minor without parental consent has been a cause for battery and assault charges against a physician, even when the treatment is successful, because the parent's (and not the child's) rights have been violated.[5]

Blackstone's *Commentaries* suggest an alternative view: the relationship between parent and child is not a property relationship at all, but a relationship resting on parental duty and obligation to the child: "By begetting them, therefore, [parents] have entered into a voluntary obligation to endeavor, as far as in them lies, that the life which they have bestowed shall be supported and preserved."[6] Rather than property rights language, the language of duty and responsibility more nearly represents our contemporary sense of what constitutes the normal parent-child relationship.

Whereas the language of property rights implies arbitrary treatment of children by parents exercising their proprietary interest, that of obligation and duty underlines the beneficent interest many parents have in the growth, development, and flourishing of their children. This distinction is important to note in examining the legal status of children, since advocacy of children's rights against parental authority or family rights frequently carries with it the underlying supposition that the interests of parents and children differ. The conclusion follows: the law must resolve the inevitable conflicts in favor of extending autonomy and rights to the minor child, and using property language to describe the parent-child relationship biases our sympathies in that direction. The language of parental duty and obligation—although it is not universally observed—more accurately reflects the spirit in which most parents exercise their authority and responsibilities. Furthermore, it implies that parents are capable of acting in the child's interest, as well as their own, and that, in fact, the two may sometimes coincide. This latter view is helpful because it potentially allows consideration, not only of parental rights, but of parental obligation—obligations to act in a realistic and helpful manner toward sexually active or pregnant adolescents.

Sex and pregnancy-related medical care for minors has traditionally been controlled by two legal conditions: (1) reaching the age of majority; or (2) demonstrating the maturity to consent to one's own medical care, or securing the proxy consent of one's parent or guardian. In *Planned Parenthood* v. *Danforth*, however, the Supreme Court set aside both of those conditions.

The plaintiffs in *Danforth*, Planned Parenthood of Central Missouri, objected to certain provisions of a state law governing abortions that had been enacted after the Supreme Court's 1973 abortion decision. In particular, they took issue with the need for "written consent of one parent or person *in loco parentis* of the woman if the woman is unmarried and under the age of eighteen years, unless the abortion is certified by a licensed physician as necessary in order to preserve the life of the mother."[7] In a related case, *Carey* v. *Population Services International* (a mail order company that sold non-medical contraceptives), a provision of the New York State education law was at issue. This law made it a criminal offense for "any person to sell or distribute an instrument or article, or any recipe, drug or medicine for the prevention of contraception to a minor under the age of sixteen years."[8]

Danforth and *Carey* raised different legal questions: at stake in the first was parental consent; in the second, state restrictions on the sale of contraceptives to minors. Despite the difference in the initial question, the effect of the Court's decisions was similar in both cases: an extension to minors of the right to self-determination in sex- and pregnancy-related medical care, or what the Court had in earlier decisions designated "privacy rights." "If the right of privacy means anything, it is the right of the *individual*, married or single, to be free from unwarranted governmental intrusion into matters so fundamentally affecting a person as the decision whether to bear or beget a child."[9]

Applying these rights in *Carey*, Justice Brennan wrote: "State restrictions inhibiting privacy rights of minors are valid only if they serve 'any significant state interest that is not present in the case of an adult.'"[10] Ruling that New York had no such interest, the Court declared the provision unconstitutional, making it possible for minors to buy nonprescription contraceptives.

In *Danforth*, the Court went further. It extended privacy rights, ruled against the absolute veto parents had over an abortion decision made by a minor and her physician during the first trimester, and implied that the physical capacity to become pregnant in itself might be sufficient criteria for extending the rights of privacy or self-determination to minors. In this last instance, by my reading, the Court seems to equate biological maturity with mental capacity to consent, although it left open in *Bellotti* v. *Baird* (1976), a related case handed down the same day, the possibility that with proper judicial intervention the mature/immature minor distinction might hold. On appeal, in *Bellotti* v. *Baird* (1979), this distinction was acknowledged by the Court, although the Massachusetts statute under review—a statute that required parental consent, or, in the absence of such consent, a court order—was found unconstitutional on the grounds that it unduly burdened the right to an abortion, thus leaving open the question of whether mature and immature minors are to be treated similarly.[11]

In *Danforth*, Justice Blackmun wrote for the majority that:

> The State does not have the constitutional authority to give a third party an absolute, and possibly arbitrary, veto over the decision of the physician and his patient to terminate the patient's pregnancy, regardless of the reason for withholding the consent. . . . It is difficult . . . to conclude that providing a parent with absolute power to overrule a determination, made by the physician and his minor patient, to terminate the patient's pregnancy will serve to strengthen the family unit. Neither is it likely that such veto power will enhance parental authority or control where the minor and non-consenting parent are so fundamentally in conflict and the very existence of the pregnancy already has fractured the family structure. Any independent interest the parent may have in the termination of the minor daughter's pregnancy is no more weighty than the right of privacy of the competent minor mature enough to have become pregnant.[12]

While scholars disagree over the meaning of the Court's argumentation about privacy rights, including the possible contradictory extension of its meaning in cases following *Griswold*, the primary question for our discussion is: even though the state may have no compelling interest in a minor's reproductive behavior and decisions, can the Court restrict the interests of others, like the family or the sexual partner?[13] As Justice White remarked in his dissent to striking the parental consent provision:

> The Court rejects the notions that the State has an interest in strengthening the family unit, or that the *parent* has an "independent interest" in the abortion deci-

sion, sufficient to justify the statute and apparently concludes that the statute is therefore unconstitutional. But the purpose of the parental consent requirement is not merely to vindicate any interest of the parent or of the State. The purpose of the requirement is to vindicate the very right created in *Roe* v. *Wade*—the right of the pregnant woman to decide "whether *or not* to terminate her pregnancy."[14]

White correctly suggests the problematic grounds on which privacy rights have been extended to minors:

> The abortion decision is unquestionably important and has irrevocable consequences, whichever way it is made. Missouri is entitled to protect the minor unmarried woman from making the decision in a way which is not in her own best interests, and it seeks to achieve this goal by requiring parental consultation and consent. This is the traditional way by which States have sought to protect children from their own immature and improvident decisions; and there is absolutely no reason expressed by the majority which the State may not utilize that method here.[15]

The extension of privacy rights to minors in *Danforth* and *Carey* resolved an ambiguity in the Court's original abortion decision, *Roe* v. *Wade*, that is, whether or not privacy rights acknowledged for adult women applied to minors. They now do, at least in the case of first trimester abortions. But new legal issues were raised by the Supreme Court's decisions:

- Can an incompetent minor consent to sex- or pregnancy-related medical care?
- Can a minor, competent or incompetent, consent to a second trimester abortion?
- Can parents be notified of requests for sex- or pregnancy-related medical care, even though they may no longer consent?

Although at one point in *Danforth* Justice Blackmun seems to imply that the physical capacity to become pregnant might be in itself sufficient reason for extending the right to self-determination, he acknowledges the possibility that some minors might not be mature enough to give consent. "We emphasize that our holding that [the Missouri statute] is invalid does not suggest that every minor, regardless of age or maturity, may give effective consent for termination of her pregnancy."

Justice Stewart in a concurring opinion suggested an alternative interpretation:

> I think it is clear that [the Missouri statute's] primary constitutional deficiency lies in its imposition of an absolute limitation on the minor's right to obtain an abortion. The Court's opinion today in *Belotti* v. *Baird* (1976) . . . suggests that a materially different constitutional issue would be presented under a provision requiring parental consent or consultation in most cases, but providing for prompt (i) judicial resolution of any disagreement, . . . or (ii) judicial determination that a minor is mature . . . or that abortion in any event is in minor's best interest. Such a provision would not impose parental approval as an absolute condition upon the minor's right but would assure in most instances consultation between the parent and the child.[16]

In *Bellotti* (1979), Justice Powell outlined the conditions for a state statute that might pass a constitutional test:

> Under state regulation such as that undertaken by Massachusetts, every minor must have the opportunity—if she so desires—to go directly to a court without first consulting or notifying her parents. If she satisfies the court that she is mature and well-informed enough to make intelligently the abortion decision on her own, the court must authorize her to act without parental consultation or consent. If she fails to satisfy

> the court that she is competent to make this decision independently, she must be permitted to show that an abortion nevertheless would be in her best interest. If the court is persuaded that it is, the court must authorize the abortion. If, however, the court is not persuaded by the minor that she is mature or that the abortion would be in her best interest, it may decline to sanction the operation.[17]

In sum, the Court in *Danforth* made certain assertions about the nature of adolescent-parent relationships, implied a connection between physical maturity and mental capacity, and carved out an area of unprecedented autonomy for minors. In *Bellotti* (1979), the Court held to the standard set in *Danforth*, allowing only that states that choose to legislate in this matter must permit the minor "to go directly to a court without first consulting or notifying her parents."

What the Court failed to directly define is the standard that ought to govern the age of majority. At what age should a child be recognized by society as independent for purposes of being acknowledged as an adult capable of assuming responsibility and relationships apart from the supervision and authority of his or her parents? As a practical matter this involves the right to marry, enter into contracts, vote, inherit property, consent to medical treatment, secure a driver's license, purchase alcoholic beverages, and be treated as an adult in criminal proceedings. Finally, parents are no longer legally or financially responsible for the actions of their offspring.

Traditionally the extension of these liberties depended on reaching majority, usually twenty-one, except where there were statutory exceptions. In recent years, following the ratification of the Twenty-sixth Amendment (1971), which lowered the voting age to eighteen, most states have reduced the age of majority. Thus, in 1975, only Mississippi and Pennsylvania retained twenty-one as the age of majority; all others were eighteen or nineteen. In most states, an individual may consent to general medical care at the age of majority; in addition, most states allow a minor's consent to medical care if she or he is married or "emancipated." Prior to the Court's decisions in *Danforth* and *Carey*, a variety of rules were in effect for minors' consent to sex-related medical care. As of 1976, most states permitted adolescents to consent to treatment for venereal disease at any age; thirty-one states allowed minors' consent to prenatal- and pregnancy-related medical care; twenty-seven allowed minor consent for contraception; and twenty-six, for abortion.[18]

To all age-based limits there have been three exceptions for consent to all medical care for minors: emergency treatment, the doctrine of the emancipated minor, and the mature minor rule. In general, physicians can treat a minor without parental consent in any life-threatening circumstance; treating serious, but not life-threatening conditions will usually depend on state statute and hospital policy.

The emancipated minor doctrine recognizes the right of an adolescent under the age of majority to act as "one who is not subject to parental control or regulation."[19] The exact conditions under which an adolescent will be recognized as emancipated or granted emancipation by courts vary according to state statute. Generally, a minor is considered emancipated if she or he is married, or living away from home and self-supporting, if his or her parents (voluntarily or involuntarily) have relinquished their rights; if a court orders emancipation; or if the minor is in military service. Some ambiguous categories here include minors attending school away from home and runaway children.

The emancipated minor doctrine largely established by statute should be distinguished from the mature minor rule that has developed through case law. Under the mature minor rule, a judge may decide that a minor had the capacity to consent to treatment, and a physician cannot be held liable for failing to secure parental consent.[20] The following criteria appear to be the crucial ones in mature minor rulings:

1. The treatment was undertaken for the benefit of a minor rather than a third party (thus excluding non-therapeutic interventions like organ donations and research).

2. The particular minor was near majority (or at least in the range of fifteen years of age and upwards) and was considered to have sufficient mental capacity to understand fully the nature and importance of the medical steps proposed.

3. The medical procedures could be characterized by the court as something less than "major" or "serious."[21]

In summary, the legal situation prior to *Danforth* and *Carey*, with respect to minor consent for medical care, could be generally characterized as one that recognized both the importance of parental interest in the care of minors and the necessity of consent for medical treatment where the family was intact—and that this interest was superseded only in life-threatening circumstances. No small consideration in this arrangement was the fact that parents were also financially responsible for paying the costs of medical care.

During the late fifties and early sixties, exceptions were made to the general rule: now minors could consent to the treatment of venereal-disease- and pregnancy-related medical care (including the minor mother's right to consent to treatment for her child). It was less likely that state statutes would allow adolescents the same liberty in matters of contraception or abortion, although until recently, no parents have successfully brought suit against a physician who prescribed contraceptives or performed an abortion without their consent.[22]

Since the last available survey of the state statutes in 1975, and as a result of the Supreme Court decisions, the consent issue has reversed. Most states now acknowledge the right of minors to consent to their own sex-related medical care in matters of pregnancy, venereal disease, contraception, and abortion.[23] The right to prescription contraceptives, like the pill or an intrauterine device (IUD) has never been adjudicated by the Supreme Court, but HEW regulations prohibit public facilities supported with federal funds from refusing contraceptives to minors. In short, it is unlikely that, having extended the right of privacy in the matters of abortion and nonprescription contraceptives, the Court would not also do so in the case of prescription contraceptives.

If the Supreme Court had not taken the turn it did in *Danforth*, it is likely that the mature minor rule might have developed further than it has in extending to adolescents the right to sex-related medical care. Although this has not happened, one standard among its guidelines needs further attention; and that is "the mental capacity to consent."

The mature minor rule requires "sufficient mental capacity to understand fully the nature and importance of the medical steps proposed"; and constitutes an important nonlegal criterion for judging competence, that is, intellectual, developmental or psychological standards by which to assess the ability to consent. Such a criterion is an important element in the notion of variable competence, which attempts to modify the single standard of chronological age as the criterion for allowing some of the liberties of majority.

Legally, variable competence refers to an individual's legal capacity to consent or not to consent; thus, state statutes take variability into account by licensing a sixteen-year-old to drive, but prohibiting the same sixteen-year-old from donating a kidney. Psychologically, the legitimacy of variable competence rests upon a relatively modern view of the child, that is, that throughout childhood and adolescence, individuals show variable rates of growth and development. Some children can be described as being quite mature at a relatively early age, say twelve or thirteen, while others appear immature even at eighteen or twenty-one.

The psychological notion of variable competence rests on the work of the Swiss epistemologist and researcher, Jean Piaget, and the American educator, Lawrence Kohlberg. Their theories cannot be examined in detail here, but the descriptions they provide of the capacities of children at various developmental stages bear not only on the issues raised by age-based competence (majority), but also on the ethical issues at stake in the decision-making process of the minor child who considers herself or himself mature and capable of acting in a morally autonomous fashion.

In *The moral judgement of the child*, Piaget tries to pinpoint the age at which children move from "moral heteronomy" to "moral autonomy."[24] Somewhere between the ages of ten and eleven (at least among the Swiss children he was studying), Piaget believes, there is some capacity for understanding facts and events in an objective manner; in addition, there may be the ability to see these facts and events in a social context, that is, in relation to their effects on others, and not simply in an egotistic fashion. A child's reasoning powers may be sufficiently advanced to enable her to understand a proposition put forward, and also to reflect upon it, to comprehend it, and finally, to understand the consequences of agreement or disagreement with it.

Piaget is the first to point out that while such a movement from heteronomy to autonomy may apply to the game of marbles (which is the area he studied), it may not apply to a range of other circumstances. Rather, every set of new rules or circumstances require a recapitulation of the whole process, until, during adolescence, a person gradually frees herself or himself from the constraining influence of others until she or he, in fact, becomes autonomous.

Lawrence Kohlberg, whose work closely parallels that of Piaget, has discussed an elaborate system of moral stages that he correlates with cognitive development. He describes six stages of moral thought that are divided into three major categories: preconventional, conventional, and postconventional or autonomous: "The postconventional level is first evident in adolescence and is characterized by a major thrust toward autonomous moral principles which have validity and application apart from authority of the group or persons who hold them and apart from the individual's identification with those persons or groups." It is at this stage that one might expect a person to demonstrate the "mental capacity to consent." According to Kohlberg, the onset of this stage is extremely variable, occurring as early as ten or eleven in some children, but never occurring at all in some adults.[25]

If Piaget's cognitive and moral categories as elaborated by Kohlberg are illustrative of the mature minor rule, then on the basis of this developmental model, a small minority of children, beginning at the age of eleven or twelve, might be capable of giving informed consent, or at least demonstrating the mental capacity to give consent. The developmental model of informed consent provides broad categories for enumerating the capacities of adolescents for giving informed consent, and legitimates the judicial thinking governing the mature minor rule.

The chief merit of the mature minor rule and the notion of variable competence in relation to consent is that each takes into account individual differences in the cognitive and moral development of adolescents. Contrast this with the inflexibility of the age-based rule, in which whole classes of children are treated equally (say, all those under fifteen, or all those between sixteen and eighteen), irrespective of their mental capacities or moral maturity.

Despite the clear benefit of treating cases on an individual basis, the flexibility of the mature minor rule has its drawbacks. There are, first of all, bureaucratic difficulties in making case-by-case assessments; it is easier from a legal point of view to treat whole classes of persons as if they were the same for purposes of voting, or giving consent to medical care, or donating an organ for transplant. In addition, there is the problem of establishing criteria sensitive enough to be revelatory in individual cases, but general enough to be usable by the courts and others who must make the crucial assessment. Ironically the people in the best position to assess the maturity of a minor child are likely to be the parents, who are explicitly excluded from the decisions surrounding adolescent pregnancy, particularly abortion. In spite of these shortcomings, the mature minor doctrine represented a flexible legal mechanism for dealing with the problems of adolescent pregnancies that protected the adolescent and provided for informed consent, while allowing a role for parents in the case of immature minors. *Danforth* truncated its potential usefulness.

The *Oxford English Dictionary* defines consent as "voluntary agreement to, or acquiescence in, what another proposes or desires." While grounded in that simple definition, the notion of consent in medical treatment and research goes far beyond it, encompassing questions of truth telling, disclosure, autonomy, coercion, and competence. Hence, in medical therapy the noun "consent" is usually modified by the adjectives "informed" and "voluntary." In our legal system, so attuned to the problems of liberty and individual rights, there is perhaps no subject in medical or research ethics about which more effort at clarification has been made, and yet about which sensitive physicians and researchers may retain a high degree of uncertainty. What constitutes free and informed consent in any given case? Uncertainty is heightened in the case of minors when "mental capacity" or competence is questionable.

There are many codes and regulations which set forth the conditions for informed consent. For example, the Nuremberg Codes state:

> The voluntary consent of the human subject is absolutely essential. This means that the person involved should have legal capacity to give consent; should be so situated as to be able to exercise free power of choice, without the intervention of any element of force, fraud, deceit, duress, over-reaching, or other ulterior form of constraint or coercion; and should have sufficient knowledge and comprehension of the elements of the subject matter involved as to enable him to make an understanding and enlightened decision.

This latter element requires that before the acceptance of an affirmative decision by the experimental subject, there should be made known to him the nature, duration, and purpose of the experiment; the method and means by which it is to be conducted; all inconveniences and hazards reasonably to be expected; and the effects upon his health or person which may possibly come from his participation in the experiments.[26]

Informed consent standards in therapy are not established by statute, but have evolved from the adjudication of malpractice suits brought by patients against physicians. The doctrine of informed consent rests on a 1914 opinion of Justice Cardozo: "every human being of adult years and sound mind has a right to determine what should be done with his own body, and a surgeon who performs an operation without the patient's consent, commits an assault for which he is liable in damages."[27]

A complicated and disputed history of the doctrine has evolved since then, although the essence of Cardozo's definition remains.[28] The complexity of informed consent belies the ease with which most surgeons and physicians secure consent for medical treatment every day; it is a routine matter in most hospitals and medical practices. Consent has taken on such importance in the case of sex- and pregnancy-related medical care for minors because the implementation of informed consent and its very "routineness" are problematic when competence is in question. Is this minor free and competent to give consent to use of the pill or an IUD? Does this seventeen-year-old really want an abortion, or is she afraid to have her parents know she is pregnant? Does this fifteen-year-old really understand the implications of giving birth and keeping her baby?

Traditionally the solution to providing consent for incompetent persons, including minors, has been to rely on proxy consent, that is, substituted consent. In the case of minors, proxy consent is commonly exercised by the parent or guardian of the child, although a court or court appointed guardian may do so. But it was precisely the issue of proxy consent that was at stake in *Planned Parenthood* v. *Danforth*, and that the Court ruled against.

What can "consent by the immature or incompetent" mean under such circumstances? In fact, one might speculate that it was precisely the immature and incompetent for whom the rulings have been made—the Court may believe that it was the incompetent more than anyone who needed easy access to contraceptives and abortions, but because of their youth and immaturity would be those most deterred by the parental consent requirement.

Whatever the Court's bias in the matter, *Danforth* and *Carey* are clearly not, in my opinion, decisions that give much attention to the question of family interest in values related to sexual activity, pregnancy, teenage motherhood, or to the capacity of minors in consenting themselves to such care. Rather the decisions seem narrowly conceived, and reflective of a strictly instrumental view of the problem. The Court appears to treat teenage sexual activities and pregnancies essentially as health problems that can best be "cured" and handled by recourse to medical advice and treatment—a view that the Court, of course, shares with many others, and implements by putting doctors in charge. Casting teenage pregnancies under the umbrella of the "medical model" minimizes the need to pay attention to other issues and values—such as the psychological, emotional, familial, and moral problems—they present. Granting the adolescent the right to make her own decisions about contraceptive use or pregnancy outcome, without the counsel and support of parents, imposes an unfair burden of decision making on many adolescents, especially younger ones; and it unjustly limits parental interests in the values and behaviors of their children.

For example, Justice Blackmun assumed that the decision to terminate a pregnancy is actually the joint decision of the minor patient and her physician. Yet, in most cases, physicians are rarely present except to perform the abortion; and group counseling is the rule rather than the exception. Justice Stewart was more realistic in his appraisal of the advice a minor may need but is not likely to get:

> There can be little doubt that the State furthers a constitutionally permissible end by encouraging an unmarried pregnant minor to seek the help and advice of her parents in making the very important decision whether or not to bear a child. That is a grave decision, and a girl of tender years, under emotional stress, may be ill-equipped to make it without mature advice and emotional support. It seems unlikely that she will obtain adequate counsel and support from the attending physicians at an abortion clinic, where abortions for pregnant minors frequently take place.[29]

He then goes on to support his last point by citing testimony in a brief submitted in *Bellotti* v. *Baird* (1976):

> The counseling . . . occurs entirely on the day the abortion is to be performed. . . . It lasts for two hours and takes place in groups that include both minors and adults who are strangers to one another. . . . The physician takes no part in this counseling process. . . . Counseling is typically limited to a description of abortion procedures, possible complications, and birth control techniques. . . .
>
> The abortion itself takes five to seven minutes. . . . The physician has no prior contact with the minor, and on the days that abortions are being performed at the (clinic), the physician . . . may be performing abortions on many other adults and minors.[30]

This picture is borne out by other observers who confirm the problematic nature not simply of obtaining informed consent under such circumstances, but also of ascertaining the quality of reflection and calculation that have gone into the decision.

> In Atlanta, one counselor shook her head in frustration at the end of the day. "I'm not sure counseling helps at all," she said. "It's all just part of the procedure that the women have to go through. They say what they think the counselor wants to hear just to get on with the routines. . . . They don't just want to open up their decision making again just before the fact."[31]

It is equally necessary, of course, to question the quality of decision making and reflection that may go into a decision to carry a pregnancy to term, to keep a baby after birth, or to place it for adoption. The point is that in many cases, adolescents, especially younger ones, would benefit from the support and advice of parents.

Ethical Issues

The ethical issues that could be advanced in examining the family impact of teenage pregnancies are numerous. But in the interests of addressing the policy issue, they will be limited to the framework established by the present law. In the absence of a consensus on what values should underlie public policy on this question, the ethical issues can be reduced to two questions, namely, Who is the competent decision-maker? and, What criteria are likely to produce a voluntary and informed decision regarding sex- and pregnancy-related medical care for minors? Three groups have interests in the discussion. The first is the adolescent and her partner; the second is the adolescent and her or his family; and the third is the public policy maker who must frame legislation, regulations, and rules governing medical practice on this issue.

Our society would like to discourage early childbearing, and so policymaking bodies and media discussions tend to treat all adolescent pregnancies as serious social welfare and health problems. It is true that adolescent pregnancies present serious and real problems; the point is that we try to remedy the situa-

ETHICAL AND LEGAL ISSUES

tion by categorizing such pregnancies only as medical problems that can either be treated by abortion or not treated at all. By failing to allocate resources or changing social welfare practices, we limit the possibilities of other solutions. From an ethical point of view, certainly, one serious problem lies in coercing a decision in one direction by limiting the resources available to the other.

In 1976, 37.4 percent of pregnancies to minors fourteen to eighteen years of age ended in legal abortions; 49 percent (197,997) resulted in live births; and 13.5 percent (54,600) ended in fetal loss. This represents an increase of about 10 percent in legal abortions over the 1974 rate, and a 10 percent decline in live births. While increased use of contraceptives may continue to bring a decline in teenage pregnancy rates, it is likely that the proportions of teenage pregnancies that end in abortion will increase.[32]

Where a pregnant adolescent may hold ethical or religious views that regard abortion as a grave offense, it may be hard not to seek one in view of the overwhelming problems she will face otherwise, especially in the absence of a supportive and sympathetic family or partner. Thus, another important ethical question facing the pregnant teenager is: how much choice does she have in either getting an abortion or carrying a pregnancy to term? That is, to what degree is her decision coerced by circumstance rather than her careful consideration of what is the right action for her to take? The decision she makes ought to rest upon the values she holds concerning the fetus, herself, her partner, and her plans for the future. Furthermore, while the values pregnant adolescents hold, as a group, probably do not differ from those held by mature women, it is likely that those values may not be as clear to minors, nor are they as likely to hold them with as great a degree of confidence. In short, it will be extremely difficult for the minor adolescent to exercise the right established in *Roe* v. *Wade*, that is, to decide whether or not to have an abortion.

Of the girl's partner, little can be said except that he has no standing in the law, and elicits little moral sympathy. He can neither legally prevent nor force an abortion. However, in a recent Nebraska case a seventeen-year-old successfully sued for custody of his child after the mother decided to place the infant for adoption. While almost nothing seems to be known about the situation of the males involved in adolescent pregnancies—in fact, like the mothers, these young fathers probably have no maneuvering room and limited resources for managing the problem. After a pregnancy actually occurs, they are usually the least powerful and least respected person in the whole decision-making process. At least in this regard, law and public policy foster irresponsibility in the male partner of a teenage pregnancy.

Given the problems and limitations both partners face, how can the decision either to seek an abortion or carry a pregnancy to term be made in a morally responsible manner? Seeking an abortion may simply be an expedient act, while carrying a pregnancy to term may reflect a continuation of the unrealistic, romantic, or irresponsible attitudes that, in many (but not all) cases, led to the pregnancy in the first place. Add to this the question of how mature or competent, in both the legal and psychological sense, the adolescent girl or boy actually may be, and it becomes clear that the extension of privacy rights may be simply one more strategy for ignoring the needs of the pregnant adolescent and her partner.

The major justification offered by the court for extending privacy rights to abortion for minors seems to rest on the view that:

> It is difficult to conclude that providing a parent with absolute power to overrule a determination . . . to terminate the patient's pregnancy will serve to strengthen the family unit. Neither is it likely that such veto power will enhance parental authority or control where the minor and the consenting parent are so fundamentally in conflict and the very existence of the pregnancy already has fractured the family structure.[33]

The Court's decision, of course, leaves a girl free to voluntarily her parents' advice and counsel; and, at least legally, they can neither prevent her from seeking an abortion nor force her to have one.[34] The view that she may be mistreated or coerced in some fashion if her parents are informed, as they would be if notification requirements were in effect, is a popular line of argument among those opposed to any legally required parental involvement in matters related to the sexual behavior or pregnancy decisions of the adolescent.[35] There is undoubtedly truth in the proposition that some parents may be shocked and respond punitively to the news of a pregnancy. Most are not likely to, although they may be confused as to exactly what they ought to do.

While some families will have different views about whether or not abortion is a morally legitimate choice at all (and individuals within families may differ), others may have grave doubts about the capacity of their adolescent daughter to be a mother; still others will attempt to force or prevent a marriage. In the case of contraception, the real parental objection may lie in the disapproval of their daughter or son being sexually active in the first place. Most parents will come to terms with sexual activity and use of contraceptives or a pregnancy. Some parents will see these activities as the first, if somewhat sad, step toward independence, and, with or without offering advice, encourage their daughter to make her own decision. Adolescents themselves may sometimes have to act without parental approval and support. But at least parents need to have a chance to influence their children's values and behavior.

Other parents, correctly or incorrectly, will not acknowledge the maturity of their child, and will act in a paternalistic manner, discouraging the autonomous decision making of their daughter to make the decision for her. (Legally speaking, they can neither prevent nor coerce an abortion, nor do they have any legal rights in relation to a grandchild, unless it is born and they are granted custody.)

While recognizing the plurality of moral views among parents and their potentially differing responses to sex- or pregnancy-related medical care, one factor unites all such parents, although some may refuse to acknowledge it. That factor is their parental obligation to act in their child's best interest. Definitions may differ about what is the best interest for any individual child, but their responsibility to discern and support that interest is clear. The ethical dilemma created by the present legal situation is that the parents may be kept in total ignorance of their child's situation, and hence, be unable to act at all—even if that only means supporting whatever decision their daughter makes.

Given the present limits established by the Supreme Court, legislation, regulations, and standard medical practice could all still recognize and support a role for parents in their adolescent children's decision making concerning contraception and abortion. The reasons for doing so are many. Society ought to support the child-rearing obligations of parents, and respect the autonomy of the family. On the question of sex- and pregnancy-related medical care for adolescents, we also ought to support a role for parents because parents have a legitimate interest in helping to form the values of their children, especially on issues that may have deep religious or ethical meaning for both generations, and may deeply affect the future course of the child's life.

That is not a self-evident claim, particularly in the case of older adolescents, fifteen to eighteen years of age, who may be considered competent in the psychological and legal sense (the latter as defined by the mature minor rule), although below the age of majority. Nonetheless, I would argue that it is in the best interests of society, the family, and the minor to require that parents be notified of sex- or pregnancy-related medical care sought by unmarried adolescents below the age of majority and living with their families.[36]

People start families and have children for many different reasons and motives. Having done so, most parents assume the pleasures and burdens of child-rearing with a degree of good-will, commitment, and responsibility that, on the whole, is unmatched by such numbers in any other effort, voluntary or not. In the course of their offsprings' childhood, parents maintain a steady commitment to feeding, sheltering, teaching, and forming their children. While some parents may be better at child-rearing than others, and some may be judged woefully inadequate by certain standards, society rightly leaves to parents, kin networks, and family friends a wide discretion in child-rearing practices—in schooling, and in inculcating moral, social, and psychological values.

Society expects commitment and effort from the family, and, with some exceptions, gets it. Nonetheless, it is in the interests of society—that is, all of us—to maintain the potential for satisfaction in parenting, which includes, for the purpose of this discussion, transmitting values. This autonomy in establishing goals and means for the family group is a prerequisite for a coherent and purposeful family life that does not simply reduce to respect for parental authority, but includes the capacity of parents and children to know and to respond to one another's values and needs.

On all the ethical grounds raised here, I would argue that the proper resolution of the problem of adolescent pregnancies lies in encouraging and fostering parent involvement, concern, and counsel, except when minors are married or legally emancipated; and in those cases where the mature minor rule can be legitimately invoked. In short, the extension of privacy rights should be limited to those who are truly capable of exercising them.

Toward a Policy Resolution

There is no easy resolution of a problem that stirs so many emotions as this one. Even if one were to stake out a position that attempted to protect a family's interest in socializing and inculcating values in its children, one is likely to encounter sturdy resistance to any efforts that appear to infringe on individual rights. Those who, on other issues, may support family autonomy in matters of child-rearing, will argue that parental involvement here will deter adolescents from seeking the services they so desperately need, thereby insuring an increase in venereal disease (because they will not seek treatment), an increase in pregnancies (because they will remain sexually active without using contraceptives), and an increase in teenage mothers (because they will delay seeking an abortion until it is too late). Still others will deny that values about sexuality or sexual activity are an appropriate component of child-rearing at all. This demythicized view, which sees sexual activity as a physical act, like eating or drinking or riding a bicycle, would deny that any values attach to sexual activity at all—other than good manners, perhaps.[37]

What would a policy toward minors and teenage pregnancies look like if it were both developed within the present framework of the Supreme Court decisions, and supported and respected the family's child-rearing role? Such a policy would have to have among its features:

1. The counseling process for adolescents in family planning clinics, abortion clinics, and prenatal clinics would have to be individualized. Social workers, counselors, physicians, and nurses who work with adolescents on sex- and pregnancy-related health care issues must attempt to act in the individual patient's best interest and not on a preconceived notion of what is best for this age group.

2. Parental notification should be required for minors requesting sex- or pregnancy-related medical care (with the exception of venereal disease treatment).

3. The notification requirement would be automatic for minors from the age of twelve to eighteen who are living with their parents, and who are judged to be too immature to give informed consent to sex- or pregnancy-related medical care.

4. Any minors subject to the notification requirement would be allowed to withdraw their request for services if they did not want their parents notified.

5. The legally established right of minors to secure abortions

or contraceptives should be protected in the face of parental opposition.

6. A public education program for parents should be instituted that, perhaps on a yearly basis and through their children's schools, would appraise them of local community statistics on sexual activity, contraceptive use, abortions, and the venereal disease rate among minors—all in a spirit that would encourage them to speak with their child about these issues in a way that would help the child think through their own values and become conscious of her or his own responsibilities.

NOTES

1. *Carey* v. *Population Services International*, 431 U.S. 2010 (1977); *Planned Parenthood of Central Missouri* v. *Danforth*, 428 U.S. 52 (1976); slip opinion cited in this paper; *T.H.* v. *Jones*, Civil no. C74-276 (D. Utah, July 23, 1975); *Bellotti* v. *Baird*, 428 U.S. 132 (1976); see also: "The minor's right to consent to medical treatment: A corollary of the constitutional right to privacy," *Southern California Law Review* 48 (1975): 1417; "Parental consent requirements and privacy rights of minors: The contraceptive controversy," *Harvard Law Review* 88 (1975): 1001; "The minor's right to abortion and the requirement of parental consent," *Virginia Law Review* 60 (1974): 305; "Minors and health care: The age of consent," *Osgoode Hall Law Journal* 11 (1974): 115; Ruth Jane Zuckerman, "Abortion and contraception: A minor's constitutional right to privacy," *Family Planning/Population Reporter* 4, no. 6 (Dec. 1975): 114–123; "The minor's right of privacy: Limitations on state action after *Danforth* and *Carey*," *Columbia Law Review* 77 (1977): 1216.

2. *Griswold* v. *State of Connecticut*, 85 U.S. 1678 (1965); *Roe* v. *Wade* 410 U.S. 113 (1973).

3. Daniel Callahan in the "Afterword" to *11 million teenagers: What can be done about the epidemic of adolescent pregnancies in the United States* (New York: The Alan Guttmacher Institute, 1976), pp. 57–59.

4. Hillary Rodham, "Children under the law," *Harvard Education Review* 43, no. 4 (Nov. 1973): 489; Sanford N. Katz, *When parents fail: The law's response to family breakdown* (Boston: Beacon Press, 1971), p. 4; Alan Sussman, *The rights of young people: An ACLU handbook* (New York: Avon Books, 1977), p. 13.

5. Angela Roddey Holder, *Legal issues in pediatrics and adolescent medicine* (New York: Wiley, 1977), p. 136; Harriet F. Pilpel and Ruth J. Zuckerman, "Abortion and the rights of minors," in *Abortion, society, and the law*, ed. David F. Walbert

and J. Douglas Butler (Cleveland: Case Western Reserve University, 1973), pp. 276–277; Andrew Jay Kleinfeld, "The balance of power among infants, their parents, and the state, Pt. 2," *Family Law Review* 4 (1970): 413–414, report in *The legal rights of children* (New York: Arno Press, 1974).

6. Robert H. Mnookin, *Child, family and state* (Boston: Little, Brown, 1978), p. 158.

7. *Danforth* (slip opinion), appendix, 32.

8. *Carey*, 2014.

9. *Danforth*, 16, citation to *Eisenstadt* v. *Baird*, 405 U.S. 453 (1972); see also *Griswold*, 1682: "We deal with a right of privacy older than the Bill of Rights—older than our political parties, older than our school system. Marriage is a coming together for better or for worse, hopefully enduring, and intimate to the degree of being sacred. It is an association that promotes a way of life, not causes; a harmony in living, not political faiths; a bilateral loyalty, not commercial or social projects. Yet it is an association for as noble a purpose as any involved in our prior decisions" (see n. 13).

10. *Carey*, p. 21.

11. *Danforth* (Stevens' dissent), 4–5; *Bellotti* v. *Baird*, 428 U.S. 132 (1976); *Baird* v. *Bellotti* (D. Mass., May 2, 1978); *Bellotti* v. *Baird*, 47 LW 2969 (July 2, 1979). For an analysis that suggests the Supreme Court went further than, by my reading, it did, see Eve W. Paul and Harriet F. Pilpel, "Teenagers and pregnancy: The law in 1979," *Family Planning Perspectives* 11, no. 5 (Sept./Oct. 1979): 297–302.

12. *Danforth* (Blackmun), 20–21.

13. The controversy concerning privacy rights in *Griswold* centers on the issue of whether the privacy rights rest with the couple (or "association," as Douglas described them in *Griswold*—see n. 9), or with the individual, as *Danforth* would imply. For discussion of this issue see David W. Louisell and John T. Noonan, Jr., "Constitutional balance," in *The morality of abortion*, ed. John T. Noonan, Jr. (Cambridge: Harvard University Press, 1970), pp. 220–260; Laurence H. Tribe, "Foreward: Toward a model of roles in the due process of life and law," *Harvard Law Review* 87, no. 1 (Nov. 1973): 33–41; Paul Ramsey, *Ethics at the edges of life* (New Haven: Yale University Press, 1978), pp. 13–18.

14. *Danforth* (White), 3–4.

15. Ibid.; see also Stevens, 3–4.

16. Ibid. (Blackmun), 21; (Stewart), 30.

17. *Bellotti* (1979). In what can only be described as the Supreme Court's ambivalence on this whole subject, Justice Powell goes on in the paragraph following to write: "There is, however, an important state interest in encouraging a family rather than a judicial resolution of a minor's abortion decision. Also, as we have observed above, parents naturally take an interest in the welfare of their children—an interest that is particularly strong where a normal family relationship exists and where the child is living with one or both parents. These factors

properly may be taken into account by a court called upon to determine whether an abortion in fact is in a minor's best interest."

18. Eve W. Paul, Harriet F. Pilpel, and Nancy F. Wechsler, "Pregnancy, teenagers, and the law, 1976," *Family Planning Perspectives* 8, no. 1 (Jan./Feb. 1976): 17.

19. Holder, *Legal issues*, pp. 139–141.

20. Pilpel and Zuckerman, "Abortion and the rights," pp. 227–278.

21. Holder, *Legal issues*, p. 146.

22. *Doe v. Irwin*, 441 F. Supp. 1247 (1977). Here, a judge of the Michigan Federal District Court reaffirmed an earlier decision that "found the Tri-County Family Planning Center practice of distributing 'prescriptive contraceptives and contraceptive devices to minor, unemancipated children in the absence of notice to, and the opportunity of consultation with, their parents' violated the constitutional rights of such parents.'" Given the drift of the Supreme Court's decision in this area, it is doubtful that the Court would let this decision stand, although from my point of view Chief Judge Fox makes a very strong case for the rights of parental notification. *Editor's note:* Since going to press the Supreme Court, in October 1980, declined to review the case.

23. At the moment, Louisiana appears to be the one exception. A state law that went into effect Sept. 8, 1978, among other measures requires: "parental consent or a court order for females under fifteen to get abortions and parental notice or a court order for unmarried women under eighteen to do so." It also mandates a waiting period of twenty-four hours and counseling by a doctor for any woman to get an abortion: "In counseling, the physician is required to tell a woman seeking an abortion and the parents of females under fifteen who are seeking abortions that 'the unborn child is a human life from the moment of conception' and that an 'unborn child may be viable' if more than twenty-two weeks have elapsed since conception." *The New York Times*, August 1, 1978.

24. Jean Piaget, *The moral development of the child* (New York: Free Press, 1965), pp. 65, 70–71.

25. Lawrence Kohlberg, Collected papers, Spring 1973 (photocopy collection); see esp., "The adolescent as philosopher," reprinted from *Daedalus* (1971).

26. Jay Katz, *Experimentation with human beings* (New York: Russell Sage Foundation, 1972), p. 305.

27. Quoted in Leonard L. Riskin, "Informed consent: Should doctors tell the truth?" *Boston University Journal* 23, no. 3 (1975): 13.

28. For some of the debate concerning informed consent, see Katz, *Experimentation*, pp. 529–534; Riskin, "Informed consent," pp. 12–20; Charles Fried, *Medical experimentation, personal integrity, and social policy* (New York: American Elsevier, 1974), pp. 18–22; Robert M. Veatch, "Ethical principles in medical experimentation," *Ethical and legal issues of social experimentation*, ed. Alice M. Rivlin and P. Michael Timpane (Washington, D.C.: Brookings Institution, 1975), esp. pp. 48–51.

29. *Danforth* (Stewart), 3–4.
30. *Danforth* (Stewart), 3–4.
31. Linda Bird Francke, *The ambivalence of abortion* (New York: Random House, 1978), p. 252.
32. See *11 million teenagers* for the 1974 figures (pp. 10–11); for the 1976 figures, see Christopher Tietze, "Teenage pregnancies: Looking ahead to 1984," *Family Planning Perspectives* 10, no. 4 (July/Aug. 1978): 206; for the increased use of contraceptives, see Melvin Zelnik and John F. Kantner, "First pregnancies to women aged fifteen to nineteen, 1976 and 1971," *Family Planning Perspectives* 10, no. 1 (Jan./Feb. 1978): 11–20. The best overall source for figures is Wendy H. Baldwin, "Adolescent pregnancy and childbearing—growing concerns for Americans," *Population Bulletin* 31, no. 2 (rev. report) (June 1980).
33. *Danforth* (Blackmun), 21.
34. Holder, *Legal issues*, pp. 246–247; see also *In re Smith* 295 A 2d 238 (Md. 1972).
35. For example, see *The New York Times*, May 10, 1978. One opponent to a parental notification bill remarked, "We are going to pass legislation like this, that attempts to create by legislation an understanding that parents have been unable to develop. . . . Its goal is impossible."
36. The argument in a recent Illinois decision gives some support to this line of thinking: "We do not hold that parents cannot be notified of their daughter's condition. To the contrary, because we believe that parents should be involved in their minor's decisions whenever possible, they generally should be informed. Nor do we hold that a minor should be free not to inform her parents merely because such disclosure may cause familial disharmony. The objectionable feature of the statute is rather that it requires that the parents be informed in *all* cases, thereby precluding an independent assessment, whether by a court or physician, that it would not be in the minor's best interest for her parents to learn of her condition" (*Wynn* v. *Carey*, no. 78-1262 (7th Cir.) Wynn 2).
37. Paul Robinson, *The modernization of sex* (New York: Harper Colophon, 1976).

9

Adolescent Sexuality and Teenage Pregnancy from a Black Perspective

June Dobbs Butts

As a black sex educator, I find it impossible to assess the problem of teenage pregnancy unless it is set in focus, against the backdrop of history. The higher fertility rate among black adolescents as compared with whites will only be elucidated when one analyzes the historical context which produced both sets of youngsters.

I believe our nation has a disease which is systemic in nature and devastating in its consequences; thus, how we approach the problem is crucial to its solution. I feel that people who design government programs and policies have been historically myopic—merely describing the symptoms of our disease rather than defining the true causative agents.

Teenage pregnancy is one fact of life which confronts all Americans whether urban or rural, rich or poor, white or black, male or female. This disturbance is creeping into our collective consciousness from quietly contained, little Midwestern hamlets just as surely as it is staring us in the face from noisily sprawling, big-city ghettoes. We see it clearly among minority groups, notably among blacks—America's largest ethnic minority—because skin color and economic impoverishment make for high visibility in a welfare-wary national economy. But the disturbance is growing steadily and stealthily also among whites—especially in the urbane, affluent class whose power heretofore has insured it privacy and protection from sensational news media coverage. So, although teenage pregnancy is a fact of modern life, it is the black teenage mother who epitomizes the crux of the problem, for it is in regard to her undeveloped, but emerging body that we find the culmination of all those abstract ideas—racism, sexism, and the stamp of despair—that are bred by grinding poverty.

And if the sight of a fourteen-year-old about to give birth is not disturbing enough, there is a convoluting problem within the problem: the offspring. What are we as a nation to do, say by the year 2000, when we are faced with a generation of unwanted, and sometimes mentally or physically defective, offspring from the kids having kids at the present?

It is my thesis that teenage pregnancy is but a vexatious symptom of a societal illness. Until America can solve the twin issues of racism and sexism, we will have a diseased country, and can expect further exacerbation of the symptoms.

I define racism as the conviction that one's own race is inherently superior to all others. The same principle applies to sexism: it is the strong belief that one's own sex is intrinsically better than the other. People who do not see other people as individuals but always view them as representatives of a particular racial group are, according to my definition, racists. And by the same token, any man who views his maleness as a reason to look down upon or to disparage all women is a sexist. And vice versa, of course.

On the personal, attitudinal level, I firmly believe that being for one group (or cause, or idea) does not imply that one is automatically against others. However, the history of our country has been permeated by such thoughts and this has led to the institutionalization of racist and sexist behavior.

I feel that the sexist bias is even more ingrained than is racism, and exists on a world wide basis. And why do men feel superior to women? I feel that men fear and/or envy the female and her ability to become pregnant, to give birth, and to suckle her young. And because of this ambivalent feeling men have historically treated women only as sex objects or as mother figures neither of which is a position of parity in the governance of society. For, if women are restricted only to the home, and men dominate outside, then each realm lacks the other's valuable perspective. But this exclusivity need not remain. Now science has given us choices. Anatomy need not be destiny for women any more than for men.

This essay will discuss several characteristics of the black experience that have relevance to teenage pregnancy. I call them principles (ideas which are valued in the black community), and urge that both the design and implementation of federally funded programs should become more sensitive to them. These principles are a sex-positive view of life, the extended family, and the historical value of fecundity.

A Sex-Positive View of Life

I believe that blacks should be studied because we have what my colleagues in the field of sex education call a "sex-positive view" of life. This is in direct contrast with the values of white society, which are essentially sex-negative. I consider what goes on in America to be a type of sexual schizophrenia, a schism between our attitudes toward sex and our sexual behavior. Why do we as a nation glorify the family, but refer to sexual activity in the pejorative? Whence do families originate, if not from sexual encounter? How can we praise the product but not the process? Our whole country is permeated with sexual innuendo—buy this product (a car, toothpaste, anything), for it will make you "sex-y"! We allow youngsters to become supersaturated with provocative sexual stimuli while telling them that the only respectable outlet for sexual expression is heterosexual coitus performed by legally married couples. The difference between what we practice and what we preach is more than a charming little deceit—it borders on the psychopathic, and the youngsters know it. We Americans are schizoid in our attitude toward sensuality, toward sexuality, and certainly, toward fecundity.

We say that sex is natural and good, but we adults panic when teenagers seek any mode of sexual expression. Adolescents today—rich or poor, black or white, male or female—feel that having sex is "in," but they seldom use contraceptives, especially for the first time. (Research studies have told us what they do, but not why.) I feel that they get discouraged by adults. I know that when I worked in New York City as a consultant in Family Life and Sex Education to the Human Resources Administration, and when teenagers flocked into the low-cost clinics (especially during the school strike, when they were bored and frustrated) asking for advice on contraception, most of the adult outreach workers did not praise them for acting responsibly—most just said, "Don't!" Wouldn't it be great if O. J. Simpson and Jesse Jackson could appear on a TV program especially designed for teenagers, and discuss the manliness of using condoms? I am serious. If O. J. can pose for magazines that deal with sex in a titillating fashion, why not use his charisma in an edifying way, by treating sex with respect and dignity? Our young people need role models who are responsible, sexually aware human beings. They need people who are not ashamed to offer some viable alternatives to the traditional chorus of voices chanting, "Don't," and, "Thou shalt not."

A clear-cut example of this sex-positive view of life can be found in the ways blacks value sensuousness. (This is different from being told by whites that we have "natural rhythm.") Distinguishable from either sex or sexuality, sensuousness is a dominant thread in the fabric of black family life. The socialization process—the many different practices involved in nurturing and raising the young—among black families is more lenient, more child-oriented, and more sensuous than is the case in the dominant white culture, regardless of the socioeconomic class of blacks. *Sensuousness* is literally the process of living in a world of sensation and perception. It means the ability to interpret the world through one's senses: sight, sound, taste, smell, and touch. The sense modality of *touch* is one of the keenest ways of interpreting stimuli and is the one that is used most in the field of sex therapy. Perhaps it is in the touching and the enjoyment of contact with human bodies that black culture is most alive, and is introduced into the life of the growing child. The fondness for touch permeates black culture from the cradle to the grave. One need only observe the highly stylized gestures and charades of black athletes, whether teenagers on the block playing basketball or pros earning a living in contact sports, to see the fondness for human touch. What is striking to me about these men is their very physicality: they handle each other freely, good-naturedly, and as an integral part of their shared nonverbal communication. One can also see the fondness for human touch—basic sensuousness without sexual overtones—that reflects much warmth and conviviality at gatherings in which blacks take part on a regular basis, such as at church meetings. For example, the slave spirituals, and later the gospel music of the black church that help to celebrate such rites of passage as christenings, marriages, homecomings, and funerals partake of sensuousness by appealing to many senses at once.

When sexual stimuli are added to other stimuli, the information is transformed beyond the level of sensuousness into what is called the *sensual*. The sexual component is the decisive factor in changing what is mere perception into a "turn on" or into a "turn off." An excellent example of sensuality in black culture is the idiom of jazz. This is a uniquely black contribution to song and dance, although whites have made far greater economic gains from their imitations of black song and dance than have the black artists whose work was original; witness the enormous adulation accorded George Gershwin, the Beatles, Elvis Presley, and recently the Bee Gees—all of whom acknowledged their black inspiration, and all of whom the adolescent culture has venerated. There is a beat and rhythm which "turns whites on," for rhythm is natural to us all, contrary to the stereotype that holds that only blacks have "natural rhythm." This was never intended as a compliment, since it was traditionally cast in the pejorative as meaning something base and denigrating; however, this is the releasing and rejuvenating quality that young whites are seeking today, most frantically in the current disco scene.

For many whites, the expression of their basic sensuality was considered anathema according to the edicts of many of their religious bodies. The equating of sensuality with sin occurred early on in Western religious thought, for things "of the flesh" could not be considered holy. Because of a difference in religious origin, we need to assess the significance of sensuality and of sensuousness in the life of the black teenager from an historical point of view. The African roots of today's black teenagers, where religious fervor and sensuality were merged, figure in their conceptualization of sensuality and sensuousness. Of course, there were strong injunctions against casual sex in early tribal Africa, which enforced strict codes that venerated fecundity and saw sex as a pleasurable means to an end, but never as an end per se. This is an important idea to fit into the conceptual framework when analyzing the strength of the black family. Given the freedom derived from this African heritage to accept and glorify in their basic sensuality, it was natural for black Americans to accept and to glorify their sexual feelings. The culture itself was sex-positive; and socialization is always facilitated by the healthy expression of one's innate sensuality. It is said that in Africa today there are virtually no people with sexual dysfunctions such as impotence or female nonorgasmic response (outside the chronically ill). And we know that experts have estimated that sexual dysfunctions occur in about half of the married populace of the United States, including American blacks. That should tell us something about the puritanical ethos of our American culture. In this country, human sexuality is not accorded respect or dignity. I personally think that the current upsurge of teenage pregnancy is a misguided, pathetic attempt to correct the situation. The kids are saying, "This is my body, and it feels good; it belongs to me." They are not thinking ahead to the future of motherhood or of fathering a family, with its constant responsibilities. They are children of a "Now" culture, and they desperately need older adults to be with them, to remind them of their roots, and to give them a sense of futurity.

The Extended Family

I feel that we, as a nation, would do well to study the survival techniques of black families. Most Americans know the manner in which blacks were captured and sold in bondage into this country, and how families were so often torn apart. Few truly appreciate the will to survive that has been nourished by the bonds of the black family and its ability to forge new survival techniques, in spite of hundreds of years of institutionalized slavery, ghettoization, discrimination, and grinding poverty.

The sense of kinship based on African tribalism has been a bulwark in the black experience. It goes without saying that the family is a major stabilizing force for most ethnic groups—so why is the black family special? The tribalism of Africa was not extinguished by the enforced bondage of slavery. The egalitarian nature of the man/woman relationship that existed among blacks during the slave days may well have been a unique example in Western civilization. Socially and sexually, black men and women were partners, equals—when permitted to live together —and they were usually very appreciative of the chance to do so in spite of the fragility of their union. Theirs was a tenuously held bond and therefore, perhaps, all the more precious; their mutual vulnerability was to be "sold down the river" at the caprice of the master. "Family" as a means of knowing who one was, and of survival itself, became an important facet of slave life. Since names were changed, families broken up, and males often sent out to stud, it was difficult to count on blood relatives for consolation and protection. Friends who were willing to see one through hard times; to bring up the offspring of a dying or a sold-away mother; who were able to learn crafts and buy their freedom, perhaps sending for loved ones; or who were willing to take into their families the ex-slaves who had made their way North—these friends became the extended black family; and there is no parallel to this type of friendship in American history: it was all purely voluntary.

The urbanization trend accelerated, and coincided with northward migration after the Civil War; it took on great impetus after World War I and II. The black family became more truncated, less "extended," but the concept has not died out by any means. It is only a bit less convenient today. Living quarters in the North were not conducive to having a flock of relatives, or even good friends, come to visit or move in for a while. So, today's young people may not have ever actually seen or lived among numerous branches of their family tree, but the concept of valuing "the family" remains quite strong in black culture.

I have seen groups of middle-class teenage black youngsters —including my own—adopt the nomenclature of family life when finding themselves in new situations—for instance, going to summer camp, or changing residences or schools. One becomes someone else's "brother," "uncle," or "mama"; and this takes the edge off inevitable disappointment when a love affair dissolves. The same phenomenon occurs with amazing regularity among black youths in prisons. Giving and receiving some type of family appellation fosters a basic sense of security, and gives purpose to one's life in unknown or trying circumstances. Thus, family provides a sense of something bigger than one's finite self—of the life force, perhaps, of which one is a part —and thus gives purpose and meaning to one's mundane travails, even when scorned by others—as when having a baby out of wedlock. The impartiality of the extended black family has traditionally bolstered up the sagging spirits of its members and flattened any inflated egos evenhandedly. The extended family has proved itself of inestimable worth in accepting and incorporating into its fold the babies of teenagers. This brings us to the third principle.

The Historical Value of Fecundity

A cursory glance at the research literature of the past generation shows that black adolescents have a proportionately higher rate of out-of-wedlock pregnancies than do white teenagers. Earlier researchers tended to write of this phenomenon in the pejorative, citing the immorality of such behavior and implying that blacks are more prone to sexual excess. Recently, the more psychoanalytically inclined researchers have dealt with teenage pregnancy from a more humane stance. Whether this is because the phenomenon is occurring in groups in which it seldom was seen years ago—that is, among richer, white groups—or because the researchers themselves are becoming more humane, is unclear in my mind. At any rate, the ambience surrounding this subject matter is one of concern now, rather than condemnation.

Nevertheless, facts show that black youngsters are becoming pregnant more frequently than whites. What does this mean when placed in the black perspective? It tells me that the researchers have counted pregnancies rather than assessing sexual activity. White teenagers engage in more types of what we in the field of sex education call nonprocreative sex. Such behavior, by definition, cannot lead to pregnancy. Nonprocreative sex means stimulation accomplished by any means other than direct genital contact. Its source can be manual, oral, anal, autoerotic, or by artificial means, such as a vibrator. White youngsters engage in all these types of sexual activity at an earlier age and for a longer portion of their lives than do their black counterparts. I do not place a value judgment on any type of sexual activity that is performed between consenting mature human beings without doing harm to either party; I only point out that some types of stimulation lead to pregnancy and others do not. It is a maladroit combination of ignorance and of innocence among black youth that encourage them to use coital patterns for "natural" sexual expression and to eschew contraceptive measures. Whites have traditionally used methods that mitigate against pregnancy, or have found it more desirable (when pregnancy not only occurred but went to term) to place the offspring up for adoption. This is a practice that is frowned upon in the black community, basically because many black people still believe in the old adage that "a baby is the future." Possibly this attitude also influences blacks' reluctance to use contraceptives effectively.

If young blacks—both male and female—today are to be persuaded to give up the myth that one proves one's worth through demonstrated fecundity, then I believe it will only come to pass when our government shows them openly and honestly that it considers them part of the nation's natural resources. They must be convinced that there is a future for them: a chance to attend school, a relevant curriculum to pursue, and a dependable chance of their finishing school and not having to drop out because of economic privation and/or unwanted pregnancy. And most important, they must be assured that the job market won't remain closed to them: that industry, the military, the arts, higher education, commerce—every branch of our country's economy counts them as an integral part of the potential labor force. When this happens, and only if it happens, our country will have gotten rid of the twin evils, sexism and racism. This, then, is my analysis of why teenage pregnancy is abroad and rampant in the land.[1] Let me now share with you the small but eloquent sample of informed opinion of black health care professionals that I garnered as back-up references offering concrete ways in which government can alter the crisis situation we now face.

The Dilemma of the Black Health Care Professional

The peculiar dilemma of the black health care professional is really no different from the dilemma of the black politician, the black school superintendent, or the black public sanitation worker: how to gain upward mobility within the system (based on one's merits and not on tokenism) while fighting to change the system.

The cruel word "genocide," which was hurled at government programs so often during the past decade and a half that the general public began to turn a deaf ear, is still heard today. The black health care professional who advocates planning and spacing one's children, who informs the public about the availability of surgical fertility control, such as vasectomy and tubal ligation, who cautions adolescents against casual sex, who upholds the rights of homosexuals, who understands the need for some people to remain "child-free" in their marriages, who sponsors and supports adoption and more stringently improved foster care networks—such a person is deeply suspect in many quarters of the larger black community. There has to be a commitment of great valor to continue working for the good of one's people in spite of frightened reactionaries.

Approximately eight years ago in New Rochelle, New York, a gang of black men were so angry about the work of a certain Planned Parenthood Center that they broke into the local office and literally, as well as figuratively, "wrecked the joint." On Monday morning, however, a group of black women who obviously respected and needed the services of the Center showed up offering to sweep and tidy the place, and get the doors open again to the public. It is counterproductive to shame or ignore the black men who were outraged. We who have had the benefit of education and some measure of success need to listen to them, interpret what the root cause of their vast rage is, and help them restore a sense of manhood—for, indeed, what they were protesting was being stripped away by an aloof white society that callously tells them that they shouldn't father any more children. Yet, the women were right also. They wanted the contraceptive services when they needed them, under their own control, not at the dictate of some organization. So, the black health care professional is much needed as liaison, as social change agent, and as an important member of the black community. And he or she must be heard by the white power structure not as a "black authority" but as a competent health care professional who happens to be black, just as he or she happens to be male or female—neither factor should create bias for or against anyone.

As I took down the comments of my colleagues, I was struck with the similarity of many of their answers. I asked them the three questions found on page fifty of the "Interim Report" published in April 1978 by the Family Impact Seminar. We spoke on the telephone, for I felt it afforded us easier dialogue than the static quality of a written letter. The questions I asked were the same for each respondent, and they were:

- Can you identify ways in which federally funded programs discriminate against certain groups—in this case, against blacks?
- Can you identify ways in which federally funded programs are insensitive to, or even do damage to, certain values and attitudes of black people?
- In what way could these programs build on the values, attitudes, resources and strengths of black people in order to encourage more effective family functioning?

Of my ten respondents, only one asked not to be identified by name. I could understand her reasons, and have quoted her materials anonymously. I am grateful for the cooperation of them all, and would have enlarged the sample, had time permitted. The people whom I quote now are candid and sex-positive men and women; I only hope their wisdom will be heard. The following are all too brief excerpts from their responses to my questions:

James Batts, M.D. The Director of the Department of Obstetrics and Gynecology at the Harlem Hospital Center in New York City, Batts commented:

> The welfare system, which encourages women to refrain from having their husbands live with them, is fla-

grant and outright discrimination. Abortion legislation is blatantly anti–poor people.

Look at the Family Planning programs—they sound good at first, but the [adolescent] child is receiving charity. This encourages children to break free of parental control and to leave home. Such programs should encourage the child to inform parents and to enlist their support. Why should only broken families receive support? Turn it around and look the other way—why not give financial support to a complete or intact family, as well as or even more so than to a family on welfare? And if a man is in the family, they should help him find a job, not get rid of him.

Kenyon Burke, M.S. Associate Director for Programs with the NAACP in New York City, Burke had this to say:

> Take the welfare program: in order to qualify for eligibility, it discourages male membership. The program as it is federally funded now is completely inadequate. What's needed is more and better day care centers, training—this is all important—for the men who are entering the labor market from the low status which has been so meager up til now, and other factors, too. More black women than white women work at this lowest level, and therefore, they're at a disadvantage. Programs for reentry (for the mature woman) are much needed. The teenager also needs work, and especially the young mother.
>
> The language of the majority group toward the black family is often insensitive. They expect and are biased in favor of two parents and their children constituting a "real" family. This is not so in the black community.
>
> The strength of the extended family in the black community is not often well understood outside of the black community. Historically we've had it, and we

must get back to that close intimacy again. We've gotten infected with that same independent, isolated feeling that infected white people: alienation! The black church could be a network to rebuild that sense of "family."

William A. Darity, Ph.D. Darity, Dean of the School of Health Sciences at the University of Massachusetts at Amherst, said:

> Yes, there is discrimination. To be specific, there's an insufficient number of black researchers and administrators.
>
> Most of these programs are designed for the majority group's needs, and not to meet specific needs of black families. Look at the Cancer programs. The funding for studies on the black family goes to white researchers. The Family Planning programs too often are designed to impose values on the recipients, that is, limiting family size, marital status, etc. There's never been real recognition of the validity of a one-parent family, particularly when that mother has never been married. Often religious impositions are made on individuals too.
>
> Family Planning and social welfare programs do damage to the kids, by branding them as "illegitimate," which is terrible. The economic issue plays a major role in all of this. Whites have the means, the economic means to either adopt or in some way to get rid of any evidence of sexuality; blacks don't. Those programs need black input and black implementation!

Ramona Edelin, M.S.W. Executive Assistant to the President of the Urban Coalition in Washington, D.C., Edelin said:

> Look at the welfare reform business going on now. The Medicaid-abortion issue restricts funds for poor

women severely. It is obvious that ultimately it is the children who are the ones being discriminated against.

Having the man in the home! There is a reform piece of legislation coming up pertaining to this. Newer legislation now permits another wage-earner to live in the home. There are some attempts being made which help: the Head Start program could pull the family into the picture. Also, Jesse Jackson's EXCEL (Push for Excellence) program speaks to the involvement of the family—it's too late once the kids reach adolescence. We need health recreational and all other kinds of preventive services (like after-school, as well as in school, programs). We could look at each governmental department and ask what they can do for the black family. They could all be asked for help.

Helen Dickens, M.D. She is Associate Dean of the School of Medicine and Professor of Obstetrics and Gynecology at the University of Pennsylvania in Philadelphia. Her comment is:

Children do not receive their fair share of the tax dollar. The total amount of funds to children and youth through Maternal and Infant Care (MIC) programs are funded annually, but if you have more patients than their amount of dollars covers, either you can't see them all or they have to pay out of pocket. MIC funds are only for high-risk obstetrics—like the teens (or at least about two-thirds of them) whom I see. Family Planning funds—for nonpregnant teenagers—are grossly inadequate.

Often the staff members are inadequate, and often they do not represent the black community at all. There may be a token or two of black representatives on the staff of these programs, but the entire programs don't reflect the thinking of the black community. Example: not paying for abortions of poor women—the

Governor of Pennsylvania vetoed this during his "lame duck" session, and effectively stalled it until the next Congress.

Most of these programs aren't funded to [build on the strengths of black families]. Their personnel don't understand or can't work with black families. There is no economic support for middle-class teenagers who become pregnant; so, often they marry even if they don't stay together long. For poor kids who get pregnant, often the male can't work or if he does, he can't earn much—so the female gets welfare, and then sometimes they just don't even marry. There could be changes in the way these programs are being mandated.

Elizabeth Graham, M.S.W. Graham, the Supervisor of Social Services in the Department of Obstetrics and Gynecology and Co-Director of Young Parents' Program at Columbia-Presbyterian Medical Center, New York, said:

Aid to Families of Dependent Children (AFDC) really divides families! The whole system fails to promote the growth and development of black family members; it creates generations of dependents instead. No "self help" is built into the system. It's always the system against them. Day care programs have long waiting lists and often a fee schedule is unreasonable. There aren't enough "family day care" programs where a two-month-old infant can be cared for. They could provide a neighborhood woman to help so that the mother could go back to work. Mothers need help with their own development, life is turbulent enough.

Any program has peaks and valleys. No program that I can think of right off the bat is blatantly insensitive, but the implementation and the monitoring systems leave a lot to be desired in most of them.

> So many of these programs are just designed to deal with the problems and to ignore the strengths! Some of the teenagers have great resources, and many programs could encourage and foster their strengths instead of fostering a continued sense of dependency.

Naomi T. Gray, M.S.W. Gray, the Director of Naomi Gray Associates in San Francisco, California, said:

> Agencies are indifferent, don't provide for minorities to serve on their boards of directors, for example, or in similar higher decision-making capacities. The federal government hasn't monitored these agencies well at all. They simply file contracts and grants—and that is not spending wisely. And the end result is that black families aren't being served well.
>
> Most of these programs don't understand the cultural values and the particular life styles of blacks—in fact, very few do. Most of them need black input into the planning and organizing phases of their programs, as well as during the implementation of such programs. And blacks should be paid for their advice!
>
> The ultimate consumers of these services should be placed in peer relationships—in other words, GIVE THEM JOBS.

Mary S. Harper, Ph.D. She is Assistant Chief, Center for Minority Group Mental Health at the National Institute of Mental Health in Rockville, Maryland. Her comments included:

> [Services] are fragmented—meaning there is no central theme or committed effort. Right now each branch has gone its own way, piecemeal. Therefore, government programs which help the black family really haven't yet been focused.
>
> We need an "Inter-Agency Committee on the Family," just as we have one on children. The federal gov-

ernment should collaborate with private organizations (concerned with families). There are over 150 of them. Why not bring them all together and work on ways in which they can conceptualize what's going on with families, with what research is needed to improve things? Blacks would be represented in all these organizations.

Robert Staples, Ph.D. An author and Associate Professor in the Department of Social and Behavioral Sciences at the University of California at San Francisco, Staples said:

> The program Aid to Families of Dependent Children (AFDC) may actually be encouraging teenage pregnancy. Also, it's a bit hazy why there were so many sterilizations in Alabama in a governmentally sponsored program a few years ago. Black input is needed! The ban on federal funds for abortion is especially bad. Black women need this option because of their economic dependence. Blacks also need more sex education in our schools—more availability of contraception, etc. One-third of blacks are now being born to teenagers! What is the future of these children?
>
> [Programs] don't, as a rule, recognize that black families need support systems. This fact portends bad things for the next generation.
>
> Somehow the role of the black man has to be strengthened through a variety of good outreach programs which are community based.

Anonymous Administrator in a large, Northern, federal program. This health care professional said:

> In Family Planning there's a large segment of the black population which earns just above the poverty level now held as the cut-off point for receiving federal assistance and services. Regionalism makes a difference

in how far one's money can be stretched. Rearing a family of four in Austin, Texas, is a lot easier than caring for such a family in Harlem, with its over-inflated rents, food, transportation, weather differences for clothing, etc. There should be a relative adjustment made for the relative cost of living.

The government is pushing voluntary fertility control without giving any consideration to other economic, social, and dental aspects of general and comprehensive health. The total person has to be considered, or it's genocide.

Community people should be employed as staff for such programs.

Just as the lives of individual men are often enriched when they can listen without bias to the observations of concerned women, so can the quality of life in white society be greatly improved when the insights of its minority members are respected and incorporated.

NOTES

1. Those interested in exploring some of these themes further may want to consult the following references: Phyllis Greenacre, *Emotional growth*, vol. 1 (New York: International Universities Press, 1971); Calvin Hernton, *Sex and race in America* (Garden City, N.Y.: Doubleday, 1965); Robert B. Hill, *The strengths of black families* (New York: National Urban League, 1971); Joyce A. Ladner, *Tomorrow's tomorrow: The black woman* (New York: Doubleday, 1971); Kenneth Little, "Some urban patterns of marriage and domesticity in West Africa," *The Sociological Review* 7 (July 1959); L. P. Mair, "African marriage and social changes," in *Survey of African marriage and family life*, ed. A. Phillips (London: Oxford University Press, 1953), p. 1; ed., Robert Staples, *The black family*, rev. ed. (Chicago: Wadsworth, 1978)—see especially chapter by Alan P. Bell, "Black sexuality: Fact and fancy"; and Charles V. Willie, B. M. Karmer, and B. S. Brown, eds., *Racism and mental health* (Pittsburgh: University of Pittsburgh Press, 1973).

10

The Impact of Adolescent Pregnancy on Hispanic Adolescents and Their Families

Angel Luis Martinez

An Hispanic Perspective

First generation. Pete Morales, seventeen, was born in Texas. His parents were born in Sonora, Mexico. They speak mostly Spanish. He speaks mostly English: "There ain't no jobs; school sucks; everywhere we go they lie to us. So we get high and mess around. If somebody gets pregnant, at least you have some excitement."

Newcomer. Juanita Cabrera has two children, lives alone, and is unemployed. She arrived from the Dominican Republic three years ago and speaks English with apparent distaste and difficulty. She is nineteen.

Second generation. Nadine Ayala doesn't speak Spanish. She takes it in school. All of her friends speak English and her boyfriend's family has never known Spanish. Her parents were born in Denver, and the family now lives in Berkeley. She is fifteen and pregnant.

In order to discuss adolescent pregnancy in the Hispanic family and community, it is necessary that we ask what we know about Hispanics, in general, and about Hispanic adolescents, in particular.[1] There are more than twelve million persons of Spanish origin who live in the United States.[2] Of these, approximately 7,200,000 are Mexican, 1,800,000 are Puerto Rican, 700,000 are Cuban, and 2,400,000 are considered "other" Hispanics. The estimate of all Hispanics, including undocumented persons, is nineteen million. (See Tables 6 and 7.)

Hispanic adolescents represent approximately 24 percent of this total, compared to a 20.3 percent adolescent population for the general population.[3] (These figures do not include the Bureau of Census estimate of three million people living in Puerto Rico who are American citizens.)[4]

More precise numbers are difficult to arrive at because of poor available sources, and because no figures exist on the number of "undocumented" or "uncounted" Hispanics in this country—adult, adolescent, or child. Within this population, a Nadine Ayala may have more in common with a Marie Osmond than with a Juanita Cabrera. In reality, we know very little about either Nadine or Juanita, or even how many of each there are in the general population. However, when Hispanic young people are spoken about, when they are considered by social service agencies, or when they are deplored in the media, they are usually spoken of generically.

The stereotypical adolescent is a media creation. A preponderance of printed media and of television programming, dealing with adolescents or adolescent concerns, focuses basically on problems: alcoholism, prostitution, runaways, pregnancy, and status offenders. Teenagers as able, responsible, and talented people are not often seen.

Behind the overall negative image of adolescents lie the images of minority adolescents. Hispanic youth, who, with black youth, are made media-visual as problems whenever they gather in groups of more than one, are also generally portrayed as linguistically maladroit and morally deficient.

The programs providing services to Hispanic young people that attract media attention are, of course, the ones that deal with problems. As a result, the picture that America gets is one of drug addicts that need rehabilitation, pregnant girls that need care, and troublemakers who seem to be in the news all the

TABLE 6
POPULATION OF SPANISH ORIGIN, BY SEX AND TYPE OF SPANISH ORIGIN (for the United States, March 1978; numbers in thousands)

Type of Spanish Origin	Both Sexes		Males		Females	
	Number	Percent	Number	Percent	Number	Percent
Mexican	7,151	59.4	3,528	60.3	3,623	58.5
Puerto Rican	1,823	15.1	825	14.1	997	16.1
Cuban	689	5.7	342	5.8	347	5.6
Central or South American	863	7.2	396	6.8	467	7.5
Other Spanish	1,519	12.6	758	13.0	761	12.3
Total	12,046	100.0	5,850	100.0	6,196	100.0

Source: Department of Commerce, Bureau of the Census, Current Population Reports, *Persons of Spanish origin in the United States,* ser. P-20, no. 328, table 2 (Washington, D.C.: GPO, March 1978), p. 5.

TABLE 7
TOTAL AND SPANISH ORIGIN POPULATION, BY AGE AND TYPE OF SPANISH ORIGIN (for the United States, March 1978)

Age	Total Population	Total	Spanish Origin					Not of Spanish Origin*
			Mexican	Puerto Rican	Cuban	Central or South American	Other Spanish	
Under 5 years	7.2	12.6	13.9	11.3	5.7	9.4	13.4	6.8
5 to 9 years	7.9	11.5	11.8	13.6	6.8	9.2	10.6	7.7
10 to 17 years	14.5	17.7	17.3	21.1	13.4	14.8	18.9	14.4
18 to 20 years	5.8	6.2	6.6	5.2	5.2	5.8	6.1	5.8
21 to 24 years	7.1	7.8	8.4	6.2	5.4	6.7	8.1	7.1
25 to 34 years	15.4	15.7	16.1	16.4	11.4	21.2	12.4	15.5
35 to 44 years	11.1	11.0	10.2	11.5	14.4	16.6	10.0	11.1
45 to 54 years	10.8	8.4	7.8	8.2	15.3	8.1	8.6	10.9
55 to 64 years	9.6	4.8	4.2	4.4	9.2	5.1	5.8	9.9
65 years and over	10.5	4.3	3.7	2.3	13.3	3.1	6.1	10.9
18 years and under	70.4	58.3	57.0	54.0	74.1	66.7	57.1	71.1
21 years and over	64.6	52.1	50.4	48.8	68.9	60.8	51.0	65.3
Median age (years)	29.5	22.1	21.3	20.3	36.5	26.8	21.5	30.0
All ages (thousands)	214,159	12,046	7,151	1,823	689	863	1,519	202,113
Percent	100.0	100.0	100.0	100.0	100.0	100.0	100.0	100.0

Source: Department of Commerce, Bureau of the Census, Current Population Reports, *Persons of Spanish origin in the United States*, ser. P-20, no. 328, table 2 (Washington, D.C.: GPO, March 1978), p. 5.
*Includes persons who did not know or did not report on origin.

time. It is a bleak and distorted picture. And the created myopia has become a real deficiency of discernment. We know so little, yet we make so many judgments.

Within every group of Latin American people in the United States there is a heterogeneous adolescent population—newcomers, oldtimers, and the degrees in between. We know that as a whole they are the least employed, earn the least when they are employed, are the least educated,[5] and have conflicts with legal authorities out of proportion to their numbers.

But we know very little about their lifestyles. We don't know whether recently arrived Puerto Rican, Mexican, or other Hispanic young people have more in common with each other, or with members of their own nationality who have either lived in this country for years or were born here. We don't know or understand how they are affected by cultural displacement, or the conflicts they experience between their families' cultural expectations and external values of American society.

Economics

> If I don't go to school, I can't work,
> if I work I can't go to school. What
> are you, crazy, or what?
>
> —Pete, seventeen

Almost one-half of Hispanics are under the age of eighteen;[6] and one out of three lives at or below poverty levels. About one-half live in the inner cities of America. One-half have completed high school; one out of five holds a white collar job.[7]

Families headed by Hispanic women are twice as likely to have incomes below the poverty level as those headed by Hispanic men; and Hispanic women are less likely to participate in the labor force than are men. Hispanics account for about 5 percent of the total population, 4 percent of the civilian labor force, and 6 percent of the unemployed.[8]

The situation for Hispanic youth is even more precarious. Although youths account for only one-quarter of the labor force, they represent half of all unemployed persons![9] It is almost impossible to do any real economic analysis on Hispanic youth unemployment because there are only poor, misleading, and discriminatory data available. A recent example is the report published by the Congressional Budget Office entitled *Youth unemployment: The outlook and some policy strategies*. For Hispanics, the data are not very useful because in the report, "unless otherwise noted, the term 'white' applies to Caucasians including those of Hispanic heritage. The term 'non-white' applies to blacks (which may include some persons of Hispanic heritage), American Indians, and Orientals."[10] Result: no data on Hispanic youth.

In June 1976, Public Law 94-311 was enacted; it directs federal agencies to expand the collection, analysis, and publication of statistics that will indicate the social, health, and economic conditions of Americans of Spanish origin or descent. The Departments of Labor and Commerce were given major responsibility for the collection and analysis of labor force and population data.

In May of 1978, the Commission on Civil Rights published a report entitled *Improving Hispanic Unemployment Data: The Department of Labor's Continuing Obligation*, which charged that "eighteen months after enactment of the law [P.L. 94-311] most of the Department of Labor's efforts were in the planning stages and the department did not know when it would publish the expanded data. . . . Moreover, it did not plan to publish Hispanic unemployment data monthly, as it does for blacks and whites. It planned to separate Hispanic unemployment data for only a very few states and for no local areas with large Hispanic population."[11]

By the mid-1980s, it is expected that Hispanics will represent the largest minority population in the United States. Without accurate data for all economic, social, and health indices to reflect the true situation of Hispanics, no comprehensive action can be taken to identify strategies that will address any of the problems faced by this population, including teenage pregnancy.

The Hispanic population in America is a very youthful one, the median age is 20.5, as compared to 28 for the overall population. In addition, the percentage of youth under eighteen within the Hispanic population is 44.2 percent, compared to 42.3 percent within the black population, and 33.2 percent within the white population. By contrast, the percentage of elderly (sixty-five years and older), within the Hispanic population is only 4.4 percent, as opposed to 7.0 percent within the black population, and 10.3 percent within the white population.[12] Hence, while the overall declining birthrate in America means a future decline in youth unemployment generally, the Hispanic youth population will continue to increase over the next decade, and, by extrapolation, will account for a larger percentage of unemployed youth, and of adolescent problems generally.

As Jones and Placek have pointed out, major sources of data relating to adolescent fertility do not separately break out pregnancy and births to Hispanics (which are included in the "white and other" category). Furthermore, there are virtually no research reports on Hispanic adolescent fertility in the United States. Thus, a discussion of teenage pregnancy in the Hispanic community has to rely on anecdotal impressions, experiences, and conjecture.

It seems reasonable to assume that the fertility rate among Hispanic teenagers is at least comparable to that of white youngsters, and may be as high as blacks. The extent of the problem of teenage pregnancy among Hispanic populations is partly indicated in the report of some preliminary analyses of new data collected from the 1979 National Longitudinal Survey on youth. These data indicate that Hispanics drop out of school much more frequently than whites or blacks; and among the major reasons cited are pregnancy, getting married, and home responsibilities. (Only 6.9 percent of whites ages eighteen to twenty-two are school dropouts who left school for these reasons, while the number for blacks is 14.7 percent, and for Hispanics, 19.6 percent.)[13]

Furthermore, there are serious implications in the high youth unemployment rate and poor employment prospects of Hispanics. Clearly, Hispanic youth, already at a socioeconomic disadvantage, will be further victimized by pregnancies. With one out of three already living in poverty, the chances for socioeconomic betterment will be limited, at best. A Hispanic child born of a teenage pregnancy has a very high likelihood of being locked into poverty.

The Hispanic youth who decides to bear and raise a child is likely to live below the poverty level. The young Hispanic parent is probably poorly educated, lives in the inner city, and lacks job skills, and in general, will exert pressure on existing family resources. She will be even less job-ready than her white American counterpart, because Hispanic women with children are less likely to work. The social cost, still unmeasured, is borne directly by the Hispanic family.

Old Traditions and New Pressures

. . . The moral bit, you know. My mother said, "You've got to get married. You can't disgrace the family.
—Rosa Maria, sixteen

Although Hispanics in the United States are not a homogeneous population, many cultural, linguistic, and traditional values are held in common. If we are going to attempt to influence Hispanic young persons' sexual and reproductive behavior, we should keep in mind that the evidence is that the educational and health programs for Hispanics that have been tried so far show that we have failed rather miserably.

Some of the causes lie in our lack of knowledge and understanding of the cultural world in which Hispanic adolescents live. For most white Americans and for a majority of blacks, the old traditions are *old* traditions. For them, "old traditions" is a term used to recall those values that are perceived almost as historical relics rather than active values. One example might be the family; within the old traditional values, this meant a nuclear grouping with a working male head, and concern for and care of the grandparent generation. Another "oldie" is the preeminence of parental authority over all matters affecting their children. These and other traditional values have changed radically in America, so that now their mention is generally within a context of wistfulness, or of a return to times gone by.

For large numbers of Hispanics, however, most of these traditional values have not changed; the modifier "old" does not apply. It is important to note that Hispanic families are more likely than either whites or blacks to be two-parent, male-headed families (78 percent, as compared with 77 percent and 63 percent in 1969, respectively).[14] Furthermore, there exists a sense of *familia* that encompasses an extended family (e.g., grandparents, aunts, uncles, and cousins), and identifies the older adults as persons with family position, authority, and relevance. If you're an Hispanic teenager, and a relative arrives from "over there" to live in your home, your life changes. When you go to visit "over there," your life changes. It happens because they are *familia*. The fact that the traditions and values are active can be seen in the threat that some parents use with teenagers who are not "behaving"; they are told that if they don't shape up they'll be sent "over there." For the parent this implies that cultural sanctions will have a stronger impact there. (Somewhat similar to the black youngster being sent "down South.") The school, the law, other adults, all receive more respect in Latin America by teenagers than they do in the United States.

The slow but generally continuous contact that occurs between Hispanics in the United States and relatives from Latin America acts as a protector and promoter of values, among them sexual values, that differ from the current values in the United States. It is not within the scope of this paper to document these differences—bibliographies are available. However, Hispanic teenagers are easily recognizable as being the group most "on the line" in this conflict of values. They identify as Latins, as coming from a distinct national group, as newcomer or oldtimer, as family; and as teenagers caught between these cultural roots and the barrage of images, ideals, and models presented sometimes by their American schools, sometimes by their surrounding community, and always by the media.

We do not know how all these experiences affect Hispanic adolescents. Or how in turn these adolescents affect their families and community. We do know that the attitudes and values in the United States regarding adolescent sex, sexuality, and parenting are contradictory, dishonest, and, at times, immoral. If we are to reach Hispanic adolescents and provide them with the skills, values and education necessary to help them make personally responsible sexual decisions, there is much that needs to be considered.

The Hispanic family has traditionally been, and is, what much of the Anglo family in this country has ceased to be. The intrinsic values of an Hispanic family are difficult to understand for anyone who exists in a milieu that has essentially disavowed the value of intergenerational living and the emotional strength of the extended family.

It would be irrational to base policy or programs aimed at Hispanic families on data gathered from non–Hispanic populations. For example, where the male in the American family plays an increasingly nebulous role, this cannot be said of Hispanics. This issue alone has major implications that affect not only the man's role but also those of "wife" or "mother." In a study of the reasons for, and consequences of adolescent pregnancies, these issues are not to be easily dismissed.

In a social milieu where parenting is increasingly being called an "alternative optional lifestyle," the Hispanic woman lives in a context in which the role of mother has an extremely high social value. When contrasted to an existence of high unemployment, inadequate education, and low social value, which is the lot of so many Hispanic adolescents, that so-called "alternative" may become a highly desirable one.

Family Relations

Wilma Montanez of the San Francisco General Hospital Perinatal Unit has conducted interviews with Hispanic adolescent women, their parents, siblings, and friends. The following comments are excerpted from her notes:

> The really interesting sight is that of grandmothers walking arm in arm with their teenage granddaughters who are obviously pregnant. It's easy to tell that she is proud that she will be a great-grandmother soon. At the same time it is clear that she is confused and somewhat bewildered at the new morals and the new configurations that her family is taking in the United States. Yes, she was pregnant when she was a teenager, but she was married first.

The confusion of the grandmother is often shared by her daughter, the teenager's mother. Doris was forty when the second of her teenaged daughters became pregnant.

> I never thought of it happening to me. I let them have boyfriends at a young age so they wouldn't have to sneak around behind my back. I figured if I gave them permission they wouldn't have sex. When the two got pregnant, I was hurt and very embarrassed at the same time.

The family, Montanez states, provides the basic support system for the pregnant Hispanic adolescent. If there is no supportive sister, the next in line is the mother. However, even here some teenagers find walls. For example, Eva, fourteen years old, confessed: "I waited for her to ask me. I had the feeling that as my mother she knew all the time. I knew she was going to be hurt, but it never crossed my mind that she would say, 'You've got to get out of the house.'"

Montanez found that most of the girls she interviewed expressed that fathers left it up to the mothers to handle the situation—fathers were the least supportive.

> Rosa Maria said, "When I went home and told my parents I was pregnant, my father, he really blew it. He asked me if I was going to get married. I said no and he didn't speak to me for about four to five months after that. That was pressure on me during that time. He was completely ignoring me. I still had to respect him and serve him. My older brother blew it too. He threatened me and said, 'You get married.'"

Younger brothers, however, tend to be more supportive in these situations. Eva shared how her brothers played a dad role for her child and her sister's. "They babysat our babies, they changed diapers. They even got sick like us during our pregnancies."

The male partner in adolescent pregnancies generally plays an uncertain role. Most do not know what they can do or what is expected of them. Socially they're seldom given any direction, nor is there a sense of what the role is, besides contributing to conception, that they are to play as males. The images are confusing, to say the least. When asked how he felt when he first found out that his girlfriend was pregnant, a seventeen-year-old Hispanic replied, "One half of me said 'Wow,' and one half said 'Oh shit.'"

"He was hurt and embarrassed. Mostly hurt," says a teenage boy's mother. Lorena, fourteen, says of her seventeen-year-old boyfriend: "He just got happy and didn't say nothing. That's all. He keeps calling every day. He wants to take me to my clinic appointments. He just wants to help me."

There can be no doubt, however, that the most profound impact of an adolescent pregnancy is on the pregnant young woman. She is ultimately alone in the shock, the amazement, the unknown. She has to confront decisions—perhaps for the first time in a lifetime where decisions have always been made for her, at times even the decision to have intercourse:

> Lorena, fourteen: "At first I was happy. When it was too late, I thought, 'What do I want a baby for?'"
>
> Rosa Maria, sixteen: "I just felt very stupid, hopeless. I was mad at my parents. I was totally restricted. They were scared of reality."
>
> Cookie, sixteen: "I always had problems with my period. So I thought at first that it was a problem with my period. When I felt kicking I knew it wasn't no period."

All of these young women are Hispanic; the information being gathered from them and their families will do much to help us understand how Hispanic families are affected by the occurrence of an unplanned pregnancy of a teenager. It will then be possible to provide the services most needed. There are obvious needs for education and preventive services—much of the current intervention, however, comes after the fact.

Educational Concerns

"Pregnancy," says Alfred Moran, Executive Vice President of Planned Parenthood of New York City, "is the major factor in the dropout rate among junior and senior high school girls."

We do not have data for the incidence of pregnancy among Hispanic girls in junior and senior high schools. However, we do have evidence that many do not finish high school.[15] Whether they are dropouts or pushed-outs, these young women, if they are not pregnant, become very much at risk of pregnancy. Where school provided at least some sort of structured time, unemployment offers no such benefits.

Hispanic adolescent boys and girls find themselves in an educational system that offers them very little in terms of realistic education or preparation for life. Reports from national organizations representing Mexican-Americans, Puerto Ricans, and other Hispanics all point to the fact that schools are simply not meeting the basic needs of Hispanics.

Rosemary Samalot, a New York City social worker and pregnancy counselor, states:

> They all get wasted. The boys don't know what to do with themselves and neither do the girls. They end up being trapped into playing house. Inevitably the girl gets pregnant and the cycle has been completed and started again. The status for both the male and the female is then essentially settled. He is unemployed and ill educated—she is even less so. For the female, the status evolved binds her to raising a child and, almost invariably, getting pregnant again.

Josefina A. Card and Lauress L. Wise found that the repercussions of teenage childbearing are long lasting: "The young parents acquire less education than their contemporaries; they are often limited to less prestigious jobs, and the women to more dead-end ones.[16] Their marriages are less stable than those of their contemporaries who postponed childbearing." For the Hispanic family—with low education, income, and unemployment—the combined problems of dropout and pregnancy among adolescents present some major concerns.

Postscript

"Implicit in many discussions by political leaders, human service professionals, and the media—and explicit in some—is the assumption that teenage pregnancy is a problem because adolescents are acting 'irresponsibly,'" states the 1976 annual report of the Alan Guttmacher Institute (AGI).[17] However, in a recent television program about teenagers, a writer quit and a minor flap ensued when he divulged that the network's censors would not allow a teenage boy to use the word "responsible" in reference to birth control. "This is not something a fifteen-year-old should think about," said the network censor. What are we telling young people?

The AGI report adds, "A recent statement on adolescent health and pregnancy by an agency of the HEW described sexually active unmarried teenaged women as 'acting out,' which is a professional term for deviant, if not pathological behavior. Since 35 percent of unmarried teenage women are sexually active, the description has two immediate results: it defines more than one-third of United States teenagers as sick, and it implies that the problem of teenage pregnancy is largely insoluble."[18]

If there is confusion for the adolescent, it seems that it merely mirrors that of their adult counterparts. For Hispanic families, the realities of the impact caused by adolescents remain family secrets. The lack of common information regarding major issues affecting their lives limits the possibilities of action. It seems likely to remain that way unless strong action is taken to enact considerable economic, social, and attitudinal changes in this society.

Having considered the factors which may affect Hispanic adolescents and their families—population, traditions, social pressures, stereotypes, economics, family relationships, and education—and the lack of information about them, it is clear that few, if any, conclusions or recommendations can be drawn regarding the impact on Hispanic families of adolescent pregnancies.

However, in addition to the suggestions presented earlier, we can list the areas on which we need information or action:

- We must strive to understand the impact of a very young and fast-growing population in Latin America on the Hispanic population in the United States.

- We must secure information on the knowledge, attitudes, and opinions of Hispanic children and youth, and their families regarding sex, sexuality, parenting, and general health issues. We need to carefully examine significant differences and similarities among Hispanics with different national origins.
- We must make policy studies that accurately reflect the effect of minimum wage laws and tax incentive initiatives on Hispanics. Through these, manpower plans can be developed that deal with the group with the highest unemployment rate—youth.
- We must improve access to health careers for Hispanics. (The United States Statistical Abstract for 1977, detailing American Medical Association licensure statistics for health professionals, offers no data on the number of Hispanics in health professions.)
- Churches must provide avenues for data and for educational leadership. James R. Brockman, S. J., associate editor of *America* magazine, has written that from one-fourth to one-third of the Catholic Church's members are Spanish-speaking and of Hispanic culture.
- We must know the extent of involvement of United States Hispanics with the Roman Catholic Church. Are they influenced more by the Church and its doctrines than the total United States Catholic population? If so, what are the implications regarding birth control, preventive services, and educational programs? The recent papal visits to Latin America and the United States, and their consequences have not been lost on the Hispanics. (During recent private discussions in Mexico City, the author learned that officials are still evaluating the impact of the Pontiff's visit on family planning efforts. It may serve us well to monitor their findings as useful indicators for American policy and programming of family planning efforts for Hispanics.) Essentially, it would be counterproductive to ignore the influence of the Church and its revitalization in the world of *Latinos*.
- Programs for teenage parents, such as the New Futures School in Albuquerque, where Hispanics represent more than

one-half of the enrolled population, must be adequately evaluated so that they might serve as planning models for similar ventures in areas of high Hispanic population.
- Studies must also be performed which address the following questions:

1. What are the causes of adolescent sexual behavior among Hispanic young people within their cultural context?
2. What are the consequences of this behavior in terms of education, health, economic, and social status?
3. How do the differing cultural attitudes regarding sexual behavior and expectations affect Hispanic young people? How are these reconciled? How do they affect parenting? Pregnancy?
4. What are the relationships between Hispanic unemployment, school dropout, and drug or alcohol use, and adolescent sexual behavior?
5. What are the prevailing attitudes toward abortion among Hispanic young people, compared to practice?
6. What are the immediate and long term effects of early parenting and/or marriage on these young people?
7. What percentage of women of Hispanic origin have children? What is their age breakdown? What are their national origins?
8. To what extent are Hispanic families changing or moving away from extended families?
9. What programs and policies should we develop to provide adequate health and education programs for Hispanic young people?

We can provide education that is honest and significant to the needs and questions of young people—but in order to do this we have to prepare ourselves as parents, teachers, health care providers, and human beings. Simply saying, "You're too young to know that," has not worked. To say in its place, "We can't talk about that, but there's a contraceptive brochure in the library," I fear, would be equally dishonest. We must not fall into the trap of trying to find simplistic or purely technological (i.e., contraceptive) solutions. We must provide the kind of education and example that takes into account not only the minority who "get in trouble," but also the majority that do not, and give them support when they choose to say, "No, I'm not ready yet." Basically we should live our lives as an example to young people of what we say we believe.

NOTES

1. This paper was prepared in collaboration with: Wilma Montanez, Health Educator, San Francisco General Hospital; Arturo Riera, OBECA Arriba Juntos, San Francisco.
2. Department of Commerce, Bureau of the Census, Current Population Reports, *Persons of Spanish origin in the United States*, ser. P-20, no. 328, table 2 (Washington, D.C.: GPO, March 1978), p. 5.
3. Ibid.
4. Commission on Civil Rights, *Puerto Ricans in the continental United States: An uncertain future.* (Washington, D.C.: GPO, Oct. 1976), p. 5.
5. Commission on Civil Rights, *Improving Hispanic unemployment data: The Department of Labor's continuing obligation.* (Washington, D.C.: GPO, May 1978), p. 12; Commission on Civil Rights, *Puerto Ricans*, table 27, p. 93.
6. Department of Commerce, *Persons of Spanish origin*, p. 1.
7. Department of Labor, Bureau of Labor Statistics, *Workers of Spanish origin: A chartbook* (Bul. 1970: 1978), chart 31, p. 46; chart 2, p. 6; chart 5, p. 9. See also "MexAmerica," *Washington Post* (5-pt. ser.), March 26 and 30, 1978; Department of Labor, *Workers of Spanish origin*, chart 19, p. 29.
8. Department of Labor, *Workers of Spanish origin*, chart 23, p. 34; chart 6, p. 10; summary indicators, p. 1.
9. Congressional Budget Office, *Youth unemployment: The outlook and some policy strategies* (Washington, D.C.: GPO, April 1978), p. xiii.
10. Ibid., p. ii, n.
11. Commission on Civil Rights, *Improving Hispanic unemployment data*, letter of transmittal, p. ii.
12. Bureau of the Census, *Census of Population: 1970*, vol. 1, Characteristics of the Population, Pt. 1, Section 1, U.S. Summary, chap. C, "General Social and Economic Characteristics," Negro Population 1970, PC(2)-1B, Persons of Spanish Origin 1970, PC(2)-1C, and U.S. Summary, Detailed Characteristics 1970, PC(1)-D-1 (Washington, D.C.: GPO, 1972).

13. Barbara Gomez-Day, "Hispanic youth and education", chap. 4 in *A profile of Hispanic youth*, Youth Knowledge Development report 10.2, Office of Youth Programs, HEW, April 1980.

14. Bureau of the Census, final report PC(1)-C1, United States Summary.

15. Department of Commerce, *Persons of Spanish origin*, table 5, p. 7.

16. Josefina Card and L. Wise, "Teenage mothers and teenage fathers: The impact of early childbearing on the parents' personal and professional lives," *Family Planning Perspectives* 10, no. 4 (July/Aug. 1978): 199–207.

17. Alan Guttmacher Institute, "Annual Report: 1976" (Washington, D.C.: Alan Guttmacher Institute, 1976), pp. 3–5.

18. Ibid.

# 11

Bringing in the Family: Kinship Support and Contraceptive Behavior

*Frank F. Furstenberg, Jr.,
Roberta Herceg-Baron,
and Jay Jemail*

Though social programs are usually based on a presumption of empirical knowledge, it is no secret that research typically follows, rather than precedes efforts at social intervention. More often than not, social scientists are called in to assess the impact of an existing programmatic initiative, and are asked to render a judgment about the wisdom of a particular course of action *after the fact*. Only rarely do they take an active part in planning the experiments that they evaluate.

The case study presented in this paper represents an exception to this general rule. We shall review the development of an experimental program to involve family members in the provision of family planning services to female adolescents. The program, "Kinship Support for Adolescents Enrolled in Family Planning Programs,"[1] grew directly out of research conducted by one of the authors and reported on at the Conference on Teenage Pregnancy and Family Impact, sponsored by the Family Impact Seminar in 1978. Because it is too early to talk about results, this paper will trace the intellectual origins of the Kinship Support Program, and provide some preliminary observations on its implementation. We will relate some of the incipient and unanticipated findings about a program that:

- modifies the conventional family planning service setting to allow more opportunities for counseling and other supportive services for adolescents;
- implements a prospective evaluation design within the family planning setting; and
- enhances family planning counselors' skills to work with families and broadens their counseling roles.

The Origins of the Program

As described elsewhere in this volume, awareness of the influence of the family on adolescents' contraceptive behavior initially emerged from a longitudinal study of adolescent childbearers in Baltimore a decade ago. One of the first findings of the Baltimore study[2] was that most adolescents took great care to conceal their sexual activity from their parents. The adults, in turn, professed ignorance that their daughters might be engaging in sexual relations, even though they acknowledged that most adolescents in their neighborhood were sexually active. Thus, it seemed as though many mothers and daughters entered a mutual "agreement of nonrecognition" that was violated only when the teenager became pregnant. In accord with this pact, most teenagers regarded intercourse as spontaneous and uncontrollable ("It's something that just happens"); and parents provided little in the way of preparation for the eventuality of coitus ("Be sure not to mess around.").

When families departed from the strategy of concealment by openly acknowledging that relations were occurring, and accordingly made some effort to impart information about contraception, there was a noticeable improvement in the teenager's use of birth control measures. Adolescents were more likely to use contraceptives and had greater success in delaying conception when their mothers knew that their daughters were sexually active and talked to them about using birth control.[3] Recent research, most notably work by Greer Litton Fox (see Chapter 3), has provided evidence corroborating this finding. (See also the perceptive ethnographic study by Rains.)[4]

In 1978, at the conference sponsored by the Family Impact Seminar, papers presented by both Furstenberg and Fox noted the paradoxical effect that occurred when parents restrict communication about sex (whether due to discomfort or disapproval); there was a marked increase in the risk that their daughters would not use contraception when they engaged in sexual intercourse. Both researchers observed that sex education and family planning programs that do not allow for parental participation may be removing an important influence on the adolescent's sexual socialization. In their summary of the conference proceedings, Ooms and Maciocha conclude by advocating that public and private agencies make parents "full partners in both preventing and coping with teenage pregnancy."[5]

During the same period that the final report of the conference was being prepared, Furstenberg served as a consultant to the Family Planning Council of Southeastern Pennsylvania, a private nonprofit organization that coordinates family planning programs in the five-county Philadelphia area. Under the direction of Dorothy Mann, Executive Director of the Council, a plan was developed to improve family planning services through selective research and training projects. In the course of working out some of the details of the plan, Furstenberg participated in a series of meetings and conferences in which family planning service providers and researchers exchanged observations and ideas. The tenor of these meetings was invariably frustrating. Practitioners looked to researchers for effective ways of serving the adolescent population; researchers had little to offer in the way of practical suggestions.

In the spring of 1979, Furstenberg approached the Council with the idea of designing a program to counteract the tendencies of families to isolate the sexually active teenager. With

Furstenberg's assistance and input by several staff members, Roberta Herceg-Baron, research analyst at the Council, drafted a proposal that was submitted to the Office of Family Planning at the Bureau of Community Health Services within the Department of Health, Education and Welfare. Three months later, the Kinship Support Program was funded.

Program Design and Objectives

The primary objective of the program was to build family support for contraceptive use among young adolescents, those under age eighteen, who enrolled in family planning programs. We need to clearly state at the outset that we were only interested in obtaining family support with the voluntary agreement of adolescent clients. We, as a team, do not believe that informing the adolescent's parents should be a required condition of receiving services at family planning clinics. The proposal described a two-stage process for reaching this objective.

First, experienced family planning counselors from participating agencies would be trained to work with the families of adolescents who sought family planning services. It was recognized that most counselors would probably not feel comfortable or competent to work with families (particularly parents) unless they were given a background in family counseling. Thus, the main objective of the training program was to provide skills for family planning counselors who had previously worked individually with adolescents, enabling them to reach out to family members who might provide support to the adolescent who sought contraceptive services. The basic assumption was that the adolescent's family could become a significant support system, enhancing her ability to use contraceptives successfully if they accepted her sexual behavior and reinforced her decision to use birth control. We recognized that peers, health, and other social service agencies, and other socio-cultural factors also play a significant part in the adolescent's sexual development. Even so, in the training program, we emphasized the family network as being capable of attenuating or accentuating the impact of these other factors on the adolescent's life.

In the second stage, after counselors had completed the course of instruction, a carefully designed research program was to be implemented in each agency. The purposes of the research program were to: (1) measure the amount of support provided to the adolescent seeking contraception by various family members; (2) determine whether family support could be enhanced by having discussions first with the adolescent alone and then together with designated family members who might be able to provide assistance to her if and when she encountered difficulties using birth control; (3) ascertain whether contraceptive effectiveness was improved when barriers to sexual communication within the family were reduced; and (4) determine whether secondary effects such as improved contraceptive use and reduction of unwanted pregnancies among other members of the family might result from their participation in the program.

Details of the research design have been described elsewhere[6] and will only be summarized briefly in this paper. We planned to recruit enough staff to provide services to 300 families. After an initial session, the adolescent and at least one member of her family would meet with the trained counselor for up to six sessions to share problems relating to sex and contraception. The aims of these sessions were to deal with potential conflicts, reduce the atmosphere of secrecy, and devise strategies for rendering assistance to the adolescent in the event such aid was required. Two types of "control" services were developed to provide a baseline for measuring the independent effects of the program. A group of 150 adolescents would receive frequent telephone contacts by clinic staff for a similar period (about six weeks) to assist the adolescent in her use of birth control, but with no specific encouragement to guide communication with the family. A third group of 150 adolescents would receive no additional support services aside from those provided through the conventional services offered in family planning programs for teenagers. Assignment to the three groups would be random, and all adolescents would receive the conventional family planning services upon first entering the clinic. Research assistants would interview each adolescent seeking birth control, and agreeing to participate during her first visit to the clinic. A series of follow-up interviews would be conducted six, twelve, and twenty-four months after enrollment. By comparing the groups of adolescents who received family support counseling to the groups who were exposed to the two "control" services, we hoped to determine the relative effectiveness of each of the three programs on the adolescent's contraceptive experiences and her ability to avoid unwanted pregnancies.

Selection of Program Sites

Using public funds from state and federal sources, the Family Planning Council of Southeastern Pennsylvania supports and coordinates comprehensive family planning services provided by twenty subcontracting family planning agencies. From this pool of agencies, six were selected for the program. The agencies included two hospital-based programs, two freestanding clinics, a community health center and a public health service. Selection of these agencies was based on the following criteria:

- *size of teenage population*. We sought to include programs that serve a large adolescent population. Adolescents under eighteen years old comprised 15–25 percent of the client load in each agency.

- *type of clinic*. We wanted to include a variety of agencies so that the results of our study could be generalized to various service settings that are supported in whole or in part by public funds.

- *characteristics of clientele*. By establishing a multi-site project base, we expected to find a good distribution of potentially relevant characteristics in the research population such as socioeconomic and racial status, variations in family structure, and pregnancy experience.

- *experienced counselors*. We required that programs selected for participation have one or two experienced family planning counselors available for the intensive twelve-week training program in intergenerational family counseling skills. Our interest was to upgrade the skills of these family planning counselors so that they could provide the service components we wished to evaluate.
- *interest in the project*. We selected programs where there was an interest in developing a family involvement program for adolescents. Many of the selected sites had experienced an increase in the number of family members accompanying adolescents to the clinic.

Recruitment of Agencies

A letter describing the project and inviting participation was sent to administrators at each of the six agencies. The letter described several direct benefits of the project to the agencies:

- One or two staff members from each agency would receive training, supervision, and experience in the techniques of family counseling. Agencies could thus provide this service to adolescents even after the study was completed.
- Since the design of the study would be longitudinal, the agencies would have data on their adolescent clients over a two-year follow-up period. The data would be useful in understanding the effectiveness of a variety of support services for adolescents, as well as providing important information on what happens to adolescents during the two-year period following the first clinic visit.

The administrators all responded to the invitation with great interest; and a meeting was arranged to discuss the program.

Introducing the Program—Concerns of Clinic Administrators

The response of the administrators was encouraging but tempered with several areas of concern: (1) how to involve family members in counseling sessions with adolescents; (2) barriers to implementing the program in family planning clinics; and (3) problems associated with conducting on-site program evaluation.

Involving the Family

In listening to the perceptive observations and apprehensions of the administrators, we were compelled to recognize the delicacy and difficulty of the project we had undertaken. The following comments are typical of the concerns which the administrators brought to our attention:

- To what extent should family planning agencies get involved with a program that not only advocates the family's knowledge of the teen's visit to the clinic, but attempts to bring about parental involvement as well?

- Is it possible that teens won't come to our clinics once word is out that we're asking them to bring their mothers or aunts or grandmothers?

- Is it realistic to expect that teens will even want to bring their families to these counseling sessions? After all, six weekly counseling sessions represent a big investment of time—not just ours but theirs too.

These comments originated in part in a legitimate concern for the privacy of adolescent clients. Although minors residing in Pennsylvania can receive medical services and contraceptives from family planning programs without the consent of their parents, the issue of parental consent requirements for family planning and abortion services is being heatedly debated throughout the country today. Within this context, it is not surprising that family planning service providers would worry about preserving the adolescent's free access to contraceptive services. Historically, family planning advocates have fought difficult battles to increase general public acceptance of birth control services. From their perspective, the latest battle lines have been drawn to protect the adolescent's access to these services.

Thus, some of the clinic administrators raised the possibility that our program might not only be unpopular with adolescents, but might be perceived by adolescents as requiring parental consent to receive services. This concern led us to develop careful procedures to ensure that adolescents not feel coerced to participate in the program. Hence, the Kinship Support Program was designed to be an optional support service that the adolescent would be offered upon her initial visit to the clinic. Her participation in the program would be strictly voluntary.[7]

There were other reasons as well for reassuring that the program would not have an undesirable impact upon adolescent recruitment into the clinics. First, not all adolescents would be offered the family counseling services; rather, half would be offered one of the two "control" services, thereby limiting the total number of teens invited to participate in the family-oriented service. We would not insist that adolescents randomly assigned to receive counseling services bring a member of their household to the counseling sessions with them. If they objected to the idea of including a close family member, they could instead designate a surrogate, such as a distant relative, a friend, a neighbor, or a boyfriend, to attend the sessions with them. Thus, a family member or some other support person would become involved in the counseling only at the invitation of the adolescent. The family planning counselor would be trained to facilitate this process of recruitment by the adolescent. Should no support person attend the sessions, the counselor would meet with the adolescent and counsel her individually, but with a focus on the social resources and support systems currently available to her.

In response to the administrators' questions regarding the acceptance of the family counseling program among adolescents, we could only point out that we, too, were unsure of its success. Research studies indicate that this program might be an appropriate service option for some adolescents. How many and for whom, we did not know; the program was designed to explore this question. Unless they were put to the test, we would never be able to ascertain the extent to which family support systems might be utilized to help prevent unwanted pregnancies among adolescents.

Modifying Services

Other administrators helped us to see the barriers that might mitigate against implementation of the program in their agencies:

- Sure, we want to expand our services for teens, particularly if we can offer them more counseling, but can we really fit an expanded program into the way we now give our services?
- We can't spend a lot of time counseling the teen because she has to get services not just from our counselors, but from the medical staff as well.
- There's really no time to do additional counseling during the clinic and certainly there's no space.
- This program would mean redefining the job responsibilities of our family planning counselors so they can do the more indepth counseling required by the program. Is this type of program really feasible in our clinic settings?

Essentially, the problem they raised was one of limited resources (particularly time, space, and personnel) for modifying family planning service delivery to include more in-depth counseling. The resistance to service expansion of the type we proposed was partly a result of the way services have traditionally been provided in family planning programs. Contraceptive services are provided in a context that is based on a medical model of service delivery. Clients are offered short-term medical services and counseling assistance with the expectation that the "treatment" (dispensing a contraceptive method) will result in long-term benefits (avoidance of an unwanted pregnancy). However, there is little flexibility in this type of medical service program for client follow-up outside of medical emergencies. The service routine typically does not provide for ongoing contacts with clients unless initiated by the client. Ordinarily, efforts are not made to maintain relations with the client once it has been ascertained that they have not encountered medical problems in using contraception.

Our program was predicated on the assumption that follow-up was essential to effective service delivery. Thus, it was necessary to negotiate separately with each of the administrators how to integrate the proposed program with the medical service model at their clinic, since resources, patient flow, and clinic schedules varied among the sites, thus generating different implementation problems.

The administrators tactfully reminded us that they were under considerable pressure to meet the external demands of large patient loads, to juggle personnel to respond to staffing needs, and to attain other service priorities. Consequently, the program we designed could not make excessive demands upon staff time and clinic space.

As the process of planning for the program evolved, it became apparent that one of our tasks was to convince agencies, accustomed to the medical model of service delivery, that some reorientation was necessary and desirable. Ultimately, this redirection required that administrators weigh the trade-off between increasing the size of their client population and the efficacy of the services rendered. The case for reexamining the medical model rests on the assumption that adolescents, particularly those in their early teens, face a number of severe obstacles in using birth control. Unless client routines are modified to take into account the problems that teenagers encounter once they are equipped with contraception, there is strong evidence that services will have a limited impact on the adolescent's contraceptive behavior.[8]

The administrators who became involved were responsive to this argument, and showed some inclination to build up the follow-up component of their program. Yet, it often proved difficult to modify established client routines even when wisdom dictated otherwise. One of the lessons we have learned, which we will refer to again in the conclusion, is that programs must be restructured to promote long-term follow-up. This requires additional resources as well as a strategic reorientation on the part of professional staff.

Evaluating the Program

Administrators also brought to our attention the inevitable disruptions a research program would pose to their clinic routine.

- Let's say we do get involved with the training program and our counselors do some in-depth counseling as described in your program, we don't know if we can see as many teens as you need for research purposes.
- As part of your research, you need to interview the teens when they come into the clinic. Won't that mean they have to spend more time waiting in the clinic than they already do?
- We don't have enough space in our clinics for our own staff; where will we put the research assistants so they can do their interviews with the teens in private?

We responded to these concerns with our assurance that we could work to make the research elements as unobtrusive as possible and that we could remain flexible with our procedures in order to avoid bottlenecks in the clinic patient flow. We also stated our interest in fitting our interviews into existing "waiting" times that the adolescents were already experiencing in the course of their visits to the clinic, thus minimizing the possibility that adolescents participating in the program would spend more time at the clinic. We suggested that adolescents might find our interview an acceptable alternative to the time they would ordinarily spend in the waiting room. In fact, this turned out to be the case. The interviews, which last about twenty to twenty-five minutes, have been carried out with only minimal changes in clinic routines.

Regarding their participation in the program, the clinic administrators suggested that since the training program for the counselors was twelve weeks in length, plans for the implementation of the research program in each agency could develop concurrently with the training program, and during that time agencies could commit themselves to the research program or withdraw. Thus far, most agencies have shown a commitment to implementing the program by freeing up additional counseling time for their staff involved in the training program and by working within their institutional settings to find appropriate space for the counseling program and research assistants.

The Training Program—Overcoming Barriers to Family Involvement

Fourteen counselors were selected by the six clinic administrators to participate in the training program, which was conducted by Jay Jemail, Ph.D., an experienced family therapist on the staff of the Philadelphia Child Guidance Clinic. The counselors were broadly representative, in their age, experience, and educational background, of counselors employed in family planning clinics. Their ages ranged from twenty-three to forty-nine. Regarding their experience working in the clinics, the least experienced participant had been counseling in the family planning setting for one and one-half years and the most experienced, for fourteen years. Educational degrees held by the participants ranged from high school diplomas to a master of social work degree. A few of the trainees held supervisory positions in their agencies. Most had had little or no previous exposure to, or training in, family counseling techniques.

Initially, the participants were skeptical about involving family members in their counseling of adolescents. This is understandable, given that family planning clinics are generally designed to deliver services to the individual adolescent. The adolescent is typically treated as if she were isolated from her relatives. Our training program challenged the counselors to assume a posture antithetical to that of the system they worked in. They were to intervene with adolescents in ways different from those used by co-workers in their agencies.

The counselors were asked to approach the project, at least hypothetically, with the premise that inviting a relative of the adolescent to the session was a positive step. Although there would be cases where clinical judgment justified seeing the adolescent alone, the counselors were asked to regard cases where a relative would be excluded from services as the exception rather than the rule. This, of course, was a significant departure from the approach commonly employed by family planning practitioners.

This new role was obviously not an easy one. There was no reason for us to expect that families would necessarily be ready to participate in a support system for adolescents enrolled in the program. As explained earlier, parents often act as if their teenage daughters are not sexually active. Similarly, some parents prefer to be ignorant of the adolescent's contact with a family planning clinic, and other parents clearly oppose that contact. Therefore, the counselors were asked in the training to devise techniques that might eventually involve some of these parents in supporting the adolescent's decision to use contraception. The trainees first had to convince themselves that the family's support might be important and helpful, then convince the adolescent, and finally convince her family.

The exercise of devising ways to bring family members into the counseling was a significant departure from the counselors' routine. Family planning counselors had developed very sophisticated schemes to protect the adolescent's confidentiality. Unfortunately, these were, at the same time, ways to exclude the adolescent's relatives from any possible involvement in the deliberations. For example, the participants in our training program described how they called the teen's home under an assumed name or identified themselves as friends who needed homework. They carefully made their calls at times when the teen was supposedly able to speak in privacy. Needless to say, the identity of the counselor was occasionally discovered, and these efforts annoyed some of the teen's parents or other relatives. When this occurred, the result was to alienate an adolescent further from her family. Such incidents placed the agency staff in a coalition with the adolescent, and, unfortunately, in an adversary relationship with the family.

Yet, the training had to deal with the problem of confidentiality. Counselors were encouraged to explore ways to respect confidentiality, but still seek to include family members in a constructive and supportive way. For example, the counselors were encouraged to allow the adolescent to tell her mother about her contact with the clinic. In this way the adolescent was free to disclose to her mother as much or as little information about her visit to the clinic as she chose. Hopefully, the counselor would then be able to form a trusting relationship with both the mother and the daughter, and encourage more constructive sharing of information between them rather than building an alliance with one or the other.

Some of the trainees' skepticism about including the adolescent's relatives resulted from previous experience with family members. Parents who brought adolescents or sent them to family planning clinics often expected the counselor to assume a surrogate parent role. Frequently, their expectation was that the practitioner would convince the adolescent to choose an abortion, bring a pregnancy to term, or use a particular birth control method. Counselors were asked by parents to dissuade the adolescent from becoming sexually active or even to influence the adolescent's choice of a sexual partner. In the past, these family planning counselors had dealt with domineering or intrusive parental figures by excluding them from the counseling session. Our training program attempted to show that, by excluding family members, the counselors had given up an opportunity to change the communication and transactional patterns of the adolescent and her parent. Moreover, the professional had assumed responsibilities that were more appropriately assumed by a parental figure.

Individual counseling of adolescents forced these family planning counselors to adopt a surrogate parent role. In our training, participants described how they had to call the adolescent before her clinic appointments, or provide support through a difficult decision about a pregnancy. Some teens, particularly the younger and less mature ones, looked to the professional to make choices for them (e.g., about whether or not to become sexually active or about which contraceptive method to use). The counselors worked with a handicap because they lacked information about the adolescent's resources and her social support system.

The willingness of family planning counselors to assume, if only temporarily, this surrogate parental role was not surprising; other health professionals also share in this role. Physicians, psychologists, social workers, and others working with children, the handicapped, and the elderly frequently assume that parents and other family members are incapable or unwilling to provide guidance and support when needed. These assumptions are rarely tested by the professionals. Consequently, family planning counselors pass up many opportunities to involve a sister or other relative by working exclusively with the adolescent.

There were other reasons cited by the counselors for excluding family members from counseling. The conditions in which contacts took place were usually poor. Sessions were frequently conducted in small cubicle-like offices where two people could barely sit comfortably, let alone three or more. Their offices were sometimes not soundproof. The counselors had very limited time for their sessions, and the flexibility required by an ongoing relationship with a client was rarely available prior to this program. These family planning practitioners were expected to provide effective counseling in one fifteen-minute session. The trainees also pointed out that in order to do counseling with family members, sessions would need to be held in the evenings. But, most of their appointments were scheduled during the day. The counselors were not enthusiastic about rescheduling their working times from day to evening hours unless they were appropriately compensated for the changes in hours and additional professional responsibilities. In order to implement the program we had to negotiate more time for counseling, more private space, and compensatory time for evening hours.

Expanding the Counseling Role

Through the training, the program challenged a commonly accepted definition of the counseling role and of the kind of interventions family planning practitioners should use. Counselors have usually been told what they are not—they are not psychotherapists, nor are they educators. Their functioning in the educational role, however, has been more acceptable than their tampering with "therapy." The counselors' functions traditionally have been to provide information, guidance and support to the adolescent during her visit to the clinic. If the adolescent's needs extended beyond this brief contact, she was generally referred elsewhere in the social service system. Expanding the counselor's role, of course, was potentially threatening to others, for example, psychologists, social workers, physicians and those who engaged in "real" therapy. Unfortunately, these limitations in role definition too often served to inhibit the family planning counselor's behavior and thus limited the potential for effective intervention. Our training program attempted to broaden the counseling role beyond its educative aspects.

The training attempted to expand the family planning counselor's skills to fit this new role. In general, the trainees were experienced at working with individuals or peer groups, but lacked the skills required to work in concert with the adolescent and her family. They needed to develop skills to work together with parental figures, siblings, and multiple generations. The participants in the program were clearly adept at forming therapeutic alliances with teens. However, for this program, they also needed to join with parental figures. It was important to illustrate for them how some interventions they commonly used could serve to link them with one generation, but alienate others.

For example, take the case of an adolescent who comes into a family planning clinic for the first time. Within the traditional, individualized counseling approach, the following scenario would unfold. The adolescent meets the counselor and indicates she has been forced by her mother to come to the clinic. Her mother is convinced that the teen is pregnant. The mother is described as being a very intrusive and domineering person who buys and counts the adolescent's sanitary napkins and thus monitors her daughter's menses. The adolescent is angry because she is not sexually active, yet her mother keeps sending her for pregnancy tests. The adolescent confides that the mother does not believe her. She describes her frustrated attempts to communicate with her mother and her anger because her mother treats her like her seven-year-old sister.

Using a role-playing technique, the counselor tries to prepare the adolescent to go home and deal with her mother. The practitioner assumes the mother's role, and their dialogue is as follows:

> Counselor: Your mother will say, "Well, are you pregnant?"
> Adolescent: Yes, she will say it just like that.

Counselor: And what will you tell her?
Adolescent: That I'm not. That they told me at the clinic I couldn't have a pregnancy test because it was too close to my period. My mother won't believe it—that I couldn't have a pregnancy test.
Counselor: [steps out of role] I keep hearing you say that the clinic wouldn't give you a pregnancy test. Maybe you could say more about that to your mother.
Adolescent: See, I told her when my last period was. She told me I was lying, and she'll say I lied to you, too.
Counselor: In that case, maybe you can tell her that the counselor at the clinic accepted everything you were saying.

The problem with this approach is that the counselor is assuming a very supportive role with the adolescent but is setting the stage to alienate the parent. Encouraging the adolescent to tell her mother that the counselor agrees with her is a mistake. The professional has involved herself in a coalition with the adolescent that she will have a hard time getting out of. Approaching this scenario from a family system perspective rather than an individual perspective, the counselor could instead suggest that the adolescent ask her mother to come to the clinic so they can all talk together about the situation.

Skills for Planning Successful Interventions

To plan successful interventions with the adolescent and build support among family members, the professional must learn to assess the strengths and weaknesses of the adolescent's family system. The counselor needs to identify what factors in the family system encourage or discourage the use of contraceptives. For example, an adolescent who is living with her mother and a pregnant teen sister is going to have a difficult time using contraceptives effectively. This kind of information is important to consider when advising the adolescent.

The training encouraged the participants to formulate more hypotheses about how the adolescent's family functions. For example, Who assumes the parenting role? Who provides support for the adolescent? What are the rules about communication within the family?

In this way, the trainees learned to expand their assessment skills. The training focused on sharpening their ability to observe interactions among family members. Prior to this training, the counselors had been taught to be very good listeners. This new role demanded that they become competent at observing process and interaction as well. They were instructed to widen the angle of the lens through which they looked at adolescents. They had had some previous experience with assessing individuals; their new role demanded that they develop skills to assess family systems, as well.

Let us consider the following example, approaching it, again, from the traditional, individualized counseling perspective before suggesting an alternative family systems approach. A fifteen-year-old girl walks in to see the family planning counselor after a negative pregnancy test. The counselor finds she had pills but that she did not take them. In the session, the teen expresses dislike for foam and a diaphragm. The counselor clarifies myths and provides more birth control information. The teen casually mentions that her friends are getting pregnant and she would not like to get pregnant. They discuss contraceptive methods again. She resists any of the methods presented by the family planning staff. She indicates the problem is keeping them hidden from her father and mother. The professional, who is genuinely concerned about confidentiality, asks if it was a problem to write to her home. "Did your mother discover our letter reminding you of your visit?" The adolescent responded, "No, she looked at the letter and put it down in my room. I think my mother knows but is trying to ignore it." The counselor then suggests that an intrauterine device (IUD) is the most unobtrusive method of birth control. With some hesitancy, the adolescent agrees to return to have an IUD inserted. Assuming the reason she is taking the risk of becoming pregnant is because she lacked an unobtrusive method of birth control, this adolescent will probably return for the IUD. However, many adolescents go through similar steps and still become pregnant.

Approaching the same encounter from a family systems point of view, a pregnancy could mean many things to this teen and to her family. Exploring this with the adolescent could help identify her ambivalence about contraceptives and the attractive features or substantial burdens of a pregnancy for her and her family. With this information, the counselor could plan interventions to encourage the use of contraceptives and help the adolescent introduce the subject of sexuality to her parents. The parents or another support person could be invited to discuss their response to the adolescent's initiatives for preventing a pregnancy. Thus, the choice of an unobtrusive birth control method might become less relevant. Widening the angle of assessment could allow a broader range of interventions by family planning counselors working with adolescents. With this wider perspective, practitioners could identify and mobilize the resources in the natural support system of the teens that would encourage their responsible use of contraceptives.

Accepting Challenges

The program made obvious demands upon the agencies and family planning counselors, particularly those that participated directly in training programs, demands which forced them, and us, as well, to look at how services are being provided. Out of six agencies selected as program sites, four agencies are now offering the counseling services described here. Midway through the training program, two agencies withdrew because they felt that the demands of the counseling program were too much for their institution to undertake at this time. We are currently training counselors from two other agencies so that we will be able to offer the program in a total of six agencies, as originally planned.

Conclusion

At this stage in the study, it is too early to foretell the outcome of the Kinship Support Program. We cannot predict whether teenagers and their families will accept the services we are offering them, or whether these services will have a noticeable impact in promoting contraceptive use among sexually active teenagers. Indeed, it will be several years before a firm judgment about the efficacy of the program can be made.

This preliminary report assesses the process of implementing what we knew from the start to be a controversial and complicated undertaking: building social support within the family for contraceptive use among sexually active adolescents. Both the ideology and social organization of family planning services provide formidable barriers to involving the family.[9] For years the family planning movement has had to contend with adult opposition to programs for teenagers who are, or are about to become, sexually active. Parental consent requirements and parental notification have become the banner of resistance to liberal policies for extending services to teenagers at the risk of having unwanted pregnancies. Consequently, family planners cast a jaundiced eye on efforts to involve the teenager's family members, fearing that such a practice will discourage teenagers from seeking contraceptive services.

We sympathize with this sentiment and share the view that mandatory family involvement would do more harm than good by frightening adolescents away from clinics. However, preliminary data from our study indicate that a majority of the adolescents report that family members (usually parents as well as siblings) know of their visits to the family planning clinic; and others indicate that they plan to communicate this information to additional family members after their initial visit; and still others report that, even though they have not transmitted the information directly, they suspect that parents and/or siblings know that they are sexually active. In short, only a minority of the first hundred or so adolescents we have interviewed report that their sexual activity is completely clandestine. Consequently, the potential for involving family members without violating the teenager's privacy is great. Most teenagers we have interviewed consent to the idea of participating in counseling sessions with one or more family members, although it remains to be seen if we will actually be able to implement the service. It is important, of course, to recognize that the Kinship Support Program is located in the Philadelphia area; other regions of the country may be more or less receptive to the idea of promoting family participation.

Regardless of whether or not family members actually are included in services, it seems clear to us that there is a need to reorient the individualized approach of family planning programs. To most service providers, it seems so obvious and logical that adolescents who want to prevent pregnancies should use birth control that they hardly stop to consider the many obstacles that teenagers face in using contraception successfully. Apart from the very real problems inherent in the various methods available, teenagers often face a climate of ambivalence, if not outright opposition, to having sex from their families. So long as contraception is required to be a clandestine activity, teenagers are likely to find it extremely difficult to use birth control regularly, especially if they elect to use a method that may be discovered by family members. It requires considerable energy to guard the secret, adding to the existing complications of maintaining a steady supply of contraceptives or managing adverse side effects.

We do not believe that all families can become agents of support for teenagers who begin to use contraception. However, at present, the family is virtually an untapped resource. We do not underestimate the difficulty of involving family members, many of whom prefer "not to know." Even if family planning counselors are not able to reach the family directly, we think that they should be able to help prepare the teenager to accept that what she is doing may be regarded as a subversive activity in the home. We do believe that the family's position is often unresolved. Several of the adolescents in our study remarked that their parents wouldn't be happy knowing they were sexually active, but would approve of their using birth control. Parents, as well as teenagers, may welcome the opportunity to discuss their feelings about sexuality, sometimes as a precondition for coming to terms with the sexual behavior of their adolescent.

Sex educators, family planners, and health professionals have been remarkably unsympathetic to the plight of parents caught in the vortex of rapid cultural change. Practitioners have shied away from working directly with parents for fear of getting caught in the crossfire of generational differences over sexual behavior. Yet, by dodging the issue, the providers of family planning services may undermine the effectiveness of the very services they offer.

In trying to reverse this trend, we have noted a number of obstacles that lie in the path of organizational change. Family planning counselors see themselves as purveyors of information to individuals, not as persons capable of bringing about change in the community. This restricted mandate minimizes the potential for conflict in their role but also limits their effectiveness as educators of their limited clientele, let alone the wider community. The Kinship Support Program has raised the question of what the scope of the counselor's role should be. If this role were to be extended beyond its present boundaries, what kinds of training and preparation should be offered to individuals who become family planning counselors?

In initiating this project, we have also been reminded of the unrealistic nature of the medical model on which most services are predicated. Some years ago, in discussing the approach of most family planning programs, Furstenberg[10] noted that there is among health professionals an "ideology of inoculation." Almost magically, service providers believe that short-term assistance will have long-term effects. However, there is overwhelming evidence that family planning programs that provide little in the way of follow-up have limited effectiveness in preventing unwanted conceptions.

Of course, there are obvious and compelling reasons for the lack of follow-up. First, far more credit is given for intake figures than for continuation rates. New clients demonstrate the vitality of programs. Second, considerable time and energy are required to follow up clients, especially teenagers who are extremely mobile and often elusive. Finally, programs may be uncertain how to perform effective follow-up. Like parents, some professionals may prefer "not to know" that their efforts at prevention are ineffective.

While by no means the only stratagem available, bringing in the family offers some conspicuous advantages to programs interested in strengthening follow-up services. Because the family is involved in the first place, it becomes far easier to recontact the adolescent over time. More important, the family becomes part of the follow-up procedure, reenforcing the teenager's resolve to use contraception and helping to bring problems in contraceptive use to the attention of program personnel, if and when such problems occur.

As pointed out repeatedly throughout this paper, we do not discount the problems of involving the family nor do we believe that this approach will always, or perhaps even usually, be practicable. Yet, if we have overstated our case for bringing the family in, we have done so knowingly, for we believe that there is great value to be gained in redirecting the attention of professionals toward viewing sexual behavior and its consequences not merely in the context of individuals but also in the context of family systems.

NOTES

1. This study was funded by a grant from the Bureau of Community Health Services, HSA/PHS/DHEW, no. FP-R-000005-01-0. We are indebted to Dorothy Mann, Barbara Plager, and Albert G. Crawford for their comments on earlier drafts.

2. Frank F. Furstenberg et al., "Birth control knowledge and attitudes among unmarried pregnant adolescents," *Journal of Marriage and the Family* 30, no. 1 (1969): 34–42; and Frank F. Furstenberg, "Birth control experiences among pregnant adolescents: The process of planned parenthood," *Social Problems* 19, no. 2 (1971): 192–203.

3. Ibid.

4. Prudence Rains, *Becoming an unwed mother* (Chicago: Aldine-Atherton, 1971).

5. Theodora Ooms and Teresa Maciocha, *Teenage pregnancy and family impact: New perspectives on policy*, preliminary report (Washington, D.C.: Family Impact Seminar, June 1979), p. 43.

6. Roberta Herceg-Baron and Frank F. Furstenberg, "Kinship support for adolescents in family planning programs," proposal submitted to the Bureau of Community Health Services, Rockville, Md., July 1979.

7. Our consent procedures call for the adolescent to be informed by the research assistant at the time of the initial contact that: her participation in this experimental program is voluntary, and has no influence on the regular clinic services she will receive regardless of her decision to take part in the study. Consent forms are written in language comprehensible to adolescents, informing them of the purpose of the project and the extent of involvement expected of them. Each adolescent is given a copy of the form after the research assistant reviews its contents with her. The adolescent is also told that she has the right to withdraw at any time without jeopardizing her access to clinic services in the future. In fact, early experience with the consent procedures indicates that all but a very few adolescents have elected to participate in the study, although a good number may not actually avail themselves of the family counseling service.

8. Frank F. Furstenberg, *Unplanned parenthood: The social consequences of teenage childbearing* (New York: Free Press, 1976).

9. Frank F. Furstenberg, et al., eds., *Teenage sexuality, pregnancy, and childbearing* (Philadelphia: University of Pennsylvania, 1981).

10. Frank F. Furstenberg, *Unplanned parenthood*.

12

Family Involvement, Notification, and Responsibility: A Personal Essay

Theodora Ooms

Both families and government have a responsibility to address the range of problems associated with teenage pregnancy. Both have been much readier to assist after the fact—once the teenage girl is pregnant—than to help her and her partner avoid pregnancy in the first place.

The federal government's major investment has been in the teenage mother and baby, with the provision of financial aid and medical care. In terms of prevention, federal funds for family planning services have been substantial; yet support of sex education activities for the majority of teenagers who are not (yet) pregnant has been minimal. Furthermore, the government has demonstrated little recognition of the broader social factors contributing to adolescent fertility. The new federal grants program targeted on teenage pregnancy is an important but largely symbolic gesture of federal concern. State governments have, with few exceptions, given even less attention to this issue. Two

Note: This chapter presents a personal summary of the policy implications of a family impact perspective on teenage pregnancy. Although I have been greatly influenced by the ideas in the previous chapters, the particular themes I select for discussion, my conclusions, and the recommendations themselves are my responsibility alone.

recent surveys of state policies reveal that written policies and funded programs are few, coordination rare, and efforts at prevention virtually non-existent.[1] In general, state governments function simply as a conduit for federal funding of welfare programs, medical services, and a few social services provided to parents of all ages, including teenagers.

Similarly, most parents have been uncertain about their role in prevention of teenage pregnancy. (As with the government, their role has seemed clearest once pregnancy, and especially birth, occurs). The revolution in sexual mores in recent decades has undermined the old accepted codes of behavior; those emotions which once served to inhibit at least some teenage sex—fear, guilt, and shame—have largely disappeared. These codes, which some term "sexual scripts," are culturally determined and expressed through the attitudes, expectations, and behavior of others.[2] Since parents no longer have a ready script at hand, adolescents are more prone than ever to the influence of other sources: the messages of their own earlier maturing sexual drives, for example, and of the tantalizing media, which romanticize sex and glamorize motherhood. Yet, it is also possible, as John Gagnon says, that many adults, including parents, are assuming that young teenagers' biological drives are stronger than they really are, and, consequently, may enhance the likelihood that teenagers will engage in early sexual activity.[3]

We need to examine closely the various messages and expectations our culture is teaching the younger generations about sex, and to identify who is, and who should be, helping to write the "sexual scripts." Parents' own uncertainty about their role is only underscored by the message they seem to be hearing from the law and medical and educational institutions, namely, that adolescents' sexual behavior is too private an area for parental responsibility. And many parents may be only too relieved to hear that they can abdicate this role.

The focus in these pages on the family context of teenage sexual behavior, pregnancy, and parenting calls into question the wisdom of this trend away from parental responsibility. Perhaps the book's main conclusion is the idea that government should view parents as at least equal and, preferably, senior partners, in efforts to prevent teenage pregnancy and provide care for teenage parents. The specific questions that follow are: How can such collaboration be achieved? and How can the roles and responsibilities of both partners be clearly differentiated?

Based on the findings of the contributors, I developed a list of eight family impact principles that may serve as a guide to evaluating existing policies and making recommendations for change. These principles are especially designed to help assess whether the policies and programs concerning teenage pregnancy are supportive of, and sensitive to, families.

Principle 1. Policies of prevention and care should be designed to take into account the multiple causes and consequences of teenage pregnancy.

Principle 2. Policies should seek to help families help their teenagers avoid too early pregnancy and childbearing.

Principle 3. Policies should recognize that an adolescent's pregnancy and childbearing can have profound effects on other members of her family, and that the family, therefore, has an interest in being consulted about the decisions she makes about her pregnancy.

Principle 4. Policies should seek to help families assist their teenager to cope with early childbearing and avoid incentives that may encourage teenage parents to become prematurely independent and isolated from their own families.

Principle 5. The responsibility for pregnancy is not the adolescent girl's alone; thus, policies should encourage male responsibility and involvement in prevention and services.

Principle 6. Policies should reflect an understanding that families with adolescents are in a stage of transition in which parents' and children's roles and responsibilities undergo a process of negotiation and readjustment. Some disputes between them are to be expected as a natural part of this process.

Principle 7. Policies should be sensitive to the different needs and values of teenagers whose families represent different kinds of socioeconomic, religious, racial, and cultural backgrounds.

Principle 8. Programs should identify those adolescents who are seriously estranged from their families and plan to meet their special needs, including those for continuous, community-based relationships that can serve as surrogates for family support.

The discussion of policy recommendations that follows is guided by these family impact principles.

Prevention of Teenage Pregnancy

Any overall policy aiming at lowering the rates of teenage fertility should take into account the broader ecological context that contributes in both direct and indirect ways to teenage pregnancy. Thus, as several contributors point out, governments at all levels need to consider that improving the quality of high school education and increasing the availability of jobs, especially for lower income youngsters, should help to provide more attractive alternatives to the career of premature parenthood. Also, although government policy cannot directly affect the messages provided teenagers today through the entertainment media, it can attempt to counteract its more negative influences by mobilizing and educating public opinion on the issue — sometimes using the media's own channels more constructively.

This book, however, examines in detail only preventive policies that affect teenage fertility through providing information and access to medical services, namely, sex education programs and family planning services. Thus, these are the only preventive policy areas discussed in this chapter.

Sex Education

The time has certainly come for government at every level to exercise stronger leadership in promoting awareness of the problems of teenage pregnancy and the need for more, and better, sex education. The targets for such efforts need to be parents and community leaders just as much as the children themselves. This is because the "inoculation" model, traditional to public health, will not work in an area of such complexity and sensitivity. Whatever initiatives are chosen, the government's efforts and those of other experts need to proceed closely in collaboration with parents, adolescents, church, business, and other community leaders, and especially the media to ensure that the need for sex education is appreciated and the approaches used are acceptable. Since different approaches will need to be designed for different communities, the federal role should be primarily to stimulate, promote, and support state and local efforts. Peter Scales, in Chapter 6, suggests several specific steps the federal government can take, including an information clearinghouse, increased research and teacher training, and possibly a legislative initiative similar to those established in the 1976 Education Amendments, which revised vocational education laws with regard to sex bias and discrimination. New state initiatives could involve new legislation, conferences to stimulate awareness, and development of model curriculum guidelines. Scales emphasizes, however, that at least two other elements are needed for sex education policies to be successful: resources to adequately train teachers, and the consultation and involvement of parents and community leaders at each stage of development and implementation. Effective approaches to involving broad segments of the community in planning and implementing programs exist and need to be used. (As described briefly in Chapter 6, these approaches deal with the problem of the undue degree of influence sometimes wielded by a very small number of concerned citizens who are opposed to schools playing any role in sex education.) The parent and community involvement, however, must be more than token in order to dispel some of the genuine parental doubts and uneasiness that greet the enthusiastic plans of many sex education advocates.

Two of the touchiest issues for parents are the nature of the curricula and the qualifications of teachers. Sex educators may be correct in criticizing programs that do not include family planning information and that are only offered to a small percentage of the students or for a single session or two. Parents, however, must also be respected when in some communities they may fear that much sex education curricula may, somehow, condone sexual activity for young teenagers, or when they feel that many teachers do not have the sufficient skills, or are not the right kind of people, to be handling this kind of subject matter. Teachers also, even with training, may not feel comfortable teaching sex education. One result of parent and community participation may be, for example, the approval of curricula that include the need to delay sexual activity as one effective method of birth control,[4] or that omit discussion of homosexuality.[5] It may also lead to offers of valuable help from experienced members of the community—health personnel, ministers, youth workers, many of them parents themselves—who have the interest and experience to teach some parts of the courses. Finally, among the most promising curriculum developments in sex education are courses that provide homework assignments that involve parents. These may indeed help to bridge the distrust between home and school, increase parent-child communication, and, most important, reach those parents who are not able, or are not motivated enough, to come to school meetings to review the curricula, or attend courses themselves.[6]

Family Planning

This book did not aim to review the effects or adequacy of federal or state family planning programs; and discussion of family planning services addressed only the local program level. At any level, however, programs offering information and services about birth control must also be addressed to the adolescent male. A recent study on male involvement in family planning sharply criticizes the current female orientation of family planning services, and says that ignorance about the importance of men's role in family planning and decision making has resulted in actual prejudice against, or outright rejection of, men who attempt to become involved.[7] Assumptions about the best methods for birth control for teens are being questioned. Some feel that we need a shift from reliance on the pill (a female method) back to barrier methods that involve the knowledge and cooperation of both partners, because they are act-specific, and because they better suit the sporadic, irregular nature of adolescent sex. Others feel that all existing methods have some disadvantages for adolescent use and thus look forward to development of new more appropriate methods for teenagers.

We know that information about and access to contraceptives are not sufficient to ensure their regular use; motivation is critical. In Chapter 11, Furstenberg and his co-authors describe an interesting approach for training family planning counselors to appreciate the family context of their teenage clients and, when possible, to involve members of her family, or even peer group, in her clinic visits. The purpose of such an approach is to encourage the young girl to openly acknowledge her sexual activity, and get some recognition and support from those close to her for using contraceptives responsibly. One further point is often forgotten. Not all teens who come to a family planning clinic are convinced that they should be sexually active.[8] Family planning counselors are quite often unprepared to offer the kind of advice that would support delaying their becoming sexually active. (Yet, there are some interesting booklets published by Planned Parenthood and others for teenagers on how to resist the pressures to have sex and learn that it's "okay to say no.")

Government Programs for Teenage Parents

At present, there is little knowledge and much confusion about the ways that federal and state governments are presently attempting to help teenage parents. Kristin Moore in Chapter 5 identifies forty-three federal programs that potentially may affect teenage pregnancy: but there is little information on how many pregnant teens or teenage parents are served, the dollar amounts expended, or what effects these programs are having.

The estimates of government money already expended on the problems of teenage pregnancy are sufficiently large ($8.3 billion per year) to justify a strong recommendation that teenage pregnancy be placed high on the policy agenda of several government agencies. Strong federal and state leadership is needed to ensure that agencies give priority within present budgets to the needs of young parents. For although such priority may mean expanding present programs or initiating new ones, the first step should be to examine more critically what is presently being done and whether federal and state programs are complementing each other's efforts or working at cross purposes. For example, the Office of Youth Programs at the Department of Labor is now making teenage parents a priority for youth employment and training programs and has plans to waive some of the eligibility requirements.[9] However, there is little evidence that these plans drew upon the research and program knowledge available in certain divisions of HEW, or that they are being developed at the community level in coordination with other kinds of related services such as daycare.

Coordination is an easy catchword in policy circles. At the federal level, the new, small Office of Adolescent Pregnancy established in 1978 in the Assistant Secretary for Health's office has been given a legislative mandate to coordinate government policies. But unless imaginative ways of rewarding cooperation are developed and methods devised to share information and resources and hammer out the necessary interagency agreements, coordination will remain a commitment on paper only. At the state level, the National Association of State Boards of Education's recent report identifies as a minimal step the designation of one focal person or unit in the government to be responsible for leading such efforts for teenage parents.[10]

As Moore suggests, many decisions are made and actions taken at the state level that substantially affect which services and benefits are available and who is eligible for them. The particular package of welfare assistance and medical care available may, unwittingly, provide incentives to encourage teenage parenthood rather than prevent conception or childbirth. Do policies discourage marriage or discourage paternal responsibility? Do they encourage the adolescent parent to move out of her family's home? Do they compete with families' own helping resources, instead of complementing them? We don't know the answers to these questions, and we need to find them out. The evidence presented in this book strongly suggests that any policy—such as AFDC benefits—found to provide economic incentives to young parents to move away from their own family's support should be changed.

Various chapters in this book suggest some of the other critical questions that need to be asked about present federal programs:

- What effects does the Child Support Enforcement Program have on unmarried teenage fathers? Does it encourage or discourage their assumption of parenting responsibilities?
- Federal funds assist day care provided by institutions or nonrelatives for the children of young mothers; yet, are there federal incentives or support to help grandmothers or other relatives provide the infant care that is critical to enable the teenage parent to return to school or receive job training?
- Do welfare assistance and day care policies, as presently designed, discourage or encourage teenage mothers' completion of high school, receiving job training or obtaining employment?
- Are present efforts to fund comprehensive services designed to differentiate adolescents of varying levels of need, and to carefully target limited resources? Do they assess and complement resources already available within the family and community?

The Controversial Issue of Parental Notification

Recent Supreme Court decisions have determined that parental consent is not necessary for minors to obtain sex-related medical care such as abortion or prescription contraceptives. However, the question of whether parents have the right to be notified by the physician that their minor daughter is pregnant —and considering an abortion—has not yet been settled by the Court. The *Bellotti* v. *Baird* decision of 1979, as discussed in Chapter 8, has left this issue somewhat up in the air.

Notification in Pregnancy

The Court agreed to review in the 1980–81 session a Utah Supreme Court decision—*H.L.* v. *Matheson*—that upheld a law which requires parental notification of a minor's request for an abortion when physically possible; and this forthcoming decision may settle the constitutionality of this issue.* Meanwhile, although most state laws and clinic policies do not require parental notification, the issue is being actively debated in state legislatures, and caused considerable controversy at various forums connected with the White House Conference on Families. Data on the question is scarce but the general impression is that considerable numbers of young (and older) adolescents are making the decision about their pregnancy without their parents being informed.

I shall discuss this important and sensitive issue in some detail here, because it illustrates how a family perspective confronts us, head on, with the extremely difficult task of balancing the rights of different family members and maintaining the interest they and society have in family privacy and autonomy.

I shall present both the arguments for and against required parental notification. Since the arguments against such a policy have been widely discussed in professional journals (such as

*On March 23, 1981, the Court did uphold the Utah law in this case but left many questions open.

Family Planning Perspectives), I will summarize them only briefly. On the other hand, in my view, the reasons for notification have not been given careful consideration. (Those who advocate notification are too often dismissed on the basis not of their arguments, but of their political affiliations.) I draw upon some of the legal and ethical concepts presented in much more depth by Steinfels in Chapter 8. However, the legal concept of a "mature" or "immature" minor I do not allude to, because the legal criteria for determining maturity are not clear, nor are suggested procedures very suitable to the situation (and time-frames) of pregnant adolescents, who need to make a decision quickly.

Professionals working with pregnant adolescents are almost unanimous in opposing required parental notification, although many of them do urge that the adolescent be strongly encouraged to inform her parents and seek their counsel. Their position rests both on issues of principle embodied in our legal framework and on concern for the possible consequences of notification. The main arguments against required notification, as I understand them, are as follows:

- Minors should have the same constitutional right to both privacy on sexual matters and control over their own bodies that adult women have. This right must have priority over any competing rights of parents.
- If parents are routinely informed about their daughter's pregnancy, they may exert such heavy pressure on her that the decision will no longer, in effect, be hers. Thus, notification might be tantamount to consent, which the Supreme Court has already declared unconstitutional.
- A pregnant teen, scared of having her parents notified, may avoid getting the necessary prenatal care. Or, instead of obtaining an early and safe abortion, she may turn to back room or do-it-yourself abortions. Notification would thus serve as a serious barrier to appropriate medical care.
- A further undesirable result is that some parents may become so angry and upset when confronted with evidence of their

daughter's sexual activity that they lose control, become seriously abusive, and do her real harm (physical or mental).

The case for required parental notification also rests on issues of principle and on concern about the consequences, as follows:

- A basic principle of the law governing medical care is that of "informed consent." Thus, an adolescent, in terms of her own best interests, should not consent to any procedure or treatment without being "fully informed" as to what is involved, that is, the possible risks and consequences of going ahead with the care or of not doing so. Yet, if a pregnant adolescent does not inform her parents, she may be making the decision (whether it be for abortion or for carrying the pregnancy to term) on the basis of incomplete information; and thus, she cannot truly be said to have given her informed consent.

The decision about a teenage pregnancy is not solely or even primarily determined by medical considerations. Ethical, social, economic, educational, and family factors all need to be weighed by the adolescent and those consulting with her. A young teenager may make the decision to continue with the pregnancy and keep her baby on the basis of some very unrealistic assumptions about her own capacities to be a parent or her family's ability or willingness to help her. Other young women, as some recent research corroborates, are motivated to choose abortion primarily because they cannot face having to admit to their parents that they have been sexually active. They are also unwilling to confront their parents' hurt and angry reaction and believe that their parents will reject them.[11] In both cases, a physician or counselor is handicapped in advising the pregnant adolescent if he or she does not have direct personal knowledge of the teenager's family situation. The best sources of information about the family's reaction to her pregnancy, their willingness or refusal to help her, and what financial and other resources they are able to provide her for whatever option she chooses, are her family members themselves. It is also her family that is most likely to have some knowledge of her competence to be a par-

ent, or what effects the responsibilities of parenthood are likely to have on her future. They may also be able to remind her of the values, beliefs, or ambitions that have up until then been most important to her.
- Parents themselves have legitimate interests in being informed and consulted about a decision that may affect them and other members in the family very deeply, most especially if their daughter decides to keep her baby.
- There is a general presumption in all other areas of the law that parents have the right to control and guide their children's behavior up to the age of majority. In return, society expects parents to be responsible for the care and nurture of children. These parental rights and responsibilities are considered by many to be fundamental, based on common law and integral to our political system. They are also generally considered to be *plenary*, that is "prevailing over the claims of the state, other outsiders, and the children themselves. There must be some compelling justification for interference."[12] (Historically, there have always been some limits set to parental power, most recently in the expansion of child abuse and neglect laws.) The Supreme Court clearly regards the case of a minor's pregnancy to be such a "compelling justification," since it denied parents their normal rights to consent to, or veto, medical treatment for their child. The Court, in balancing the rights of one family member, the minor adolescent, against those of others, the parents, decided that the interests of the adolescent must have priority. Yet, to go one step further and deny parents even the presumptive right to have any influence on the decision or the chance to support and counsel her, is regarded as undermining the concept of parental autonomy too deeply and to be an unnecessary interference with the integrity of families.
- Although the legal presumption should be that parents, once informed, can and will deal with the news of pregnancy constructively, some proponents of notification agree that provisions should be made in any notification requirement to allow for the exceptional situation, when indeed the adolescent needs

to be protected from parental abuse or when the minor is considered to be legally emancipated.

An admitted consequence of notification may often be conflict between parents and their daughter. Yet, in no other area of life is it the duty of professionals to protect minor children from disputes with their parents. Disagreements and conflict are a natural and often quite necessary part of family life with adolescents. The critical point is to ensure that provisions in any notification requirement permit its waiver in certain exceptional situations. Equally critical is to provide guidelines to help counselors distinguish between family conflict and parental abuse.

Underlying these arguments for and against parental notification is the veiled issue of abortion, which is seldom explicitly discussed. Most actual or proposed laws require parental notice only when the minor requests an abortion. Hence those on both sides of the abortion issue at times implicitly argue as though we know that parental notification would result in fewer abortions being performed. But we do not know this to be true. Especially if parents were notified of the condition of pregnancy itself, their reaction will vary from family to family and community to community. It is as likely that some parents will urge their daughter to have an abortion as that others will urge that she should not. If more parents were notified of their daughter's pregnancy we do not know whether abortion rates would rise or fall nationally.

It is important to note that the contributors to this volume, all of whom share a family perspective, find themselves on different sides of the notification controversy. As for myself, I am quite torn. With regard to the arguments of principle, I am impressed with the symbolic nature and teaching function of our laws. I believe that if the law should presume that parents need not be informed, one more regrettable step will have been taken in symbolically eroding parental authority and responsibility. Also, as a parent, I find many of the other reasons for informing parents quite persuasive.

On the other hand, regarded as an empirical issue, my professional view is that it may be premature to take this position in the absence of information about what consequences would follow. Regrettably, at present we have quantitative evidence neither about the effects of policies which do not require parental notification nor about those that do. Empirical research on these questions might help to settle the debate one way or another for at least some of us. Unfortunately, the Supreme Court will make its decision without the benefit of such findings.

Required parental notification is considered by many to be a means towards the goal of encouraging family involvement in a minor's pregnancy. It is not, however, the only means available. For those who believe that it would be better if, in general, parents were told about their daughter's pregnancy, the debate centers largely on a question of appropriate policy strategies. What is the best way to help clinics and individual physicians inform and sometimes involve parents? On the one hand, there is the view that without a legal requirement there would be no effective pressure on, or incentive for, busy and overworked physicians and clinic personnel to take the time and trouble to inform parents and deal with some of the delays or disagreements that may be a consequence. On the other hand, there is the view that the best way to get increased family involvement is to build positive incentives into program funding such as money for training counselors, and payments for family sessions and even home visits. Such incentives, together with strong policy statements from professional associations, would serve to encourage agencies to inform parents on a voluntary basis, and such an approach, although possibly slower, has the great advantage of avoiding the negative effects on some adolescents of required notification.

On balance, I believe that the best policy is to require that parents be informed of their minor's pregnancy in most cases. Thus, any such policy must include implementation guidelines that are sensible, practical, and flexible so as to identify and safeguard the adolescent who may need special protection.

Guidelines for Family Notification and Involvement

It is seldom that laws relating to notification address themselves to the question of how such notification is best carried out. Indeed, whether informing parents is a matter of legal requirement, or simply voluntary agency policy, it is clear that the task can be carried out either routinely and clumsily—such as sending a standard form letter in the mail—or in ways that are constructive and supportive. Clinics or individuals who plan in general to inform parents of a minor's pregnancy should, in my view, develop clear guidelines as to how such a policy can be applied with flexibility and sensitivity. To my knowledge, no such set of guidelines exists. Thus, I offer below some preliminary ideas about how best to attempt to involve parents and yet still safeguard the teenager's welfare.

As an example, I use the case of an unmarried pregnant minor requesting services from a clinic, where her primary contact will be a counselor (who may be a trained professional, paraprofessional or even volunteer), but the steps would also apply to a private physician.

Because of the complexity of parent-adolescent relationships on such a sensitive issue as pregnancy, notification should be regarded as a process consisting of several steps. These may occur over a number of days or even weeks.

Step one. After confirming the girl's pregnancy, the counselor will review with her what her choices are regarding the pregnancy and her legal right to make the decision. The counselor will ask whether she has already told her parents about her pregnancy, and, if not, will explain why they need to be informed. She will be given the option of informing her parents herself first.

Step two. The counselor will need to then talk with at least one parent either on the phone, in the office, or on a home visit, to confirm that they know about their daughter's pregnancy, and to offer any help to the family. This contact should be made within a set time limit, such as within two weeks of the confirmation of pregnancy.

The counselor, in talking with the adolescent, and notifying her family, should make him or herself available for additional sessions with the young girl, her parents, and possibly her boyfriend over the next few days to answer any questions or help mediate any serious tensions that may arise. (Pregnancy to a minor is usually a crisis for her and her family, and thus, crisis counseling techniques should be available.)

Step three. The counselor will be prepared to waive the notification of the parents only if there is clear evidence presented by herself and another third party, preferably a member of her family, that this is essential to prevent her from being seriously harmed, or that both parents are unavailable.

(Situations do arise when physical violence or serious mental abuse is a real threat: alcoholism or drug abuse may be a factor, the pregnancy may be a result of incest, or the teenager may be living away from home for a while and, for legal purposes, is considered emancipated.) The difficulty is how the counselor can determine whether the teenager's presentation of her family situation is accurate or exaggerated. Many teenagers will say, and believe, "My father will kill me if he finds out . . . my mother will throw me out of the house . . . my brother will beat up my boyfriend." In this case the counselor should ask the adolescent to bring in some other adult member of the family (older sibling, aunt, grandparent) or adult friend (neighbor, minister) who may be more understanding but who knows her family situation first hand.

Step four. If this person confirms the need to waive parental notification, she or he will be asked to act as a surrogate parent, in helping the adolescent think through her situation along with the counselor.

The idea of asking another family member (or adult friend) to be consulted when it is considered inadvisable to inform the parents is comparable to a suggestion made by adolescent rights advocate and lawyer Harriet Pilpel in an article in 1979.[13] (It seems far preferable to the suggestion made by the majority opinion in *Bellotti* v. *Baird*, that the adolescent appeal to a judge.) Indeed, it might be appropriate to rename a parental notification policy "family" notification, with the understanding that parents normally, but not always, would be the family members informed.

If a parental/family notification were the rule, there is no doubt that skilled people would be needed to carry it out, guidelines would need to be developed and special training instituted. This, in turn, would require additional funds and changes in administrative practice and procedures. It may, for example, require that staff be reimbursed by third-party payors for home visits or family sessions. These facts are cited by some as obstacles against such a policy; many have pointed out that counselors who presently help pregnant adolescents frequently have little special training or time to offer for protracted counseling or work with the family. This is not a sufficient reason to discard a policy that is otherwise desirable, but rather serves as a cautious reminder that such a policy should not be adopted without careful planning and resources allocated to implement it.

This kind of approach to working with adolescents and the families is often used by staff of mental health counseling centers and runaway youth centers—in the analogous crisis situation of a teenager running away from home. Indeed, the act providing federal funds for the runaway youth programs requires parental notification within seventy-two hours. Staff of the centers support the adolescents when they call their parents to tell them where they are, and frequently mediate family conflicts in order that the adolescent can return home.

Notification for Contraceptive Care

In October 1980 the Supreme Court, in refusing to take the case, let stand the Michigan court of appeals decision in *Doe* v.

Irwin (1980), which declared that parents had no right to be informed of their daughter's request for contraceptive care. However, the question of the constitutionality of any state law requiring contraceptive notification remains open: we do not know why the court refused to hear the case, and no Michigan law was at issue.

In practice in recent years, most birth control clinics, and many physicians, have not considered it necessary to inform parents when a minor child is prescribed contraceptives (although, again, some physicians encourage such communication, especially when a young teenager is involved). This position also rests on arguments about adolescents' right to privacy and the belief that parental notification would serve as a barrier to teenagers seeking and using contraceptives.

It is indeed, quite consistent to be persuaded that parental notification is desirable in the case of a minor's pregnancy, but believe it to be a serious mistake when prescribing contraceptives to a minor. In the latter case the stakes are less high, and the rights and interests of parents and other family members are much less profoundly involved.

The ethical and legal arguments for and against contraceptive notification are similar to those concerning pregnancy notification. It is worth noting, however, that two kinds of prescribed contraceptives—the pill and the IUD—can incur side effects and involve slight risks of medical complications which can be serious. These medical consequences suggest to me that as a practical matter most parents should be informed when these contraceptives—and only these—are being considered for minors. Again, this is an area where family planning clinics need to be encouraged to involve family members more than they do at present, especially for girls of school age, as suggested in Chapter 11. And certainly the question of the extent to which parental notification for prescribed contraceptives is a barrier to teenagers' use of contraceptives needs further, high-quality research (see Fox, Chapter 4).

Service Programs to Teenage Parents

The discussion and suggestions made in the following sections could be equally applied to public and private agencies. They concern ways to reorient present services in order to involve family members more in the delivery of services to pregnant adolescents and adolescent parents. As Forbush, Maciocha, and Furstenberg and his co-authors mention, there are many factors that influence the way services are delivered: basic administrative decisions about allocation of space, funds, reimbursement mechanisms, hours of services, how staff spend their time, as well as the values, attitudes and skills of agency staff. Any attempt to implement an approach that would involve families more closely may necessitate changes in any or all of these elements, some of which will definitely cost extra money (such as more in-service training). The following suggestions are based on experiences already underway in teenage parent programs, or agencies providing other kinds of services. For the most part, however, they have not yet been carefully evaluated.

Family Planning, Prenatal, Maternity and Postnatal Services

These programs need to be flexible about which significant family members should be invited and encouraged to accompany the teenage girl to her appointments and join her in discussions with medical personnel. Family support is also critical during her labor (and delivery) and her stay in the maternity ward. Some programs are now willing to involve the teenager's boyfriend and/or her mother, sister, aunt, or even a girlfriend. Unfortunately, many still do not. Such practices are essential for the adolescent to get support, but may also be critical in ensuring that medical advice and recommendations are followed through regarding her own care or that of her child. It may also lead to a discovery that the clinic's and her own mother's advice are in conflict, or that the new grandmother and mother have not yet worked out an acceptable way of sharing child care responsibilities. The meetings may also help the grandmother learn to be a more effective teacher to her daughter.[14]

Services to Teenage Parents

During the intake process, and later as well, staff should collect information about the teenager's family situation: to what extent the families (hers and/or her partner's) are able to provide shelter, economic assistance, and other infant care; to what extent other family members share in the care of the baby; whether the sharing of responsibilities creates much stress and conflict or is relatively harmonious. This kind of information is usually best obtained not only from the adolescents but also from talking with the other family members themselves, who should be asked to join in the interviews. The teenager's parents, grandparents, siblings, and close friends should all be considered as potential sources of information, support, and help in planning what the agency's own role and services should be.

Such an assessment of the client's family context is often best made in a home visit; yet, agency policies, neighborhood factors, and reimbursement practices tend to discourage such visits, which years ago were considered routine. Interviews with the teenager and other family members may also take special skills and require training for those who have the experience of working only with individuals. Agency staff should be trained to assess when a family situation is so disorganized, chaotic, or in such turmoil that specially trained help is needed, and when referral to agencies more experienced in therapy and preventive work with families is needed.

The Estranged Pregnant Adolescent or Adolescent Parent

Information in a client's case record (if, for example, she is referred from some other social service agency) may alert the agency to the adolescent for whom no family resources or support are available. Such information should emerge from the intake process. The adolescent may be fleeing from a home with serious abuse, alcoholism, or mental illness.[15] Yet it may still be worth exploring with the client whether other relatives or adults in the community are a possible resource, even if her closest relatives are not.

These teenagers will usually need a much more comprehensive array of services, including, for instance, housing, foster care, group home, or independent living. Serious consideration also needs to be given to identifying some community people or organizations that may serve as surrogate families or role models to the young parent. They can serve a purpose that no formal program or agency counselor can fulfill.

Family Participation in Agency Policy

Agencies should actively seek to involve parents, adolescents, and other family members in the community to serve as members of boards, advisory, and planning committees, either as volunteers or as paid paraprofessional staff. Their ideas are needed on issues of program design and policy, particularly when the program staff are from a different socioeconomic, racial, or ethnic background than their clientele. This kind of community and consumer input, according to Forbush and Maciocha, is rare in services to adolescents, although it has been a required element in many educational programs such as Head Start. (The new teenage pregnancy grants program encourages this kind of participation.) Another way of obtaining continued feedback is to hold discussion meetings with groups of teenage clients, grandmothers, and so forth, and ask for suggestions of ways to improve agency practices.

Evaluation

Increasingly, service program personnel realize that in order to build a case for receiving private or public funding they need to increase their efforts to evaluate what they are doing. Unfortunately, most agencies have neither the expertise nor the resources to plan and undertake such evaluation. Funding sources that impose evaluation requirements on programs without providing the additional funding or technical assistance to carry them out are self-defeating. Moreover, since goals, service characteristics, and community settings differ so much from program to program, it may be quite unrealistic to expect that a standard evaluation model leading to comparisons between programs can be applied (such as seems implicit in the Title VII of the new legislation). More promising are management models of evaluation that help the program staff be clearer about their goals, make realistic plans about data collection, and provide the kind of continuous feedback that leads to program improvements during the course of the evaluation.[16] As evaluations are planned, it is important to collect information on family backgrounds and on the kind and degree of assistance adolescents receive from their families. (Regrettably, evaluation models that presently exist do not appear to include this kind of information.)

Adolescent Father Involvement

Many agencies are, at present, confused about how to involve adolescent fathers and whether it is in the best interest of the teenage girl and her baby to do so. We know so little about teenage male needs, roles, and attitudes. To date, many people have felt that the teenage girl is better off if the father does not become involved. Fears of having to pay child support or of paternity suits seem to keep many fathers from openly expressing interest.

Slowly we appear to be reevaluating this exclusion of the adolescent male. Small bits of evidence indicate that he is more present in the teenage mother's life than was once thought.[17] And his role is being recognized as critical to the couple's responsible and consistent use of contraceptives. I would suggest that as part of an overall assessment of each teenage client's family context, the staff person assess with her the extent to which her male partner needs to be involved either to meet his own needs (for example, for employment counseling) or to help support her.

Research and Evaluation

The contributors to this volume have made many suggestions and raised substantial questions that need further research or evaluation. I will select from among these a few of the crosscutting themes that seem to have the most relevance to policy:

- Fertility-related data for each year of age through twenty are needed at federal, state, and local levels, and, whenever possible, on a county-by-county basis, to pinpoint areas of specific need. Findings should also be reported by year of age.[18]
- Research needs to be focused on teenage sex and pregnancy as they occur in different contexts—in families of different income levels, racial, ethnic and religious backgrounds, and different types of neighborhood (rural, suburban, urban).
- Research is needed on the many ways in which families—and other informal support systems—provide assistance to teenage parents and their children. This is important to the intelligent planning of services.
- More careful assessments are needed of the ways in which the organization and delivery of services may conflict with the ethnic or religious values, attitudes, and practices of clients.
- Longitudinal studies are urgently needed to determine how well teenagers function as parents over a number of years, relative to other parents. We need to learn what the problems or successes of their children are. What are the particular stresses and difficult times for teenage families? What kinds of teenage families have the most difficulty? What conditions or supports are necessary for teenage families to cope successfully?
- Parents of teenagers need to be asked their views on their

children's needs, on the needs of the family as a whole, and on their perceptions of services to their teenage children. This is very rarely done.[19]
- Research and evaluation studies to determine the most effective program approaches should include an examination of service delivery issues, such as the question of parental notification and other kinds of involvement of families in abortion and family planning clinics, and in programs that serve teenage parents.
- In order to understand the complexity of family functioning, the ecological setting, and the impact of programs on families, we can no longer rely on standard research methodology that was developed primarily to do research on individuals (such as large sample surveys, elaborate controlled experimental designs, and standard program evaluation). We may need to borrow from anthropological and clinical sciences and begin to rely on in-depth interviews with several family members together, group discussion meetings, or use methods of observation. And, instead of program evaluations or quantitative policy analyses, we may need to undertake qualitative, consumer-oriented assessments of service delivery.[20]

Conclusion

This book has stated the case for bringing a family impact perspective to bear on an important social problem, that of teenage pregnancy. It has based its case essentially on three propositions. First, a family and ecological perspective can provide a sound social scientific basis for policy decisions. Our Constitution asserts the primacy of individuals for legal purposes, but our lives attest to the complex web of interacting dependencies, and policy needs to reflect this fact. Second, public policy founded on a family perspective should lead to a more efficient use of resources and result in programs that are both more efficient and more effective. This statement is proposed largely as an hypothesis that emerges both from the conceptual framework and the evidence presented in this book, but which still needs to be tested, since few programs have yet to incorporate these family elements systematically.

Finally, public policy founded on a family perspective is sound politics. We are in an era when there is considerable concern about the strength and stability of families, and also some distrust of government programs and professionals. It is imperative, then, to find the ways in which government and the professions can help individuals through supporting and empowering their families.

NOTES

1. See Sharon J. Alexander, Cathlene D. Williams, and Janet B. Forbush, *Overview of state policies related to adolescent pregnancy* (Washington, D.C.: National Association of State Boards of Education, 1980), pp. 10–13. For a recent discussion of written sex education policies in thirty states, see Asta Kenney and Sharon J. Alexander, "Sex/family life education: An analysis of state policies," *Family Planning/Population Reporter* 9, no. 3 (June 1980): 44.

2. For an exposition of the sexual scripts theory, see John H. Gagnon and W. Simon, *Sexual conduct: The social sources of human sexuality* (Chicago: Aldine, 1973).

3. John H. Gagnon, "The creation of the sexual in early adolescence," in *Twelve to sixteen: Early Adolescence*, ed. Jerome Kagan and Robert Coles (New York: Norton, 1971).

4. As an example, a comprehensive model of a sex education curriculum has been developed by the Center for Family Studies, Freemen Institute in Salt Lake City, Utah, called *Decision-making, choices, and outcomes of teenage sexuality, pregnancy, and parenting*. This curriculum includes a nine point segment entitled "A rational case for abstinence." The course, taught at Parent Education Resource Centers in the community, starts with the premise that parents, schools, churches, media, and community are all "life support systems" for youth.

5. George Thoms, principal, George Mason High School, McLean, Va., and Mary Lee Tatum, teacher/director of their successful and well-accepted sex education program, pointed out at the Seminar's October 1978 conference that their personal judgment of the value of including homosexuality in the curriculum was overridden by the need to respect the values of the parents in their community who did not want this topic addressed.

6. Planned Parenthood of Santa Cruz County, California, gives homework as-

signments that involve parents and are developing a parent involvement handbook as part of their Family Life Education Program Development Project. A similar idea is being developed by Martha Roper, sex educator for the school district of University City, St. Louis, Mo., who, in addition, often asks for a parent's signature on the sex education homework assignment. A highly developed sex education package, *Reverence for life and family*, in extensive use throughout the St. Paul–Minneapolis Archdiocese, also incorporates a high degree of parental involvement.

7. Diana Oresky and Elizabeth Ewing, *Male involvement in family planning: A review and annotated bibliography*, Jan. 1978, p. 5. This report was performed under contract by the National Institute for Community Development, Inc., in Arlington, Va. Copies of the report, which was part of a wider study, can be obtained from Office of Family Planning, Bureau of Community Health Services, Health Services Administration, 5600 Fishers Lane, Room 7-49, Rockville, Md., 20857.

8. Catherine Chilman, *Adolescent sexuality in a changing American society: Social and psychological perspectives* (HEW pub. no. [NIH] 79-146; Washington, D.C.: GPO, 1979) p. 298.

9. Stephen Boochever, *Improving services to young parents through CETA*, 1980 report by National Association of Counties Research, Inc. (Washington, D.C.: National Association of Counties Research, 1980); available at 1735 New York Avenue NW, Washington, D.C. 20006.

10. Alexander et al., *Overview of state policies*, p. 11.

11. Raye Hudson Rosen and Twylah Benson, sociologists at Wayne State University, are presently researching pregnancy resolution in a sample of teenagers in a rural county in Michigan. One of the many factors influencing teenagers' decisions is the direct and indirect role of parents. Preliminary results of the sample of ninety-nine under-twenty-year-olds who became pregnant indicate that of those who chose abortion (and had not told one or both of their parents) almost three-quarters did so for fear of hurting them or for fear of parent-imposed sanctions. This fear may account for the interesting finding that a higher percentage of Catholics chose abortion than Protestants. See their paper presented at the annual meeting of the Society for the Study of Social Problems, Aug. 1979, "Help or hindrance? Preliminary findings on pregnant teenagers' relations with parents."

12. Chief Judge Fox of the Michigan Federal District Court in his opinion *Doe v. Irwin* (1977), cited in Judith Areen, *Family law: Cases and materials* (Mineola, N.Y.: Foundation Press, 1978), p. 906. Judge Fox quotes extensively from an important article by Bruce C. Hafen, "Children's liberation and the new egalitarianism: Some reservations about abandoning youth to their 'rights,'" Brigham Young University *Law Review*, 1976, pp. 606–658.

13. Eve W. Paul and Harriet F. Pilpel, "Teenagers and pregnancy: The law in 1979," *Family Planning Perspectives* 11, no. 5 (Sept./Oct. 1979): 301.

14. An alternative approach to family sessions is to offer parallel group ses-

sions to grandmothers. A few programs, including the well-known Johns Hopkins program, offer groups for grandmothers to provide them with opportunities to discuss issues of shared responsibility and intergenerational conflict.

15. The plight of the alienated pregnant adolescent is discussed in a recent article by Sylvia B. Perlman, "Pregnancy and parenting among runaway girls," in *Journal of Family Issues* 1, no. 2 (June 1980): 262–273.

16. An example of this management model of evaluation is currently being applied by SWRL Educational Research and Development Inc., Los Alamitos, Calif., under contract to the Mott Foundation, to six of the Mott-funded Too Early Childbearing programs.

17. Leo E. Hendricks, "Unwed adolescent fathers: Problems they face and their sources of social support," paper originally presented to the American Association on Marriage and Family Therapy, 37th Annual Meeting, Oct. 1979; accepted for publication in the journal *Adolescence*.

18. In several of their recent articles in *Family Planning Perspectives*, Kantner and Zelnik are still reporting the results of their two surveys aggregated for women aged fifteen to nineteen; see, for example, "Reason for non-use of contraceptives by sexually active women ages fifteen to nineteen," *Family Planning Perspectives* 11, no. 5 (Sept./Oct. 1979): 289–296.

19. *Family planning and the teenager*, a service delivery assessment report (Office of the Inspector General, Department of Health and Human Services, 1979) is the only study I am aware of that obtained from individual interviews and group discussions the views of parents about family planning services to adolescents.

20. Since 1978, the Office of the Inspector General, HEW, started conducting service delivery assessments on HEW programs. (Forty had been completed by June 1980.) These assessments are assigned by the Department Secretary, and findings presented to the Secretary in a personal briefing. The assessments, usually completed within three to five months, are conducted by regional teams of HEW staff that collect information directly from consumers, providers, and others. They emphasize qualitative aspects of service delivery that cannot be readily quantified.

Afterword

Family Impact Analysis

This book is the product of one of the Seminar's three case studies in family impact analysis. Each study was designed to test the substantive, administrative, and political feasibility of family impact analysis. We hoped to learn if it was possible to identify the impact of policies on families in ways useful to policy makers; to define methods for use in family impact studies; and to determine the funds and personnel needed for adequate studies.

Although they share a basic conceptual framework, the three studies differ considerably in scope, design, and methodology. Whereas the other two case studies' point of origin is a specific policy or program, the teenage pregnancy study begins with a broad social problem. And where the flexitime and foster care studies were conducted by Seminar staff, and involved survey methodology (flexitime) or detailed examination of policy implementation (foster care), the adolescent pregnancy study, developed and coordinated by myself and Teresa Maciocha, drew substantially on the commissioned papers of twelve other experts, and the discussions at an invitational conference.

What Is Family Impact Analysis?

Family impact analysis is a relatively new term. Several academic centers and policy organizations around the country are undertaking quite varied kinds of activities which can be called family impact analysis.[1] Thus, it is important to first provide the Seminar's definition.

Family impact analysis is a process of critically assessing the past, present and probable future effects of public (and sometimes private) policy on families. Its purpose is to help make policy more sensitive to, and supportive of, families. In contrast to policy-oriented research that is experimentally designed and conducted over many years, family impact analysis is designed to meet the needs for practical policy recommendations in a relatively short period of time and to use modest financial and technical resources.

Family impact analysis is generally considered to be one form of policy analysis. Yet, in important ways it differs from most policy analysis, and has elements in common with program evaluations, social impact assessments, service delivery assessments, and policy-oriented research. The methodology of family impact analysis is broad and eclectic, drawing on the knowledge and tools of many different disciplines and professions. It nearly always involves collecting new information from families themselves. Its unique combination of elements can be summarized as follows:

- Family impact analysis is guided by an explicit conceptual framework that treats the family in its ecological setting as the central unit for analysis;[2]
- Family impact analysis defines *public policy* to include the basic laws, regulations and appropriations, and the details of implementation, such as service delivery characteristics, that are not often considered by policy analysts.[3] Family impact analysis is interested in assessing how programs actually work from the perspective of those most clearly involved and affected—the providers and families themselves.
- Family impact analysis places central importance on the need to recognize and discuss the cultural and ethical values inherent in policy that are so often "driven underground" in policy discussions.[4]

The Ecological Perspective

Policy analysis needs to be rooted in some kind of descriptive map of how the world operates and how a particular policy problem fits into this general picture. Policy analysts talk in terms of models, but to many, the term *model* connotes a scientific, predictive capacity that is seldom attainable in the field of social policy. The terms *framework* and *perspective* seem more appropriate. A sound framework is one that accounts adequately for available facts and helps describe observable relationships.

The core assumptions of the ecological perspective—which serve as the framework for this study—are the interdependence of the individual with those in the immediate environment, usually family members, and the reciprocal interactions between the family system and other systems and institutions in society.[5] The guiding principle of this framework is that an individual should be understood and helped in relation to his or her context. (By contrast, what is often called the medical model views an individual in isolation, paying more attention to the person's biological and intrapsychic functioning, and targeting services or treatment to the individual almost exclusively.)

Several contributors in this book refer to the medical model implicitly underlying present policy concerned with teenage pregnancy. Although the model is not discussed at length, it is manifest in the strong emphasis on providing better health-related information and services to the individual adolescent girl—and her baby. In recent years, this model has been called into question as being too narrow. It is now recognized that information and service availability are a necessary but *not* sufficient condition for effective contraceptive use; that the social and economic consequences of teen parenthood are perhaps more pressing than health problems; and that other persons in the adolescent's immediate environment appear to be more critical to her effective functioning and use of medical services than professional health care providers.

Introducing the ecological perspective to the topic of teenage pregnancy (or to any topic) adds greater depth and complexity. To adapt a metaphor from Salvador Minuchin, a Seminar member, it is like shifting from a black and white still camera with a fixed focus lens, to a color movie camera with a zoom lens. This complexity, as several contributors point out, makes research considerably more difficult to plan and carry out. It also leads to re-evaluating the present focus and design of service programs.

The Framework Tables

The complex interacting relationships implicit in an ecological perspective appear at first to discourage any unravelling into separate strands. To aid this task, the Seminar developed two framework tables that, as two-dimensional tools, schematically simplify and categorize the relationships potentially involved in any family impact study. A review of all the different elements and relationships within a table, and of one table to the other—almost as one uses a checklist—ensures that all possible factors are considered. Those particularly salient for the study are then identified for further exploration and development. The tables are presented below, with a word of caution first about their usefulness and limitations.

We find the process of family impact analysis to be a richly reiterative one and difficult to describe sequentially. We continually move back and forth between the various aspects of family functioning and contexts and the different components and characteristics of policy.[6] Thus, the framework tables have flexible use: at several points in time a quick review of one table or the other, or separate segments of one, can be helpful in illuminating new relationships and further questions. The tables are of most help in drawing up an extensive list of family impact questions, but by themselves do not determine which questions are salient. Criteria such as availability of data, immediate relevance for policy, and so forth normally influence this decision. Moreover, it is quite clear that a two-dimensional static table cannot adequately convey the dynamic nature of families, policy, or a real sense of how families experience the impact of policy.

The tables are presented here as originally developed, with some minor modifications.[7] The contributors' names are noted on the tables indicating the topics they explored.

Figure 6: Public Policy Dimensions

The public policy table addresses the question, What do we mean by policy? It systematically lays out the various components and levels of policy implementation that need to be reviewed in family impact analysis, including service delivery characteristics at the local level. The vertical columns are for the different levels of government that affect the way a policy is carried out or that themselves initiate the policy. The Value Assumptions and Theoretical Framework column is to be regarded as an overlay on the whole table. It reminds the analyst to search for the theoretical and value assumptions underlying decisions at every level: assumptions which may not be explicit and which may, of course, be conflicting or confused.

Five contributors' chapters in this book aim to describe and analyze a range of federal, state, and local policies that affect adolescent family formation and functioning. Moore's descriptive inventory focuses primarily on federal laws, regulations and funding but mentions how critical state-level decisions are to the ways federal programs are implemented. Scales' chapter on sex education examines the multiple roles of federal, state, and local governments and private organizations, as well as parent involvement. Forbush and Maciocha describe programs at a local level, as well as their historical development and various service delivery characteristics. Steinfels critiques the ethical assumption underlying recent landmark Supreme Court decisions regarding the delivery of health care to minors. Furstenberg, Jemail, and Herceg-Baron describe a new demonstration program that challenges many of the assumptions and practices of family planning counselors and of the clinic settings where teenage clients are served.

Figure 7: Family Impact Dimensions

The family dimensions table attempts to answer two questions. What aspects of family functioning are affected by a pol-

FIGURE 6
EVOLVING FRAMEWORK: PUBLIC POLICY DIMENSIONS

Implementation Components	Value Assumptions & Theoretical Framework	Levels of Government		
		Federal	State	Local
Historical background		*Forbush*		*Forbush*
Laws:				
• Act(s), amendments, ordinances, Court interpretations	*Steinfels*	*Moore* *Scales*	*Scales*	*Scales*
Regulations		*Moore*	*Moore*	
Appropriations:				
• Funding levels, allocations, terms (incentives, disincentives)		*Moore* *Scales*		
Administrative practices:				
• Standard procedures, guidelines			*Moore* *Scales*	*Scales*

Implementation characteristics

- Auspices: private/public (school, hospital, agency, workplace) — *Forbush, Furstenberg/Baron/Jemail, Scales, Forbush, F/B/J*
- Staffing: professional/bureaucratic (orientation, training, affiliations, unions)
- Convenience and Accessibility to families (hours, location)
- Coordination (with other programs) — *Moore, Scales* ; *Forbush*
- Sensitivity to families' needs and realities — *Butts, Martinez, Steinfels, F/J/B*
- Nature of relationship with family — *Butts, Martinez, Forbush, Scales, F/B/J*

Related programs/policies — *Moore, Steinfels*

Related laws and court decisions — *Steinfels, Steinfels, Steinfels*

FIGURE 7
EVOLVING FRAMEWORK: FAMILY IMPACT DIMENSIONS

Family Types and Immediate Contexts	Family Functions			Background Data Relating to Problem/Need
	Membership Functions	Economic Support & Consumer Functions	Socializing and Nurturant Functions	
		Coordinating and Mediating Roles		
Family Types				
Socioeconomic characteristic (income, occupation, education)	*Fox*	*Furstenberg*	*Furstenberg* *Fox*	
Structure:	*Fox*	*Furstenberg*	*Furstenberg* *Fox*	
• single parent/two parent				
• nuclear/extended				
• none/one/two wage earner				
• orientation/procreation*				
• primary/reconstituted**				
• de facto***				
• estranged				
Life cycle stage:	*Fox*	*Furstenberg*	*Fox* *Furstenberg*	*Jones & Placek*
• early formation				
• with school-age children				
• with children in transition to adulthood				
• with no child dependents				
• with elderly dependents				
• aging				

Family Immediate Contexts

			Furstenberg	
	Fox	*Furstenberg*	*Fox*	*Jones & Placek*

Internal relationship:
• interdependency
  (economic, psychological)
• conflicting/complementary
  rights and interests				

Pluralistic context (ethnic, religious, racial, cultural values and behavior)	Butts Martinez	Butts Martinez	Butts Martinez	
Informal social network (friends, extended family, neighbors, community groups)		Butts	Butts	
Neighborhood environment (housing, stores, transportation, recreation, municipal services)				

---

*Family into which one is born (orientation); family which one creates (procreation)
**Family of first marriage (primary); family of second or subsequent marriage (reconstituted)
***Family not defined by blood, marriage or legal adoption, but by informal or formal foster care or informal adoption.

icy? And what differences between families need to be taken into account by a policy?—differences that influence both the nature of the need or problem, and the ways that a policy attempts to remedy this need.

The three broad categories of family functioning designated in the vertical columns overlap considerably; for example, a program such as family planning will aim to directly affect family size (the membership function), but will also indirectly affect families' economic resources and ability to nurture and educate their children. The cross-cutting roles of coordination and mediation are indicated to remind the analyst of the increasing complexity of families' lives; the many institutions and services that all families relate to; and the importance of considering aspects of programs that increase or decrease stress on families in attempting to orchestrate their lives.

The horizontal columns highlight differences of socioeconomic class, structure, stage in life cycle, cultural/racial background, and neighborhood that the Seminar identifies as relevant to family impact analysis. In recent years, policy analysis has shifted from being interested only in socioeconomic differences, to paying more attention to differences of family structure. Our ecological perspective considers both of these, as well as other contextual differences. Depending on the goals and nature of the policy, certain differences will be relevant and others will not. Some may have implications for how laws and regulations are written, while others may simply affect the knowledge, attitudes, and practices of service providers at the delivery level.

Five chapters primarily address the family dimensions of teenage pregnancy illustrated on this table. Jones and Placek present the basic background data on the topic, yet are only able to distinguish between differences of race and age. (With the exception of a recent paper,[8] nationally representative data on fertility do not report other family-related differences, such as socioeconomic status or family structure.) Fox reviews how families of different structures and other characteristics affect teenage sexual behavior in ways that may lead to changes in family membership (through pregnancy and childbearing). Furstenberg discusses the various ways in which teenage parenthood can affect the economic and nurturing functions of families. And Butts and Martinez examine teenage pregnancy as it affects the social and cultural context of black and Hispanic families.

Each of the Seminar's case studies led to some minor modifications of these framework tables and improved our understanding of their usefulness, as well as of their limitations. For example, the teenage pregnancy study pointed up the important omission in the original version of Figure 7 of "estranged families." Although their numbers may be exaggerated, some adolescents, for all practical purposes, are isolated from family support and influence and are seriously estranged from their families on a temporary or permanent basis. Clearly, a family perspective must identify this group as a separate category with special needs, and for which policy may need to be designed somewhat differently. (Figure 7 is now modified to include "estranged families" under structure.)

In general, the ecological framework guided the focus and design of the study. The two tables helped to organize the complex dimensions of the study and in generating some interesting questions.

Study Design and Methodology

The study grew from a series of questions raised in a discussion on teenage pregnancy at a Seminar meeting in March 1977. Later, after a preliminary review of the literature, we decided to focus on the entire range of policies: both those that aimed to affect rates of pregnancy and childbearing (primary prevention), and those that aimed to assist the well-being of teenage parents and their children (secondary prevention). This broad scope suggested the need to commission papers from an interdisciplinary group of experts. These papers, and their discussion at an invitational conference, were used by Ooms and

Maciocha as the basis for further family impact analysis, particularly of the newly enacted federal legislation. This analysis and summaries of the papers were published in a preliminary report in June 1979. In all, the study took fourteen months, from the spring of 1978, when the experts were first identified, to the summer of 1979. Direct costs of the study were approximately forty-five thousand dollars.

The general format of a series of commissioned papers leading towards a conference is a common one. The special challenge for me, as director of a family impact study, was to help the contributors firmly maintain the family focus. Thus, in addition to selecting the original topics, I worked closely with each author in developing outlines and reviewing drafts. From this experience, however, I would now recommend that any future study with this design should include an early meeting of the contributors as a group to review the ecological and family perspective and develop the specific questions together.

In general, the contributors drew on analysis of their own research or professional experience and reviews of the literature. Where there was little or no literature, they gathered new information either through in-person or telephone interviews (with families and professionals) or through a simple survey. The conference to discuss the papers was held in October 1978; it brought together a diverse group of fifty invited experts representing different levels of federal, state, and local policy, as well as different disciplines.

Usefulness of Study Design

Two questions follow, at this point: Was this study an efficient use of time, money, and skills? And second, What type of organization under what circumstances could undertake this kind of family impact study? First, the economic questions: I would argue that, with strong staff direction, a family impact study of this type, using outside consultants to research and prepare papers, is a highly effective use of time and money. An alternative model would be to conduct the study using extra staff. However, in our experience, we would have been able to hire only one additional person (at less than full time) for the $17,000 we spent on consultants. For this amount of money, it is doubtful we could have found in one available person, the great fund of knowledge needed to cover so many aspects of teenage pregnancy. Certainly no one person, in fourteen months, could have interviewed, surveyed, or studied the great number of families or reviewed the amount of literature that the consultants, as a whole, did. The design we used thus draws upon a greater range and degree of expertise than would have been possible if conducted entirely by Seminar staff. It is, then, a model that is especially suitable for a family impact study with a broad focus.

Second, as a corollary, I conclude that this model is not well suited to low budget, community-level organizations. Apart from the question of cost, it would be difficult, although not impossible, to engage well-known scholars without the visibility and publication possibilities that a national organization can offer. It is probable that the approach could be used at state and regional levels. However, in my view, the model is best suited to the national level: to federal agencies, interagency task forces, independent commissions, policy institutes and national associations.

Some social problems, I suggest, that might be studied using this model of family impact analysis are: drug and alcohol abuse, care of the chronically ill elderly, family violence, care of the handicapped—to mention only a few. In each of these areas, the problem traditionally viewed as "belonging" to an individual could benefit from being viewed in a family context, since families are much implicated in the problems. As with teenage pregnancy, policies aimed at these problems are multiple; are to be found in several federal agencies, at different levels of government; and involve a variety of professional disciplines. The breadth and scope of the problems would necessitate involving experts from many varied perspectives. And, as the teenage pregnancy study, two overarching questions of such family impact analyses would be: Does government policy understand the ways that families are involved in, and affected by, the individual's problem? And, does government policy in this area support or undermine attempts by the family itself to cope with the individual's problem?

With a few exceptions, the impact of policies on families defies precise and objective measurement. Our three family impact studies have illustrated that, at this stage of the newly emerging field, in the absence of agreement upon desired outcomes or techniques by which we can determine and measure family impact, the best that we can hope for is to identify and describe possible or probable impact. (In so doing, we rely heavily on the felt perceptions of those who experience the effects.) The book is thus an exploratory study, generating hypotheses and questions and suggesting policy and practice changes that remain, for the most part, to be tested further.

The study laid the groundwork for detailed field studies which the Seminar has sponsored in several communities. In Boston, Children's Hospital Medical Center, with the help of a consortium of agencies, the Alliance for Young Families, conducted a study of the impact of policies relating to day care on school-age parents and their families. And the Michigan Congress of Parents, Teachers, and Students (PTA) undertook, in four diverse Michigan communities, a study of the effects of the new state sex education law—permitting the teaching of contraception in school—on teenagers and their families.

There are essentially two aspects to the concern about the political feasibility of family impact analysis. First is whether or not the process itself—the methods, activities and resources used—is understood and accepted as valid. Second is whether the products of family impact analyses—the reports and recommendations—are accorded proper consideration or are perceived as biased tools in the continuing debate about government intrusion in family life. On this issue, the teenage pregnancy study is a lightning rod. Sex education, family planning, abortion, and unmarried parenthood arouse considerable controversy. Debates on these topics all too frequently become polarized in political terms: Those *for* sex education, family planning, and related services for teenagers are perceived as belonging to the liberal wings of the political parties, and those *against* such programs as belonging to the conservative wings.

The conclusions and recommendations of this family impact study confound such a simple polarization. We found that our focus on families led to some recommendations that echo those of liberal-leaning professionals and advocates. Other recommendations, regarding parental notification and the need to involve families in sex education and services to teenage parents, echo the sentiments of those who hold a more conservative ideology.

My sense, and hope, is that the family perspective presented in these pages will help to bridge the gap between those who advocate government programs as solutions to children and youth's problems and those who fear such programs as anti-parent and anti-family. If this proves to be true, family impact analysis will indeed be useful to policy.

Theodora Ooms

NOTES

1. Some study centers consciously describe themselves as doing family impact studies; for example, the Family Study Center at the University of Minnesota, which has published a monograph by Marcia G. Ory and Robert K. Leik, *Policy and the American family: A manual for family impact analysis* (Minnesota Family Study Center, University of Minnesota, Dec. 1978); and the Center for the Study of Family and the State, Duke University, which has published *Crest Street: A family/community impact statement*, by Elizabeth Friedman (working paper no. 578, Institute of Policy Sciences, Durham, N.C.). Other policy research centers are examining the effect of specific policies on families, although they do not call these studies family impact studies; among them are the Center for the Study of Families and Children at Vanderbilt University, and the Center for Women and Families at the Urban Institute. And, of course, there are many individual schol-

ars throughout the country who are examining the effects of policy on families of the elderly, handicapped, and so forth.

2. By contrast, a recent textbook makes it very clear that, traditionally, policy analysis "regards the well-being of individuals as the ultimate objective of public policy" (p. 4) and states that the individual's welfare and trade-offs between individuals are the two building blocks of policy analyses (pp. 261, 262). See Edith Stokey and Richard Zeckhenhauser, *A primer for policy analysis* (New York: Norton, 1978).

3. See Erwin C. Hargrove, *The missing link: The study of the implementation of social policy* (Washington, D.C.: The Urban Institute, 1975); and Walter Williams, *The implementation perspective: A guide for managing social service delivery programs*, Chapters 1 and 2 (Berkeley, Calif.: University of California Press, 1980).

4. See Alva Myrdal, *Nation and family* (Cambridge, Mass.: MIT Press, 1941).

5. For a more complete statement of the ecological perspective see the Family Impact Seminar's *Interim Report* (Washington, D.C.: Family Impact Seminar, 1978), pp. 13–35. The Seminar has drawn heavily on ideas originating in fields of human ecology and social psychology, and social systems theory, especially as expounded by Seminar members Urie Bronfenbrenner, Nicholas Hobbs, and Salvador Minuchin.

6. Stokey and Zeckhenhauser in their *Primer* write, "Good policy analysis is an iterative process; rarely does it proceed in a straightforward fashion from the definition of the problem to the selection of a preferred action. Rather it works backward and forward as one's understanding of the problems deepens" (p. 324).

7. See the Seminar's *Interim Report* (pp. 25–52) for the original presentation of the framework tables and a detailed discussion of the elements indicated on each table.

8. See brief discussion of a new paper by Kantner and Zelnik, "Parents' social status found to play key role in daughters' sexual activity and contraceptive use," *Family Planning Perspectives* 12 (July/Aug. 1980): 208.

Index

Abelson, H., 225
Abernethy, Virginia, 100
Abortion: as choice of pregnant teenager, 12, 21, 109, 297; counseling on, 32, 33, 295, 296; family's attitude toward, 147; and notification arguments, 283, 284, 305 n., 384; opposition to, 13; public funding of, 31, 61, 321, 324; statistics on, 20, 59–61; Supreme Court decision on, 27, 278
About your sexuality, 234
Administration for Children, Youth, and Families, 187, 191, 195–197, 199, 205, 207, 229, 244
Administration for Public Services, 179, 180, 186
Adolescence, 10, 15, 16, 20, 111, 290, 291
Adolescent Health, Services, and Pregnancy Prevention and Care Act, 210
Adolescent father. *See* Father; Male
Adolescent mother: cost to government of, 22; economic status of, 141; health of, 65–68, 183, 184; isolation from family, 37, 266, 373, 374, 379, 391, 392, 409; residence, 136–140, 392; support by family, 136–140, 154, 390, 391; unemployment of, 21; welfare dependence of, 21, 140, 167, 168, 192, 318, 319
Adolescent parents, 165, 197, 199, 200, 339, 390, 391, 413
Adolescent pregnancy: disposition of, 59–63, 109, 146–148, 297, 397 n.; explanations for, 20, 21, 24; health aspects of, 42
Adoption, 21–23, 25, 44 n.1, 65
Adult Education Act, 198, 199
Age, study by, 69
Ager, J., 96
Aid to Families with Dependent Children (AFDC): benefits and policies, 165–175; child support payments with, 194, 195; employment services with, 203, 204; failures of, 322, 324; foster care segment, 188; legislative authority for, 186; Medicaid available with, 178, 179, 182
Akpom, Amechi C., 88, 103
Alan Guttmacher Institute, 27, 28, 33, 51, 59–61, 65, 339, 340
Alcohol, Drug Abuse, and Mental Health Administration, 197
Alliance for Young Families, 412
Alter, J., 225
America, 341
American Academy of Child Psychiatry, 33
American Academy of Pediatrics, 27, 33
American Association of Family Physicians, 27
American Association of Sex Educators, Counselors, and Therapists, 29, 236
American Bar Association, 28
American Civil Liberties Union, 28
American College of Obstetrics and Gynecology, 27
American Medical Association, 27, 341

415

American School Health Association, 223
Apgar scores, 65, 67, 68

Barglow, P., 100, 103
Batts, James, 318
Baumrind, D., 92
Beiser, Helen R., 116
Bellotti v. *Baird*, 28, 282, 285, 286, 295, 380, 388
Benziger Family Life Program, 234, 235
Bernard, Jessie, 108; *Women, Wives and Mothers*, 108
Birth control: family communication about, 90; parents' values and, 102; technological revolution in, 25; teenage use of, 12, 20, 45 n., 47 n., 55, 57–59, 64, 65, 349, 377. *See also* Contraceptive care; Family planning programs
Birth Control and Unmarried Young Women (Lindemann), 77
Birth rate, 20, 22, 49–55, 59, 61–63, 215, 332. *See also* Fertility
Black teenagers: cultural attitudes, 25, 46 n., 310–316; extended family, 313–315; fertility, 33, 50–52; illegitimacy rates, 62, 63, 315; pregnancy outcomes, 59, 60; rate of marriage and adoption, 22; sexual activity, 55, 56, 315, 316; welfare dependency of, 34, 318, 319
Blackstone's *Commentaries*, 280
Bloch, Doris, 84
Board of Education, Prince George's County, Maryland, 237
Booth Memorial maternity homes, 23, 258
Boy Scouts, 199, 231
Boys Clubs, 231
Brockman, James R., 341
Brody, Eugene B., 97
Bronfenbrenner, Urie, 119
Bureau of Community Health Services, 175–177, 183, 184, 204, 348
Bureau of Education for the Handicapped, 206

Bureau of Elementary and Secondary Education, 244, 246
Bureau of Health Education, 230
Bureau of Special Projects Program, 198
Burke, Kenyon, 319
Burt, Martha, 172
Butts, June Dobbs, 25, 28, 409
Byler, R., 226; *Teach us what we want to know*, 226

Calderwood, Deryck, 234
Califano, Joseph, 30–32
Card, Josefina A., 339
Carey v. *Population Services International*, 278, 281, 282, 284, 287, 288, 294
Catholic Charities, 33, 258
Catholics United for the Faith, 242
Center for Disease Control, 60, 61, 220, 222, 239, 244, 248
Center for Population Options, 229, 231, 235
Center for Population Research, 207
Chamis, G. C., 217, 220
Child abuse and neglect, 188, 190, 196
Child Abuse Prevention and Treatment Act, 188, 189
Child care: family division of, 151–154, 160, 161, 390, 391; family help with, 139–143; lack of federal support for, 379. *See also* Day care
Child development, 21
Child Health Assessment Program, 31, 183
Child labor standards, 204
Child Nutrition Program, 193
Child Protective Services, 190
Child support, 12, 194, 195
Child Support Enforcement Program, 194, 195, 379
Child Welfare League, 24, 33
Child Welfare Resources and Information Exchange, 246
Child welfare services, 188, 196
Childbearing. *See* Birth rate
Children, legal status of, 279–281. *See also* Minor

INDEX 417

Children and Youth Centers, 176, 184
Children's Bureau, 196
Children's Hospital Medical Center, 412
Children's rights movement, 23, 27
Civilian Health and Medical Program of the Uniformed Services, 185
Clawar, S. S., 227, 239
Coleman, J., 114
Columbia-Presbyterian Medical Center, 322
Commentaries, Blackstone's, 280
Commission on Civil Rights, 331
Commissioner of Education, 246
Commodities Supplemental Food Program, 193
Common law, 280
Communication, family, 90, 91, 93–99, 145
Community Health Center Program, 184
Comprehensive Employment and Training Act (CETA), 200–202, 247
Conference on Teenage Pregnancy and Family Impact, 345
Confidentiality, 27, 120–122, 359, 364. *See also* Privacy rights
Congressional Budget Office, 331
Consent: defined, 292; informed, 292, 293, 295, 382; parental, 11, 27, 283, 284, 352, 353, 380; proxy, 293, 294
Consortium on Early Childbearing and Childrearing, 256
Contraceptive care, 278, 282, 348, 366–369, 388, 389. *See also* Birth control; Family planning programs
Couch, Gertrude B., 93
Counseling, 23, 32, 33, 36, 162, 178, 295, 296, 302
Counselors, family planning, 357–363, 368, 369
Courts, 14, 305 n. *See also* Supreme Court decisions

Dale, G., 217, 220
Darity, William A., 320
Day care, 188, 189, 196; federally funded, 190–192; need for, 259, 271, 319, 322; and other services, 378.
See also Child care
Department of Agriculture, 192, 193, 202, 206, 208
Department of Commerce, 331
Department of Education, 198
Department of Health and Human Services, 30 n. *See also* Department of Health, Education, and Welfare
Department of Health, Education, and Welfare: Administration for Children, Youth, and Families, 187, 191, 195–197, 199, 205–207, 229, 244; AFDC, 167–175; Alcohol, Drug Abuse, and Mental Health Administration, 197; Bureau of Community Health Services, 348; Child Support Enforcement program, 194, 195; education programs, 198, 199; family planning programs, 175–181; lack of coordination with other programs, 378; Maternal and Child Health Services, 255; Office of Adolescent Pregnancy Programs, 34–39; sex education survey, 231; social services, 186–189; teenage pregnancy initiative, 30, 30 n., 31, 33–39; Work Incentive Program, 203, 204
Department of Housing and Urban Development, 199, 200, 208
Department of Labor, 200–204, 209, 331, 378
Department of the Interior, 202
Dickens, Helen, 321
Disposition of pregnancy, 59–63, 109, 146–148, 297, 397 n.
Divorce, teenage, 137, 339
Doe v. Irwin, 388, 389
Drug abuse, 197

Early and Periodic Screening, Diagnosis, and Treatment, 182, 183
Ecological perspective, 11, 37, 374, 395, 400–402, 410
Edelin, Ramona, 320
Education, 21, 29, 208, 258, 303
Education Amendments, 29, 199, 246, 375

Education Development Center, 199
Education for Parenthood, 199, 227, 230, 231
Educational achievement, 138, 139, 141, 165, 255, 271, 338, 339, 379
Elementary and Secondary Education Act, 199, 244, 247, 255
11 Million Teenagers, 28, 51
Emancipated minor doctrine, 287
Emory University Family Planning Program, 235
Employment, 165, 201, 259, 319, 323, 339, 378, 379
Employment and Training Administration, 203
Encyclopedia Brittanica Corporation, 226
Engage/Social Action Forum, 233
Erickson, Milton, 18
Erikson, Erik, 16
Ethical issues, 13, 14, 279, 296–301
Everly, K., 220
EXCEL (Push for Excellence), 321
Exploring Childhood, 199

Family: and baby, 155, 156; and baby's father, 149–151; benefits for, 154–158; costs for, 158–160; counseling of, 351, 354, 361; cultural context of, 114–123; discord in, 101; and disposition of pregnancy, 109, 146–148, 397 n.; estrangement from, 37, 266, 374, 391, 392, 409; extended, 313–315, 319, 334; formation of, 165, 166, 181, 182, 403; functioning of, 73, 74, 133, 134, 165, 166, 403, 408; Hispanic, 333, 334; involvement in programs, 119–124, 210, 263–274, 386–389, 413; isolation from, 373, 379; life cycle stages, 17, 110–114; membership, 88, 102, 103, 408, 409; military, 185; participation in policy-making, 274, 275 n., 392; relations within, 100, 101, 124, 156–158, 161; role in social control, 106–109; sibling relationships in, 105; socioeconomic characteristics of, 87, 103, 104; support of adolescent mother by, 136–140, 154, 390, 391; system, 110–114; values, 101, 102, 119, 299–301. *See also* Parents
Family impact analysis: defined, 399; family impact dimensions, 403, 406–409; framework, 402–409; methodology, 400, 409, 410; 1978 legislation, 36–39; public policy dimensions, 403–405; purpose of, 10, 399, 400; study design, 409–413
Family impact principles, 373, 374
Family Impact Seminar, 10, 133, 318, 345, 347, 399
Family life education. *See* Sex education
Family perspective, 10, 11, 14, 365, 369, 395, 396, 410
Family Planning Council of Southeastern Pennsylvania, 347, 350
Family Planning Perspectives, 27, 380
Family planning programs, 319–321, 324, 325; family involvement in, 40, 41, 146, 161, 347, 366–369; federal, 175–181; federal funds for, 25, 26; opposition to, 28, 29; recommendations for, 376, 377; and Roman Catholic Church, 341
Family Planning Services and Population Research Act of 1970, 177. *See also* Public Health Service Act; Title X
Father: effect of Child Support Enforcement program on, 379; family's attitude toward, 149, 150, 151; in Hispanic culture, 337; involvement by service agency, 36, 37, 265, 266, 272–274, 393, 394; lack of data on, 69, 161; role in decision-making, 297, 298; role in sex education, 83, 92, 123, 124; support by, 149, 150. *See also* Adolescent parents; Male; Parents
Fecundity, defined, 59
Fertility: earlier physical maturation, 16, 51; need for research on, 10, 68, 69, 207; rates, 32, 49–52, 54, 332. *See also* Birth rate
Florence Crittenton homes, 23, 258

Food Service Equipment Assistance Program, 194
Forbush, Janet, 24, 29, 30, 390, 392, 403
Foster care, 44 n., 188, 189
Fox, Greer Litton, 17, 18, 21, 40, 143, 145, 347, 389, 408
Furstenberg, Frank, 18, 21, 40, 41, 95, 102, 109, 210, 347, 348, 369, 377, 390, 403, 409; *Unplanned Parenthood*, 132
Future Homemakers of America, 230, 235

Gadpaille, W. J., 92
Gagnon, John, 18, 91, 116–118, 372
Gallup Polls, 215, 226, 227
Garfield, Mary G., 92
George Mason Junior-Senior High School, 228
Girl Scouts, 231
Gittlesohn, Roland B., 234; *Love, Sex, and Marriage: A Jewish View*, 234
Goldfarb, Joyce L., 96, 103
Gordon, S., 220
Government. *See* Family planning programs; Policies; Service agencies
Graham, Elizabeth, 322
Grandmother: aid with child care, 151–154; attitude toward baby, 156, 157, 160; involvement by service agency, 38, 266, 397, 398 n.; as primary caregiver, 265, 270, 271, 273. *See also* Family; Mother; Parents
Gray, Naomi T., 323
Griswold v. State of Connecticut, 283

H. L. v. Matheson, 380
Haley, Jay, 17, 18
Harlem Hospital Center, 318
Harper, Mary, 323
Hawkins amendments, 201
Head Start, 188, 192, 196, 321, 392
Health, mother and infant, 65–68, 183, 184, 255
Health Care Financing Administration, 178, 182, 183. *See also* Medicaid
Health care worker, black, 316–318

Health Services and Centers Amendments Act, 30
Herceg-Baron, Roberta, 146, 348, 403
Hill, Reuben, 17
Hispanic family, 69, 330, 333–340
Hispanic population, 326–329, 331, 332
Hispanic teenager: cultural attitudes, 334–336; extended family, 336–338; fertility, 332; lack of fertility-related data on, 34, 331, 332, 341; poverty level, 333; school dropout rate, 34, 332, 338, 339; sex education curricula for, 247; statistical description of, 327–329, 332
Hodgman, Christopher H., 92
Hottois, J., 225, 241, 242; *The sex education controversy*, 241
House Select Committee on Population hearings, 31, 32, 224
Housing, 199, 200
How to Help Children Become Better Parents, 230
Howard University, 232
Human Resources Administration, New York City, 310
Hyde Amendment, 61, 181

Illegitimacy, 22–24, 62, 63, 320
Impact, 239
Improving Hispanic Unemployment Data: The Department of Labor's Continuing Obligation, 331
Infant, 19, 67, 68, 154–156, 183, 184
Informed consent, 292, 293, 295, 382
Institute for Family Research and Education, 236, 238, 239, 242
Institute for Sex Research, 220, 236
Insurance, 174
Interfaith Statement on Sex Education, 233

Jackson, Jesse, 12, 321
Jacobson, S., 237
Jemail, Jay, 357, 403
Jessor, Richard, 93, 101, 106
Jessor, Shirley L., 93, 101, 106
Job Corps, 202

Job training. *See* Employment
John R. Beyster Associates, 36
Jones, Audrey E., 20, 332, 408
Joseph P. Kennedy, Jr., Foundation, 32, 33
Journal of Current Social Issues, 234

Kantner, John F., 26, 55–61, 64, 69, 74, 103, 104, 226
Kennedy, Edward, 30
Kinship Support for Adolescents Enrolled in Family Planning Programs study: design and objectives of, 348–350; evaluating program of, 356, 357, 366–369; involvement of family in, 352–354, 366; modifying services for, 354–356; origin of, 345–348; program sites for, 350, 351; recruitment of agencies for, 351; training counselors for, 357–366
Kirby, D., 225
Kirkendall, L. A., 240
Klerman, Lorraine, 262
Kohlberg, Lawrence, 290, 291
Ktsanes, Virginia K., 96, 120, 121

Ladner, Joyce, 25
Legislation, federal, 9, 25, 26, 30–39, 201
Levinson, Daniel J., 112
Lewis, Robert A., 94, 95, 100
Life cycle stages, 17, 110–113
Lindemann, Constance, 77; *Birth Control and Unmarried Young Women*, 77
Lipman-Blumen, Jean, 75
Live births, 61–63
Love, Sex, and Marriage: A Jewish View (Gittelsohn), 234
Luker, Kristin, 146

McGee, Marsha G., 103
McHugh, James, 224
Maciocha, Teresa, 24, 29, 30, 347, 390, 392, 399, 403, 410
Majority, age of, 286, 287, 383
Male, adolescent: and family planning programs, 14, 37, 38, 376, 377; need for research on, 10, 69, 124; responsibility of, 12, 26, 373; role of, 21, 22, 74, 75, 178; services for unemployed, 204; sexual activity, 72 n. *See also* Adolescent parents; Father
Mann, Dorothy, 347
Manpower Development Research Corporation, 203
March of Dimes, 230, 235
Marriage, teenage, 57, 137, 173, 174, 339
Martinez, Angel Luis, 34, 409
Maternal and Child Health Services, 175, 176, 255
Maternal and Infant Centers, 176, 184, 321
Maternity homes. *See* Residential facilities
Mathtech, Inc., 220–223, 239, 248
Maturation, biological, 15, 16, 51
Mature minor rule, 282, 287–289, 291, 292, 381
Media, 12, 16, 44 n., 222, 223, 241–243, 327, 335, 372, 374
Medicaid, 165, 169, 174, 186; coverage for adolescents, 31, 183; family planning assistance, 175, 176, 178, 179; funding of abortions, 61, 182; legislative authority for, 186; reimbursement of service agencies, 265; source of medical assistance, 182–184
Medical care, 11, 27, 281, 287. *See also* Contraceptive care; Minor; Notification
Medical model, 355, 356, 368, 369, 401
Medical perspective, 23, 26–28, 294
Menarche, age at, 16, 51, 84
Michigan Congress of Parents, Teachers, and Students, 412
Military families, 185
Miller, B., 96, 108
Milner, N. A., 225, 241, 242; *The sex education controversy*, 241
Minimum wage law, 204, 341
Minor: emancipated, 287; legal rights

of, 16, 44 n., 200, 278, 279, 283–285, 287, 302, 303; mature, 287–289; medical care for, 280, 281, 284, 287–289, 302
Minuchin, Salvador, 401
Miscarriage, 59–61
Montanez, Wilma, 336
Moore, Kristin, 22, 377, 379, 403
Moral judgement of the child (Piaget), 290
Moran, Alfred, 338
Morganthau, Joan E., 92
Mother, of adolescent, 83–91, 95–99, 101, 104, 105, 108, 112, 113, 144, 145. *See also* Family; Grandmother; Parents

Naomi Gray Associates, 323
National Alliance Concerned with School-Age Parents, 33, 256, 260, 263, 264
National Alliance for Optional Parenthood, 235
National Assessment of Educational Progress, 245
National Association for the Advancement of Colored People (NAACP), 319, 320
National Association of Broadcasters, 12, 44 n.
National Association of Counties, 201
National Association of State Boards of Education, 33, 378
National Birth Control League, 26. *See also* Planned Parenthood Federation of America
National Center on Child Abuse and Neglect, 196
National Clearinghouse on Child Abuse and Neglect, 196
National Conference of Catholic Charities, 33
National Congress of Parents and Teachers, 229. *See also* Parent-Teacher Association
National Council of Churches, 232, 233

National Council of La Raza, 34
National Council on Family Relations, 236
National Council on Negro Women, 34
National Diffusion Network, 246
National Directory of Services for School-Age Parents, 256
National Education Association, 224, 242
National Family Sex Education Week, 239
National Federation of Settlements, 231
National 4H Clubs, 231
National Institute of Child Health and Human Development, 205, 207, 244
National Institute of Education, 208, 224
National Institute of Mental Health, 205, 221, 238, 323
National Institute on Drug Abuse, 197
National Longitudinal Study, 245
National Longitudinal Survey of Young Women, 209
National Longitudinal Survey on youth, 332
National Natality Survey, 63–66, 68, 69
National Panel on High School and Adolescent Education, 245
National School Age Mother and Child Act, 30
National School Lunch Program, 194
National Survey of Family Growth, 57, 59, 67, 69
National Urban League, 34
"Neighbors in Need" project, 234
New Futures School, 341
New York City Family Living and Sex Education Student Peer Information Project, 238, 239
New York Medical College Family Life Theatre, 235
NFSEW Notebook, 239
Nix, Lulu Mae, 35
Notification of parents: barrier to

seeking help, 120–122; contraceptive care, 388, 389; court cases regarding, 282, 286, 305 nn., 306 n., 380, 388, 389; importance of, 302, 413; in pregnancy, 380–388
Nuremberg Codes, 292
Nutrition, 192–194, 208

Occupational training. *See* Employment
Office of Adolescent Pregnancy Programs, 34–36, 38, 245, 378
Office of Child Development. *See* Administration for Children, Youth, and Families
Office of Child Health, 183
Office of Child Support Enforcement, 194, 195
Office of Developmental Services, 196
Office of Economic Opportunity, 184
Office of Education, 198
Office of Human Development Services, 33, 179, 180, 186, 195, 203
Office of Indian Education, 206
Office of Management and Budget, 35
Office of Maternal and Child Health, 176, 183, 184
Office of Planning and Evaluation, 36
Office of Planning, Research, and Evaluation, 195
Office of Regional, State, and Community Affairs, 195
Office of Services for Children and Youth, 196
Office of the Assistant Secretary for Health, 33
Office of Youth Programs, 201–203, 378
Ooms, Theodora, 347, 409

Parent-Teacher Association (PTA), 229, 230, 412
Parental consent, 11, 27, 283, 284, 352, 353, 380
Parenting education, 196, 199, 244
Parents: educational level of, 104; impact on sexual behavior, 93–99; involvement in programs, 210, 265–274, 386–389; notification of, 120–122, 282, 284, 286, 299, 302, 380–389, 413; obligations of, 12, 13, 280, 281, 300, 383; rights of, 13, 279, 282, 383; role in prevention of pregnancy, 372; sexual information transmitted by, 75–84, 99, 100, 123, 124. *See also* Family; Father; Grandmother; Mother; Sex education
Parents Who Care, 241
Philadelphia Child Guidance Clinic, 133, 143, 144, 357
Piaget, Jean, 289–291; *The moral judgement of the child*, 290; theory of, 16
Pilpel, Harriet, 27, 388
Placek, Paul J., 20, 62, 63, 332, 408
Planned Parenthood Federation of America, 26, 33, 221, 229–231, 236, 317, 377
Planned Parenthood of Chicago, 235
Planned Parenthood of New York City, 338
Planned Parenthood v. Danforth, 278, 281–289, 294
Plenary rights, 383
Policies, federal: abortion, 181, 182; AFDC, 165–175; child support enforcement, 194, 195; coordination of, 378; education, 198, 199; effect on male of, 298; employment, 200–204; family participation in, 392; family perspective, 413; family planning, 175–181, 371, 376, 377; financial aid to mother, 141, 371; health care, 182–185, 371; involvement of parents, 373; nutrition, 192–194; racial discrimination in, 318–325; range of, 11; recommendations for, 41, 42, 302, 303, 373, 374; services for teenage parents, 378; sex education, 246–249, 371, 375; social services, 186–189, 390–394; teenage parents, 31, 32; teenage pregnancy, 9
Policies, state: abortion funding, 181, 182; child support enforcement, 194, 195; coordination of, 378; day care, 190, 191; family participation

in, 392; family planning, 178–180; medical care, 168–173, 182; sex education, 215; teenage parents, 371, 372, 378
Policy, public, 39, 400, 403–405
Policy analysis, 400, 401, 414 n.
Population Institute. *See* Center for Population Options
Prenatal care, 65–68, 172, 173, 185, 263
Prevention programs: primary, 11, 31–33, 35, 409; secondary, 11, 31, 33, 272, 409
Privacy rights, 279, 282–284, 298, 301, 304 n., 352, 380, 389
Project on Equal Education Rights, 33
Property rights, 280, 281
Proxy consent, 293, 294
PTA Today, 230
Public assistance. *See* Aid to Families with Dependent Children; Medicaid; Welfare benefits
Public Health Service, 184, 245
Public Health Service Act, 175, 177, 178
Public Law 92-603, 178
Public Law 94-311, 331
Public policy, 39, 400, 403–405

Quinn, J. M., 232

Race, differences in, 25, 37, 50, 51, 55
Racism, 308, 316
Rains, Prudence, 146, 347
Red Cross, 230
Reiss, Ira L., 88, 108, 114
Research and evaluation, need for, 10, 34, 68, 69, 124, 161, 207, 331, 332, 341, 394, 395
Research on teenage childbearing, federal, listed, 204–207
Residential facilities, 23, 25, 258, 264, 265, 269, 270
Richmond, Julius, 30
Rights, minor's. *See* Minor
Rights, parents', 13, 279, 282, 383
Roberts, E. J., 91
Roe v. Wade, 27, 297

Roebuck, Julian, 103
Roman Catholic Church, 29, 341
Rosen, R. A. H., 109
Rothenberg, Pearila Brickner, 85, 87, 88
Runaway Youth Act of 1974, 189, 197

Salvation Army, 23, 199, 231, 258
Samalot, Rosemary, 339
San Francisco General Hospital Perinatal Unit, 336
Sandberg, Eugene, 217
Sanger, Margaret, 26
Saxon, B., 237
Scales, Peter, 29, 40, 93, 220, 225, 375, 403
Scheuer, James H., 31
School-Age Parent Continuation Program, 260
School-age teenagers, 11, 19, 20, 29
School Breakfast Program, 194
School dropout, 29, 33, 247, 255, 332, 338
Second pregnancy, 158, 160
Secretary of Education, 246
Senate Human Resources Committee, 233
Service agencies: characteristics of, 260–262; evaluation of programs, 262, 263, 392, 393; family involvement with, 263–274, 392; funding, 259, 260, 265; lack of follow-up, 271
Sex education: church-based, 232–235; community projects, 235; defined, 216; development of curricula for, 247, 376, 396 nn., elements of successful, 235, 236; evaluation of, 39, 40, 217–222; federal programs, 32, 243–245, 252 n., 371, 374–376; goals of, 216, 217; in media, 222; opposition to, 47 n., 239–243, 248, 375; parents' attitude toward, 12, 226, 227; parents' participation in, 227, 228, 236–239, 375, 396, 397 n.; in parochial schools, 224, 250 n.; from peers, 222, 230; in private schools, 250 n.; in public schools, 44 n., 223–229, 250 nn.; number of

schools offering, 12, 13, 29; state policies, 215, 223, 224; teenagers' desire for, 93, 227; training of teachers, 236, 253 n., 375, 376; by voluntary organizations, 229–232. *See also* Family; Parents
Sex Education, 238
Sex education controversy (Hottois and Milner), 241
Sex Information and Education Council of the United States (SIECUS), 29
Sexism, 14, 308, 316
Sexual activity, teenage, 10, 45, 46 n., 55, 70 n., 72 n., 166, 215, 315, 377, 382
Sheehy, Gail, 112
Shipman, G., 116
Shriver, Sargent, 32
Shriver, Eunice, 32
Siblings, 17, 105, 152–154, 157, 159, 161, 269. *See also* Family
SIECUS Report, 236
Simon, W., 116–118
Sinai Hospital, 135
Single-parent households, 88, 89, 102, 103, 320, 330
Sklarew, B. H., 232
Smith, Eleanor Wright, 109
Social Security Act, 183, 186, 188, 189, 204
Social Security Administration, 167
Social Security Amendments of 1965, 178, 179
Social services. *See* AFDC; Medicaid; Service agencies
Sorensen, R. C., 226
Spanier, Graham B., 74, 94, 95
Special Milk Program, 194
Special Supplemental Food for Women, Infants and Children (WIC), 192, 193
Stanford Research Institute International, 22, 165
Staples, Robert, 324
State and Local Educational Program, 207

Steinfels, Margaret O'Brien, 14, 18, 40, 41, 381, 403
Stillbirth, 59–61
Supplemental Security Income, 178, 179, 182, 186
Supreme Court, decisions of, 27, 28, 278, 279, 281, 284, 288, 289, 380, 383, 385, 388, 389, 403
Synagogue Council of America, 233, 234

Tanner, J. M., 15
Tatum, M. L., 228
Tax incentive initiatives, 341
Teach us what we want to know (Byler), 226
Teen Times, 230
Teenage Health Consultants, 231, 232
Teenager. *See* Adolescence; Adolescent mother; Adolescent parents; Black teenager; Father; Hispanic teenager; Male
Thoms, G. H., 228
Tietze, Christopher, 63
Title I, 255
Title III: Division of Supplementary Centers and Services, 206
Title IV-A, 186, 188, 191. *See also* Foster care
Title IV-B, 188, 191. *See also* Child Welfare Services
Title IV-C, 191
Title V, 175–177, 183
Title V, Part A, P.L. 93-644, 188
Title VI, 30, 34, 36, 186
Title VII, 30, 34, 35, 393
Title VIII, 30, 36
Title IX, 33
Title X, 175, 177, 178, 244
Title XIX, 175, 177–179, 182
Title XX, 175, 177, 179–181, 186, 187, 189
Torres, Aida, 121
Twenty-sixth Amendment, 286

Uddenberg, Nils, 101
Unemployment, 21, 200–204, 330, 331, 341

Uniformed Services Health Benefit Program, 185
Union of American Hebrew Congregations, 234
Union of Orthodox Jewish Congregations, 234
Unitarian Universalist Association, 234
United Church of Chist, 234
United Methodist Church, 233
United States Catholic Conference, 224, 233, 234
United States Commission on Obscenity and Pornography, 225
United States Statistical Abstract for 1977, 341
United Synagogues, 234
United Way, 259
University of California at San Francisco, 324
University of Massachusetts at Amherst, 320
University of Pennsylvania, 221, 321
University of Pittsburgh Graduate School of Public Health, 263
University of Washington, 221
Unplanned Parenthood (Furstenberg), 132
Unplanned pregnancy, 64, 65. *See also* Adolescent mother
Urban and Rural Systems Associates, 120, 121
Urban Coalition, 320
Urban Institute, 36

Variable competence, 289, 291
Venereal disease, 12, 13, 27, 68, 219, 220, 245, 287
Vinovskis, Maris, 22, 31
Vocational education, 198, 244, 375
Vocational Education Act of 1963, 198

Webster School, 255
Welfare benefits: effect on establishment of household, 140, 379; emergency assistance, 168, 170, 171; and teenage mother, 13, 14; unborn child coverage, 169–173, 179; unemployed father coverage, 168, 170, 171, 174, 179. *See also* AFDC; Medicaid
"What Parents Should Know about Sex Education," 238
White House Conference on Families, 380
Wise, Lauress L., 339
Women, Infants and Children (WIC), Special Supplemental Food for, 192, 193
Women, Wives and Mothers (Bernard), 108
Women's Bureau, 202, 203
Women's rights movement, 23, 33
Work Incentive Program (WIN), 191, 203, 204
World Health Organization, 216

Young, Leontine, 23–25, 109
Young Men's Christian Association (YMCA), 258
Young Women's Christian Association (YWCA), 230, 231
Youth Act of 1980, 201
Youth Adult Conservation Corps, 202
Youth Community Conservation and Improvement Programs, 202
Youth Development Bureau, 196, 206
Youth Employment and Demonstration Projects Act, 200, 201, 247
Youth Employment and Training Program, 201
Youth Incentive Entitlement Projects, 202
Youth unemployment: The outlook and some policy strategies, 331
Youthwork, Inc., 203

Zabin, Laurie Schwab, 57
Zelnik, Melvin, 26, 55–61, 64, 69, 74, 103, 104, 226
Zero Population Growth, 235